C. G. Drake
S. J. Peerless
J. A. Hernesniemi

Surgery of
Vertebrobasilar Aneurysms

London, Ontario Experience
on 1767 Patients

Foreword by M. G. Yaşargil

SpringerWienNewYork

Charles G. Drake, OC, M.D., FRCSC
University Hospital, London, Ontario, Canada

Sydney J. Peerless, M.D., FRCSC
MERCY Neuroscience Institute, Miami, Florida, U.S.A.

Juha A. Hernesniemi, M.D., Ph.D.
Department of Neurosurgery, University Hospital, Kuopio, Finland

This work is subject to copyright.
All rights are reserved, whether the whole or part of the material is concerned, specifically those
of translation, reprinting, re-use of illustrations, broadcasting, reproduction by photocopying
machines or similar means, and storage in data banks.

© 1996 Springer-Verlag/Wien
Softcover reprint of the hardcover 1st edition 1996

Product Liability: The publisher can give no guarantee for information about drug dosage and
application thereof contained in this book. In every individual case the respective user must check
its accuracy by consulting other pharmaceutical literature.
The use of registered names, trademarks, etc. in this publication does not imply, even in the
absence of specific statement, that such names are exempt from the relevant protective laws and
regulations and therefore free for general use.

Printing: A. Holzhausens Nfg., A-1070 Wien
Cover design: Ecke Bonk

Printed on acid-free and chlorine free bleached paper

With 180 Figures in 554 Single Illustrations and 201 Tables

Library of Congress Cataloging-in-Publication Data

Drake, Charles G.
    Surgery of vertebrobasilar aneurysms : London, Ontario, experience
  on 1,767 patients / C. G. Drake, S. J. Peerless, J. A. Hernesniemi;
  foreword by M. G. Yaşargil.
        p.   cm.
    Includes bibliographical references and index.
    ISBN-13:978-3-7091-9411-9
    1. Vertebrobasilar aneurysms – Surgery.   I. Peerless, S. J. (Sydney
John)   II. Hernesniemi, J.   III. Title.
    [DNLM: 1. Cerebral Aneurysm – surgery.   2. Vertebral Artery –
– surgery.   3. Vertebral Artery – physiopathology.   4. Basilar Artery –
– physiopathology.   5. Basilar Artery – surgery.   WL 355 D761s 1995]
RD594.2.D73   1995
617.4'81 – dc20
DNLM/DLC
for Library of Congress   95-10940
                                                                              CIP

ISBN-13:978-3-7091-9411-9   e-ISBN-13:978-3-7091-9409-6
DOI: 10.1007/978-3-7091-9409-6

Every man owes it as a debt to his profession to put on record whatever he has done that might be of use to others.

Francis Bacon (1561–1626)

Foreword

It is a great privilege to write the foreword for this classical work of Professor Charles Drake. There is no doubt that intracranial aneurysms have existed since the beginning of time. This terrifying disease of the brain arteries, with its dramatic consequences for the patient, has surely been observed in all human collectives, although clear definition and description in the literature began only 300 years ago. During the last century, clinical signs and symptoms have been carefully observed and analyzed, and 100 years ago, the first attempts were made for surgical treatment, such as the ligature of external and internal carotid and vertebral arteries.

With the introduction of angiography, an entirely new dimension of diagnosis and differential diagnosis of the vascular diseases of CNS, was accomplished. In the years between 1945 and 1970, the neurosurgeon was increasingly stimulated to directly eliminate intracranial aneurysms. The most respected and avoided location, the aneurysms at the bifurcation of the basilar artery, remained as a "dark corner." Several pioneers of neurosurgery attempted to explore the interpeduncular fossa, but finally retreated. Not so Charles Drake. His vision must have been stronger than his anxiety, after experiences of initial fatalities, to persevere more decisively in this desperate fight instead of to yield. Such steadfastness requires enormous courage. But what distinguishes courage! Surgical courage is not just a fearless or unscrupulous action. Courage depends on the well calculated decision between the possible risks and the possible success of a planned action. The courageous action requires, further on, a constant balance between impeccable vision and an immaculate concept, continuously judging the applicability of each single manipulation. Finally, courage implicates the wisdom to know the right time, the right place, the right proportion, and the right significance of surgical application. Charles Drake would stay this unique, gigantic fight on 1767 cases, establishing the principles of the surgical treatment of vertebrobasilar aneurysms. In this publication, he courageously presents his experiences and unique results. His achievements are beyond any analytic and critical judgments. He illuminated the "dark corner" within the CNS, and provided a guiding light. It is evident that others are indeed following. This monumental work will remain a milestone in neuroscience.

M. Gazi Yaşargil

Preface

Until recently I have resisted writing a book on aneurysms or arteriovenous malformations since most of our experience has been published where it could be seen promptly and widely in neurosurgical journals. Having contributed many chapters in multi-authored books, I became concerned that by the time the galley proofs arrived much of what I had written was out of date or needed major change – and these were even moreso when the volume was finally published a year or so later.

But I have been persuaded by many neurosurgeons that because our experience with posterior circulation aneurysms is so large and unique and unlikely to be repeated, that it deserves summation in a book, if for no other than historical reasons. I can only hope that it will also be of value to those younger neurosurgeons who are pursuing these aneurysms to their final solution.

The operative illustrations have been updated from those featured in Clinical Neurosurgery, Volume 26, 1979. A new inclusion is the transmastoid-transpetrosal approach, an old technique used for clival tumors, which has been very useful for certain mid- and lower basilar aneurysms. Persuant to long felt convictions, the results have been amplified with description and discussion of the poor outcomes.

That the patient profiles and outcomes are in some detail is only because of Juha Hernesniemi, M.D., Ph.D., who took more than a year out of his life in Miami to put one hundred or so features of each patient into a computer data base.

The book is dedicated to these patients who with their families allowed us to approach their aneurysms under and in front of their brain stems. If only we could have back again many of those who were lost or badly hurt, for a second chance in the operating room with what we have learned.

Charles G. Drake, OC, M.D., FRCSC

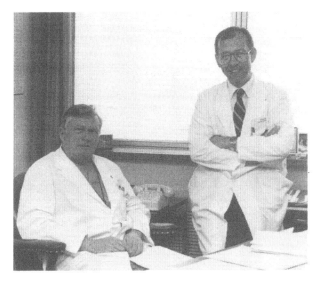
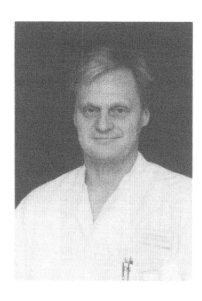

C. G. Drake and S. J. Peerless   *J. A. Hernesniemi*

Acknowledgements

The clinical material to be discussed constitutes mostly a personal series of the two senior authors who operated upon 95% of the patients. We are grateful to Drs. J. P. Girvin, G. G. Ferguson, H. R. Reichmann and S. P. Lownie to have their cases included in the series, and for their continuing and most important help in the clinical work through the years.

The referring doctors, mainly from the USA and Canada, but also from many different countries in Europe, South America, Australia, Asia and Africa, made this unique series of 1767 patients with vertebral-basilar aneurysms possible. The patients were operated upon at the teaching hospitals of the University of Western Ontario in London, Canada; at Victoria Hospital 1959–72, at University Hospital 1973–1992, and at the University of Miami/Jackson Memorial Hospital in Miami, Florida 1991–1992. Many patients were operated upon by the senior authors at other university clinics around the world as visiting surgeons and their staffs' kind hospitality remains fresh in our memories.

The work could only be done because of the team. Our neuroanesthesia was exceptional under Drs. R. Aitken, G. Varkey, A. Gelb and P. H. Manninen especially and we must acknowledge their skills in providing us with slack brains and their thoughtful originality in blood pressure control and brain protection and ceaseless vigilance over countless hours. The excellence of neuroradiology unders Drs. J. Allcock, A. Fox and their staff was a major factor in what we were able to accomplish. Not only did they insure superb imaging and expert interpretation, they were early into the endovascular story when in 1978 Dr. G. Debrun brought the latest techniques to our unit and with Dr. F. Vinuela and the rest achieved remarkable innovations over the years. We were fortunate to have neuroradiologists and anesthesiologists who thought beyond their specialty and contributed many fresh ideas to management of these complex patients.

We thank the nurses on the floor and the operating theater staff whose skills and efficiency have supported our patients, and us, day and night through the years. The medical staff, physiotherapists, occupational therapists and dieticians in the different hospitals have always given excellent pre- and postoperative care. The contribution of these many dedicated professionals to our results can never be measured, but it has been the cornerstone for the recovery of our patients.

The help of countless neurosurgeons and residents, who were educated at the teaching hospitals of the University of Western Ontario in London, Canada, is gratefully acknowledged. Many new ideas were tested, and even born, in discussions with them and with many foreign visitors. We are proud of these young people, many of whom now have leadership roles in universities around the world. That posterior circulation aneurysms are now operated upon worldwide in major neurosurgical units is in large part the result of their efforts and teaching.

The manuscript was only made possible with the personal and secretarial assistance of Ms. Heather Carter, whose skills are too numerous to be listed here. Further, the authors wish to thank Mrs. Deborah Bisnaire, Mrs. Dorothy McManus and Mrs. Lynda McMillan for their secretarial help and data collection, and to Dr. F. Gutman,

XII Acknowledgements

Mr. M. Peerless, Ms. A. Hanks and Mr. M. Halmu for their assistance in developing the database. This research was supported in part by grants to Dr. Hernesniemi from UH of Kuopio, Maire Taponen Foundation, Families Hernesniemi, Kuopio and Ruovesi, FIN, Family Ketola, Lantana, FL, and Jack'son Memorial Hospital Foundation.

Springer-Verlag, and especially Mag. Elisabeth Hunger and Mr. Raimund Petri-Wieder, deserve special recognition for their generous help, patience and outstanding production work.

London, Canada
Charles G. Drake, OC, M.D., FRCSC
Sydney J. Peerless, M.D., FRCSC
Juha A. Hernesniemi, M.D., Ph.D.

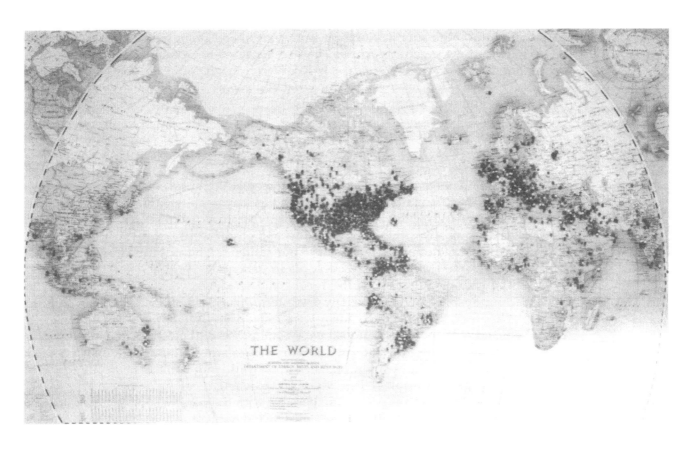

The admitting office used a pin for each case – where they come from in North America and around the world

Contents

Authors' Addresses *XVII*

Abbreviations *XIX*

List of Operative Drawings *XX*

1. Historical Notes *1*

2. Clinical Material *7*

3. Small Aneurysms at the Bifurcation of the Basilar Artery: 493 Patients *17*

Clinical Features *17*
Early Surgical Experience *17*
Anatomical Features *18*
The Subtemporal Approach *21*
Induced Intraoperative Hypotension *27*
The Transsylvian (Pterional) Approach *28*
Other Approaches *29*
Upward Projecting Basilar Bifurcation Aneurysms *30*
High Basilar Bifurcation *36*
Low Basilar Bifurcations *36*
Forward Projecting Aneurysms *37*
Backward Projecting Aneurysms *37*
Results *38*

4. Large (or Bulbous) Basilar Bifurcation Aneurysms (12.5–25 mm): 265 Patients *42*

Clinical Features *42*
Results *51*

5. Analysis of Operative Morbidity in Basilar Bifurcation Aneurysms: Small and Large (Non-Giant): 758 Patients *55*

Perforator Injury or Occlusion *55*
Final Comments on Non-Giant Basilar Bifurcation Aneurysms *65*

6. Giant Basilar Artery Bifurcation Aneurysms: 137 Cases *68*

Anatomical Features of Giant Basilar Bifurcation Aneurysms *68*
Clinical Features *68*
Treatment *69*
Explored Only *69*
Intra-Aneurysmal Occlusion *69*
Neck Clipping *75*
Vertebral Artery Occlusion *80*
Basilar Artery Occlusion *81*

7. Non-Giant (Small and Large) Basilar Superior Cerebellar Artery Aneurysms: 210 Patients *95*

Anatomical Features *95*
Clinical Features *95*
Treatment *96*

XIV   Contents

8. Giant Basilar-Superior Cerebellar Artery Aneurysms: 56 Patients   *110*

Anatomical Features   *110*
Clinical Features   *110*
Explored Only   *110*
Neck Clipping   *112*
Basilar Artery Occlusion   *112*

9. Midbasilar Trunk Aneurysms: 44 Patients   *119*

Anatomical Features   *119*
Clinical Features   *121*
Approach   *121*
Results   *128*

10. Basilar-Anterior Inferior Cerebellar Artery Aneurysms: 41 Patients   *133*

Anatomical Features   *133*
Clinical Features   *133*
Approaches   *135*
Results   *141*

11. Giant Basilar Trunk Aneurysms: 59 Patients   *143*

Anatomical Features   *143*
Clinical Features   *143*
Treatment   *143*
Neck Clipping   *145*
Parent Artery Occlusion   *145*
Trapping   *162*

12. Vertebral-Basilar Junction Aneurysms: 77 Patients   *167*

Anatomical Features   *167*
Clinical Features   *167*
Approach   *167*
Results   *174*

13. Giant Vertebrobasilar Junction Aneurysms: 39 Patients   *177*

Treatment   *177*
Vertebral Artery Occlusion   *180*
  Unilateral Vertebral Occlusion   *180*
  Bilateral Vertebral Occlusion   *180*
Trapping and Evacuation   *192*

14. Non-Giant Aneurysms of the Vertebral Artery: 181 Patients   *195*

Anatomical Features   *195*
Classification   *195*
Clinical Features   *197*
Approaches   *201*
Results   *203*

15. Giant Vertebral Aneurysms: 40 Patients   *207*

Anatomical Features   *207*
Clinical Features   *207*
Treatment   *207*

Contents   XV

16. Non-Giant Aneurysms of the Posterior Cerebral Artery: 59 Patients *221*

Anatomical Features *221*
Clinical Features *221*
Subtemporal Approach *221*
Results *228*

17. Giant Posterior Cerebral Aneurysms: 66 Patients *230*

Anatomical Features *230*
  P1 Aneurysms *230*
  P1–P2 Junction Aneurysms *230*
  P2 and P3–P4 Aneurysms *230*
Clinical Features *230*
  P1 and P1–P2 Junction Aneurysms *230*
  P2–P4 Aneurysms *230*
Treatment *232*
  P1 Aneurysms *232*
  P1/P2 Posterior Communicating Aneurysms *239*
  P2–P4 Aneurysms *239*

18. Multiple Aneurysms: 462 Patients *249*

Treatment *249*

19. Vertebrobasilar Aneurysms and Associated AVMs: 54 Patients
  With a Contribution of *J. Rinne* *256*

General Principles of Treatment *256*
Patients *262*
Treatment *262*
Summary of Poor Results *263*

20. Solitary Incidental Vertebrobasilar Aneurysms: 70 Patients *267*

21. Vertebrobasilar Artery Aneurysms in Children: 49 Patients *269*

Clinical Features *269*
Treatment *269*

22. Timing of Surgery *275*

Rebleeding: Transfer of Patients *275*
Early versus Late Surgery *275*
Final Comments on Timing of Surgery *276*

23. The Anesthetic Management of Patients During Posterior Fossa Aneurysm Surgery
  By *P. H. Manninen* and *A. W. Gelb* *280*

Preoperative Preparation *280*
Premedication *280*
Anesthesia Management *280*
Monitoring *280*
Induction *281*
Maintenance *281*
Fluid Administration *281*
Induced Hypotension, Temporary Arterial Occlusion, and Cerebral Protection *281*

XVI   Contents

Emergence and Recovery *282*
Positioning *282*
Monitoring of Brain Stem Function *283*
Complications *283*
Conclusion *283*

24. Endovascular Saccular Treatment of Posterior Circulation Aneurysms
By *S. P. Lownie* *285*

Detachable Balloons *285*
Thrombosis with Coiled Wires *287*
Experience at the University of Western Ontario, 1971 to 1994 *288*
Conclusions *298*

25. Complications of Surgery for Vertebrobasilar Artery Aneurysms and Final Comments
With a Contribution of *M. Niskanen* *300*

Factors Increasing Complication Rates *300*
Influence of Surgical Timing *300*
Complications During Anesthesia *300*
Problems in Exposure *301*
Intraoperative Aneurysm Rupture *301*
Perforator Injury *301*
Inadvertent Major Vessel Occlusion *302*
Postoperative Deterioration of Neurological State *302*
Memory Deficits *303*
Postoperative Hematoma *303*
Incomplete Occlusion and Re-Operation (Failed Aneurysm Surgery) *303*
Vasospasm *304*
Rebleeding *304*
Postoperative Infection *304*
Medical Complications *304*
Hydrocephalus *304*
Statistical Analysis for Predictors of Poor Outcome *304*
Discussion *305*
Final Comments *306*

References *312*

Subject Index *325*

Authors' Addresses

Charles G. Drake, OC, M.D., FRCSC
Former Professor and Chairman,
Department of Surgery, Division of Neurosurgery,
University of Western Ontario, University Hospital,
339 Windermere Road, London, Ontario N6A 5A5, Canada

Sydney J. Peerless, M.D., FRCSC
Former Professor and Chairman,
Division of Neurosurgery, University of Western Ontario,
University Hospital,
339 Windermere Road, London, Ontario N6A 5A5, Canada

Present Address:
Director, Mercy Neuroscience Institute,
3661 South Miami Avenue, Ste. 209,
Miami, Florida 33133, U.S.A.

Juha A. Hernesniemi, M.D., Ph.D.
Department of Neurosurgery, University Hospital of Kuopio,
FIN-70210 Kuopio, Finland

Stephen P. Lownie, M.D., FRCSC
Division of Neurosurgery, University of Western Ontario,
University Hospital,
339 Windermere Road, London, Ontario N6A 5A5, Canada

Pirjo H. Manninen, M.B., Ch.B., FRCPC
Department of Anesthesia, Toronto Western Hospital,
399 Bathurst Street, Toronto, Ontario M5T 2S8, Canada

Adrian W. Gelb, M.B., Ch.B., FRCPC
Department of Anesthesia, University of Western Ontario,
University Hospital,
339 Windermere Road, London, Ontario N6A 5A5, Canada

Minna H. Niskanen, M.D., Ph.D.
Department of Anaesthesia, University Hospital of Kuopio,
FIN-70210 Kuopio, Finland

Jaakko K. Rinne, M.D.
Department of Neurosurgery, University Hospital of Kuopio,
FIN-70210 Kuopio, Finland

Abbreviations

ACA	anterior cerebral artery
ACom	anterior communicating
AComA	anterior communicating artery
AComAs	anterior communicating arteries
AICA	anterior-inferior cerebellar artery
AV	arteriovenous or arterial venous
AVM	arteriovenous malformation
AVMs	arteriovenous malformations
BA	basilar artery
BB	basilar bifurcation
BT	basilar trunk
CBF	cerebral blood flow
CSF	cerebral spinal fluid
CP	cerebellopontine
CT	computerized tomography/computed tomogram
F	female
GDC	Guglielmi detachable coils
IBCA	isobutyl-2-cyano acrylate
ICA	internal carotid artery
ICP	intracranial pressure
LP	lumbar puncture
M	male
MCA	middle cerebral artery
MRA	magnetic resonance angiography
MRI	magnetic resonance imaging
PCA	posterior cerebral artery
PCom	posterior communicating
PComA	posterior communicating artery
PComAs	posterior communicating arteries
PICA	posterior-inferior cerebellar artery
PICAs	posterior-inferior cerebellar arteries
SAH	subarachnoid hemorrhage
SCA	superior cerebellar artery
SCAs	superior cerebellar arteries
TIA	transient ischemic attack
VA	vertebral artery
V-B/VB	vertebral-basilar or vertebrobasilar
VBA	vertebrobasilar artery
VBAA	vertebral-basilar artery aneurysm
VBJ	vertebrobasilar junction

List of Operative Drawings

3.I. A-C Subtemporal approach to region basilar bifurcation *p. 22*

3.II. A-C Initial view of entrance to interpeduncular cistern over tentorial edge *p. 24*

3.III. A-E Dissection and clipping of basilar bifurcation aneurysm *p. 26*

3.IV. A-F Use of fenestrated clips and tandem clipping *p. 32*

7.V. A-B Operative illustration for basilar SCA aneurysm *p. 96*

10.VI. A-C Subtemporal transtentorial approach to the basilar AICA and V-B junction aneurysms *p. 134*

12.VII. A-D Transmastoid transpetrosal approach *p. 172*

14.VIII. A-H Lateral suboccipital approach *pp. 202–203*

Chapter 1
Historical Notes

The first case of this series of vertebrobasilar aneurysms was operated on in January 1959 and is described in detail in Chapter 9. In 1960, at the time of the senior author's first report on the intracranial treatment of five ruptured basilar artery aneurysms, only seven other treated basilar aneurysms could be found in the literature; of these, only four had been clipped. A few operations had been reported for smaller aneurysms at the more accessible sites on the posterior circulation: vertebral, posterior inferior cerebellar artery (PICA), P2 and basilar artery branches in the cerebellopontine angle (Fig. 1.1). Remarkably, nine procedures for giant globular or fusiform aneurysms had been done, but with a high mortality (Fig. 1.2).

On the other hand, for aneurysms on the anterior circulation, some 350 intracranial operations had been reported by that time (a later report in 1969 Cooperative Study includes 151 McKissock's cases giving a total of 522) and many more had been treated by carotid occlusion or trapping.

That more basilar and even vertebral aneurysms had not been approached was probably related to three factors:

(1) their presumed rarity;
(2) the later development of safe routine vertebral angiography; and
(3) the more dangerously hidden position of these aneurysms in front of the brain stem.

Although Moniz had opacified the posterior circulation by open retrograde subclavian injection in 1934, it was Krayenbühl in 1941, using the same method, who was the first to demonstrate an aneurysm on the vertebral-basilar system. Hamby was critical of the retrograde catheter technique described by Radner in 1947, which involved sacrifice of the radial artery. For many years vertebral angiography was done through direct vertebral artery puncture in the neck anteriorly or from laterally in the sulcus arteriosus of the atlas, but only a few radiologists became routinely adept with this technique. However, with the advent of safe percutaneous brachial and later femoral artery cannulation, the retrograde catheter techniques supplanted all others, and four-vessel studies are now routine. Still, it is remarkable that as late as 1965, only about 25% of the patients admitted to the Cooperative Study had had vertebral angiography, the probable reason for the low incidence of posterior aneurysms in that study (5.5%). The recent extensive survey of Fox confirms Hamby's earlier estimate that about 17.5% of all intracranial aneurysms occur on the vertebral-basilar circulation.

Beginning with Cushing in 1915, a few giant globular or fusiform vertebral-basilar aneurysms had been exposed during surgery for presumed tumors, or in the course of the posterior fossa "tic" operation for trigeminal neuralgia. The first definitive intracranial treatment of a posterior circulation aneurysm was carried out by Olivecrona in 1932 when he trapped and excised a large PICA aneurysm which had produced a lower angle syndrome. Dandy, in 1937, actually "shelled out" a large saccular aneurysm of the vertebral artery with little bleeding, although the patient did not survive. He also reported finding 11 atherosclerotic fusiform S-shaped aneurysms of the vertebral-basilar artery during exploration of the cerebellopontine angle for tic douloureux or Meniere's disease. He believed that compression of either the trigeminal nerve (10 cases) or the auditory nerve (1 case) was the cause of the tic douloureux or Meniere's syndrome, respectively. In 1927, in a 63 year old woman with unbearable tinnitus unrelieved by left eighth nerve section, he ligated the left vertebral artery. A few weeks later, the right vertebral was compressed "not longer than 2 seconds." The patient "died instantly without another heartbeat or respiration; there could be no more rapid death or one so

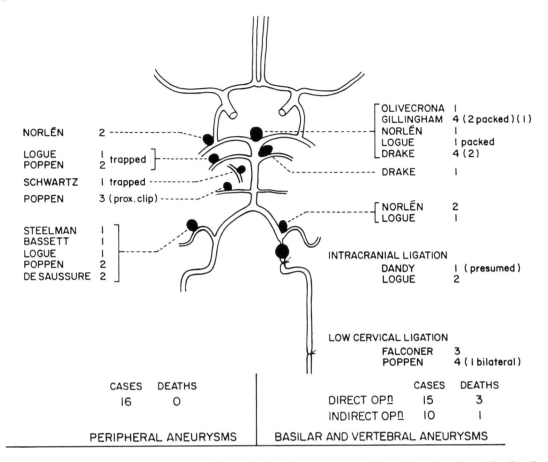

Figure 1.1. Early surgical treatment of vertebrobasilar aneurysm. Sites of ruptured vertebrobasilar aneurysms operated upon before 1960 modified from Drake 1979. ( ) = deaths

silent." In 1940, he ligated a vertebral artery between the atlas and the axis in one of the patients with trigeminal neuralgia, in the hope that it might lessen the strain on the patient's aneurysm. Tönnis, in 1937, described a remarkable surgical experience when he incised what he thought was an acoustic neuroma. The patient survived without complication after packing the interior of the aneurysm with muscle.

Even though the technique of vertebral angiography had been described at least 15 years before, it is outstanding that the first deliberate direct attacks on ruptured posterior fossa aneurysms were done without the aid of angiography. Schwartz, in 1946, explored the left cerebellopontine angle of a 27 year old woman with an angle syndrome following a hemorrhage. He found and trapped a small aneurysm arising from an unusual artery which he could not identify, coursing from the mid basilar region toward the trigeminal root. In 1947, Steelman et al. trapped and excised a 2 cm ruptured aneurysm arising from PICA under the cerebellar tonsil. Hydrocephalus and a deformity of the fourth ventricle had been discovered at ventriculography for persistent coma.

The first reported attempt to obliterate a basilar artery aneurysm was that by Olivecrona. In 1954, using a subtemporal approach, he was able to clip a ruptured, forward projecting aneurysm at the basilar bifurcation. The patient improved remarkably from postoperative hemiparesis and aphasia being capable for part-time work.

Although Dandy reported ligation of the left vertebral artery for a presumed ruptured aneurysm on that artery, he had no proof of the lesion; the 54 year old man had had two episodes of severe occipital pain with paresis of the eleventh and twelfth cranial nerves. Poppen appears to have been the first to ligate the vertebral artery for a verified ruptured vertebral artery aneurysm. In 1945, in a 40

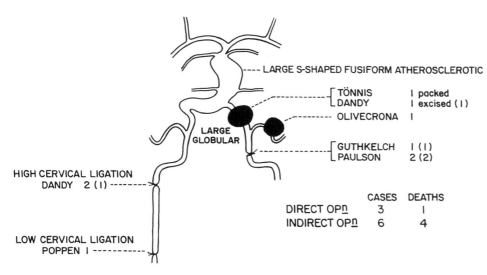

Figure 1.2. Early surgical treatment of vertebrobasilar aneurysm. Sites of giant intact vertebral and basilar aneurysms treated directly or by vertebral ligation before 1960. ( ) = deaths

year old man in coma after three hemorrhages from a right vertebral aneurysm, the artery was ligated in the vertebral triangle in the neck. Seven years later, after removal of a fourth ventricle ependymoma from the same patient, a "nonpulsating" saccular aneurysm of the right vertebral artery, 4 x 3 mm in size, was noted. Subsequently, in 1948 and 1950, he occluded the vertebral artery in two other patients; one with a ruptured vertebral aneurysm and the other with a large vertebral aneurysm which had produced an angle syndrome; the latter aneurysm ruptured fatally six months later.

Poppen was also the first to occlude one vertebral artery for ruptured aneurysms involving the basilar artery, once bilaterally. In 1951, he described the ligation of both vertebral arteries in the neck, six weeks apart, in a 57 year old man who had ruptured a large atherosclerotic "fusiform aneurysm and elongation of the basilar artery." Right hemiparesis, with cerebellar dysfunction and marked personality change all recovered after the second operation, but the aneurysm ruptured fatally six months later. His second case in the same year was also a ruptured fusiform atherosclerotic aneurysm of the "entire basilar artery." The 42 year old man was still working seven years later, after ligation of the much larger left vertebral artery. A third vertebral ligation was done for a similar aneurysm which had produced an angle syndrome, with "dramatic improvement." Logue, in 1957, occluded the vertebral artery proximal to PICA and a small ruptured fusiform vertebral aneurysm, which almost certainly was a ruptured dissecting aneurysm of the vertebral artery. A similar case was also done six months later. Both patients were temporarily disabled postoperatively with presumed brain stem ischemia.

The first deliberate occlusion of the basilar artery for ruptured aneurysm was reported by Mount in 1952. A young man sustained four hemorrhages from an enlarging basilar bifurcation aneurysm. Large posterior communicating arteries (PComAs) were shown by carotid angiography. Under hypothermia, the basilar artery was clipped obliquely between the posterior cerebral origins and one superior cerebellar artery (SCA). A stormy postoperative period ensued but recovery was complete after one year and the aneurysm no longer filled on postoperative angiography.

Up to 1960, including Drake's initial 5 cases (Fig. 1.1), 25 operative procedures had been done for ruptured basilar or vertebral aneurysms, of which 10 were proximal vertebral artery occlusions. Four deaths resulted, 3 from direct operation, but 16 aneurysms on peripheral branches had been clipped or trapped without sequelae. Nine vertebral artery occlusions had been done for large intact globular or fusiform aneurysms, with only four survivors.

In the next decade, several surgeons reported their experiences. In 1964, Jamieson was discouraged by his results in 19 cases; 10 died and only 4 of the 9 survivors were employable. About the same time, Logue et al. noted the same poor results with aneurysms at the basilar bifurcation. However, it became evident that aneurysms along the trunk of the basilar artery, on the posterior cerebral and vertebral arteries, or peripherally situated on SCA or PICA, were much more amenable to surgical treatment. Then, in 1967, Jamieson reported on a further eight cases, four at the bifurcation and four on the trunk of the basilar artery, with only two deaths. In 1968, Drake was also more optimistic after experience with another 17 patients; in 15 with non-giant aneurysms, there was only one death. In the same year, he illustrated the surgical approaches and techniques used for vertebral and basilar aneurysms and in 1969, discussed an overall experience of 43 cases, of which 70% had satisfactory outcomes.

Since then, the series of patients with vertebral-basilar aneurysms operated upon by the neurosurgical service at The University of Western Ontario, London Canada has exceeded 1760 (Fig. 1.3).

The approaches to basilar artery aneurysms worked out in the 50's and early 60's, viz. subtemporal, frontotemporal, subtemporal-transtentorial, transmastoid-transpetrosal and lateral posterior fossa, have stood the test of time. But other problems emerged related to the arterial branchings at each aneurysm site, most particularly the perforating arteries in the region of the basilar bifurcation. One or more of the cranial nerves may be intimately related to these aneurysms as well, or simply impede access to them.

Since the difficulties with dissection and occlusion of aneurysms vary directly with their size, the author's classification has continued to be used.

Small	< 12 mm	($^1/_2$ inch)
Large	12–25 mm	($^1/_2$–1 inch)
Giant	> 25 mm	(1 inch)

During the last two and a half decades, there have been remarkable advances in the investigation and operative and perioperative management of patients underoing surgery for intracranial aneurysms. In particular, modern dedicated neuroanesthesia has allowed the exact premises of the aneurysm to be revealed under slack and relatively protected brain during deep hypotension, temporary clipping or trapping. Under the microscope, all the tiny structures intimate to the aneurysm are revealed with microinstrumentation for their dissection and the exquisitely accurate application of a spring clip to the neck. Of particular significance on

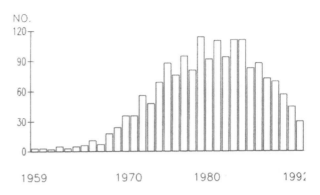

Figure 1.3. Yearly number of patients operated on in this series of 1767 patients with vertebrobasilar aneurysms in 1959–1992. The decline in numbers of patients was due to foreign government restriction on hospital reimbursement in Canada, but mostly, the education of countless neurosurgeons and residents, so that posterior circulation aneurysms are now operated upon world-wide in major neurosurgical units

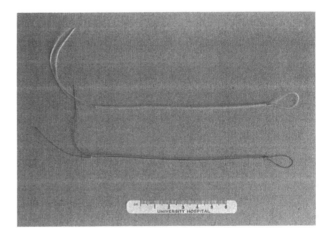

Figure 1.4. The microtourniquet: above the original made from two small sizes of polyethylene tubing PE 50 inside PE 190, below current tourniquet made from plastic suture inside PE 190 polyethylene tubing

this unit was the design of the fenestrated clip in 1968 which greatly simplified the management of large basilar bifurcation aneurysms and which has proved to be so useful in other aneurysms including the tandem techniques. With few exceptions, mostly related to size and configuration, small and large intracranial aneurysms can now be obliterated with highly satisfactory outcomes.

Hunterian parent artery occlusion proximal to giant aneurysms had to be used more often for those on the vertebral-basilar than the carotid circulation, even though the basilar artery and its branches are not very different in size. So often the neck was globular, rigid with fibrosis, atheroma and mural thrombus and the major branches and perforators arose from the base of the sacs. The mass was frequently buried in the brain stem and surrounded by cranial nerves and the narrow confines above and in front of the clivus impeded safe access to the whole of the neck. The first sight of one of these aneurysms is most impressive and for some years, in contrast to anterior giant aneurysms, opening and evacuation of the sac to promote clipping seemed very perilous. The problem for basilar artery occlusion was to be able to identify those arteries with sufficient natural collateral before commitment to clip occlusion of the artery.

The senior author was encouraged to try basilar artery occlusion after inadvertent occlusion of the artery by clips occluding the necks of large aneurysms on it but without sequelae.

The first deliberate basilar clip occlusions were done in the presence of one or two large PComAs, but when one of these patients remained stuporous and hemiplegic, some form of temporary occlusion while the patient was awake became necessary. The first of these patients, in 1973, had temporary basilar artery occlusion under local anesthesia, but even though the trigeminal ganglion was injected with local anesthetic, the patient was uncontrollably restless and squealing with pain from manipulation on the still sensitive dura of the tentorium and clivus as well as the bayonet forceps holding the artery occluded for about four minutes. Light anesthesia was induced and the artery was then occluded with a Scoville clip temporarily while the patient was re-awakened. When he seemed to tolerate the occlusion the clip was left in place and he had an excellent outcome.

In the next patient in 1975, a simple microtourniquet was improvised by placing a tiny poly-

ethylene tubing (PE-50) around the upper basilar artery and threading both ends through slightly larger tubing (PE-190) whose length was cut and left protruding about $1^1/_2$ inches outside the head after the wound closure (Fig. 1.4). The next day in the angiographic suite, the tourniquet was tightened and held by a small artery forceps and basilar artery occlusion verified by a flush injection. After the patient remained unchanged, the tourniquet occlusion was maintained by a firmly closed Weck clip and the patient returned to the observation unit with the clip-removing forceps for constant surveillance. The nurses were trained and instructed to open the clip and loosen the tourniquet if significant deterioration occurred. After 24 hours without sequela the patient was returned to the operating room where under local anesthesia the tourniquet was buried by enlarging the stab wound so that clip occlusion of the tourniquet at the level of the bone flap could be done and the stem beyond divided and removed. Later tourniquets used silk or plastic sutures inside the polyethylene tubing. The tourniquet was subsequently used on the vertebral and posterior cerebral arteries (59 times in posterior circulation) as well as the anterior and middle cerebral arteries in the treatment of giant aneurysms. It was also used to produce a severe stenosis of the artery when its complete occlusion was not tolerated. The details of these occlusions are under the respective aneurysm sites.

Inspite of considerable advances in the management of intracranial aneurysms in the last half century, some difficult problems remain to be solved. Chief among these are the prevention or treatment of the central consequences of subarachnoid hemorrhage (SAH) and the technical means to isolate most aneurysms from the parent circulation by neck occlusion, especially on the posterior circulation (Tables 1.1 and 1.2).

6   Historical Notes

Table 1.1. Non-giant vertebrobasilar aneurysms: summary of results in three different time periods

Years	Excellent	Good	Poor	Dead	Total
1959–1970	48 64.9	6 8.1	9 12.2	11 14.9	74
1971–1981	465 75.6	80 13.0	42 6.8	28 4.6	615
1982–1992	510 74.9	97 14.2	49 7.2	25 3.7	681
Total	1023 74.7	183 13.4	100 7.3	64 4.7	1370

Table 1.2. Giant vertebrobasilar aneurysms: summary of results in three different time periods

Years	Excellent	Good	Poor	Dead	Total
1959–1970	5 38.5	3 23.1	2 15.4	3 23.1	13
1971–1981	86 48.0	39 21.8	30 16.8	24 13.4	179
1982–1992	98 47.8	45 22.0	37 18.0	25 12.2	205
Total	189 47.6	87 21.9	69 17.4	52 13.1	397

Chapter 2
Clinical Material

The clinical material to be discussed is derived from a series of 1767 patients with vertebral-basilar aneurysms operated upon at the teaching hospitals of the University of Western Ontario in London, Canada; at Victoria Hospital 1959–1972 (140 patients), at University Hospital 1973–1992 (1540 patients) and at the University of Miami in Miami, Florida at Jackson Memorial Hospital 1991–1992 (31 patients). Fifty-six (56) other patients were operated upon at other university clinics as a visiting surgeon. Ninety-five (95) percent of the patients were operated on by the two senior authors.

Nine patients have been entered twice:

1. a female of 48 years had her ruptured small basilar bifurcation aneurysm in 1970 clipped with an excellent angiographic and clinical result. Thirteen years later she had headaches and examinations revealed a giant aneurysm in the same location which was successfully thrombosed by basilar tourniquet occlusion but she remained in poor condition;

2. a female of 33 had her small ruptured posterior-inferior cerebellar artery (PICA) aneurysm repaired in 1983, and three years later an incidental small basilar bifurcation aneurysm was clipped, both times with excellent results;

3. a female of 44 years had her small ruptured basilar bifurcation aneurysm totally occluded in 1976 with excellent result. Recurrent subarachnoid hemorrhage (SAH) in 1990 revealed a large aneurysm at the same site, which was repaired with an excellent result;

4. a female of 37 years had her ruptured small PICA aneurysm repaired with excellent outcome in 1975, ten years later a rebleed revealed a small aneurysm at the same site which was repaired with a good result;

5. a male of 47 years had explorative surgery for his giant superior cerebellar artery (SCA) aneurysm in 1970. He was for several years self sufficient but after decline and clipping of the aneurysm from the contralateral side in 1979, he remained in poor condition;

6. a 33 year old woman had her ruptured basilar bifurcation aneurysm repaired in 1973 with an excellent result. Seven years later, a rebleed from a giant aneurysm at the same site was treated with basilar artery clipping eight days after SAH. Another fatal SAH occurred the next day in spite of the basilar occlusion;

7. a male of 18 years had his giant ruptured basilar trunk aneurysm partially repaired in 1973 by occlusion of its waist by a silk ligature and a clip. Angiograms in 1984 revealed again a giant aneurysm at the same site which was treated successfully by occlusion of his only vertebral artery;

8. a female of 38 years had her ruptured small basilar trunk aneurysm completely clipped in 1978; an aneurysm of giant size at the same site was treated by trapping seven years later with a good result;

9. a female nurse aged 28 had her ruptured backward projecting small basilar bifurcation aneurysm repaired with an excellent result in 1971. Two years later, headache was investigated and a new superior projecting aneurysm at the same site was found. A cardiac arrest from unrecognized profound hypotension at the beginning of reopening caused severe hypoxic brain damage and she remained decorticate.

Otherwise all cases represent one patient irrespective of the number of operations or aneurysms (125 patients had multiple elective procedures in London, Ontario for the primary lesion).

The distribution and size of the aneurysms on the vertebral-basilar tree is seen in Table 2.1.

Patient ages ranged from 3–80 with a mean of 46.6 years. The female sex predominated 1140 vs 627 males, almost a 2 : 1 ratio except that 80% of vertebral aneurysms were in females. Mean age in females was three years more than in males (47.7

Clinical Material

years / 44.6 years).[1] Multiple aneurysms occurred in 462 (26.1%) and associated arteriovenous malformations (AVMs) were present in 59 (3.3%).

Saccular aneurysms predominated (Table 2.2), but 127 were nonatherosclerotic, fusiform in type, mostly in the giant series (85) and in a younger age group with a mean age 10 years younger than in other series. Four had arteriovenous fistulas, three with huge venous varixes located on PICA distally and one had a ruptured small saccular aneurysm on the fistulous artery associated with a small but separate AVM. Three had a traumatic origin; one was a false aneurysm arising from the mid basilar trunk after transsphenoidal pituitary surgery and another was a vertebral dissection, clearly related to chiropractic manipulation. The third also was a vertebral dissection occurring four weeks after a facial fracture and surgical repair.

As with those on the anterior circulation, most basilar aneurysms rupture after reaching a critical size (5–6 mm) and wall thinness, during those emotional and physical stresses in life, including REM sleep, which suddenly raise the blood pressure beyond the range normally sustained by the thinned wall at the dome. Initial, minor "warning leaks" and vicious recurrent bleeding seem to be as common as in the anterior circulation.

Most patients presented after a SAH, 924 with single and 416 after multiple bleedings. Four hundred and twenty-seven (427) were unruptured, presenting as one of multiple aneurysms, incidentally found or with mass effect. Thirty-five patients with remote bleeding (more than one year) were classified as unruptured aneurysms. Nineteen point two percent (19.2%) were hypertensive. One hundred and ninety-three (193) patients had a re-operation on their aneurysm (failed aneurysm surgery), 68 from referring institutions and 125 from our unit (5 patients operated on elsewhere had 2 or more operations in London).

Intracerebral hemorrhage occurred only in four patients.

---

[1] Twenty patients had their SAH during pregnancy or very close to the birth of the child. The practice of this unit for a ruptured aneurysm is a reasonably early repair for we have had no maternal or foetal morbidity, even using profound hypotension. Since ruptured AVMs do not carry the same risk of early repeated bleeding, their treatment has been delayed until after the birth of the child.

Every known method of treatment has been utilized (Table 2.9 and 2.10). In the early cases, only McKenzie and Olivecrona silver clips were available (Fig. 9.1). Silk ligatures were used occasionally, even until 1976 to occlude larger necks or to narrow them for the small clip. The removable replaceable spring clip was a great advance when the Mayfield clip became more widely available in the early 60's. The Scoville clip had a smaller spring and applier to apply in narrow confines.

A problem remained with large basilar bifurcation aneurysms where the P1 segment was adherent to the side of the neck and waist of the aneurysm; its dissection free of the neck for application of a clip blade underneath was difficult and dangerous for tearing of the sac. Faced with such a problem, in September 1969, Dr. Mayfield agreed to have Mr. George Kees fashion three clips with differing blade lengths over the weekend, but with a fenestration at the base of the blades in which the P1 segment could be placed intact while the blades fell

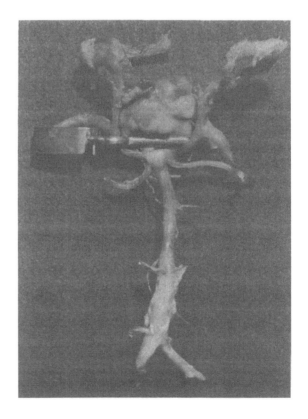

Figure 2.1. M.R., F, 59, death due to myocardial infarction on postoperative day 4 in August 1970. Specimen shows principle and application of Drake fenestrated clip with P1 intact in the aperture

across the neck of the aneurysm. This first case was a complete success and the fenestrated clip came into common use for most basilar bifurcation aneurysms (Fig. 2.1). In addition to the P1 segment, perforators and literally every other major intracranial artery and the third and optic nerves have been left intact in the aperture. Subsequently, Sugita's modification of the Drake-Mayfield clip with narrower blades and handle have been most used. In 1973, the senior author stumbled on the tandem technique using fenestrated clip blades to close the opposite two-thirds of the neck of a giant carotid ophthalmic aneurysm, whereon five long straight clips placed side by side and piggyback had failed to occlude because the thick neck in the fulcrum kept the tips apart. The fenestration left the near neck open while the blades closed in parallel on the far side. The simple addition of a shorter straight bladed clip across that portion of the neck remaining open in the aperture easily completed the occlusion of the neck. The use of this tandem principle on non-giant basilar bifurcation aneurysms was delayed until 1978 when it was realized that in spite of carefully trimmed and measured fenestrated blades, several cases had rebled because of small portions of neck remaining open in the aperture, a problem easily overcome with a short tandem clip. Since then the tandem clip principle has been used extensively on non-giant, mostly large aneurysms especially at the basilar bifurcation, and in its many variations has played a major role in clipping the necks of giant aneurysms on all intracranial arteries.

Coagulation to shrink the neck of posterior aneurysms has seldom been used, especially at the basilar bifurcation for fear of occlusion of hidden perforators.

A few unclippable aneurysms were coated with gauze, cottonoid or plastic, alone or in combination, but except for small sacs, never completely. In spite of apparent incomplete treatment, a few have had prolonged survivals probably more related to the nature of those aneurysms than the encasement.

In 1965, two giant basilar bifurcation aneurysms were treated by the pilo-injection of horsehairs through their walls. In 1971, another was filled with 16 feet of copper beryllium wire with Dr. Sean Mullan. Both pilo-injected aneurysms recurred and rebled three months and seven years later. In spite of apparent complete angiographic occlusion, the wired aneurysm enlarged again below the unchanged wire-induced thrombus killing the patient by mass effect (cf. Chapter 6, p. 69). Because of their failure, these early transsaccular occlusions were abandoned. In a fourth patient, five feet of wire was injected into a huge bifurcation aneurysm in 1987. She was poor thereafter and died one week later.

Recently a few, deemed inoperable because of grade or medical state, have been treated by transfemoral endosaccular detachment of balloons or wire coils. Any firm conclusions must await prolonged trial of these methods (see Chapter 24).

Fourteen aneurysms in 12 patients were excised; all were peripherally situated on anterior inferior cerebellar artery (2), SCA (4) or PCA (6) alone or in 9 patients associated with an AVM.

Proximal parent vessel occlusion has been used extensively, mostly for otherwise inoperable giant aneurysms, but also for a few smaller fusiform and all except two ruptured vertebral dissections. Although the basilar and vertebral arteries were most frequently involved, all of their branches have been proximally occluded too in the treatment of aneurysm.

Trapping was used electively when immediate reduction of the mass was deemed imperative either at the time or with subsequent growth above an occlusion. On a few occasions (11), trapping was used of necessity to control bleeding.

Finally, in 41 cases, the aneurysm was only explored, definitive treatment not seeming to be possible at the time, although most were giant aneurysms. As might be expected, their outcome has not been a happy one. In a group of 31 untreated giant aneurysms, 68% were dead at 2 years and by 5 years, 84% had died with the remaining patients severely disabled.

For most aneurysm sites, the grade of the patient at operation and ischemia with vasospasm account for the majority of poor results in experienced surgical hands. In this series, their impact was less because of the pattern of referral, the majority of patients being sent from greater distances in delayed fashion and in better condition; 51% were operated on between days 11 and 30 (Table 2.11). Only 10% of all patients with non-giant aneurysms arrived in poor condition (Grade 3 or worse, Table 2.3). The Botterell classification has been used throughout the series. It is nearly identical to that of

Clinical Material

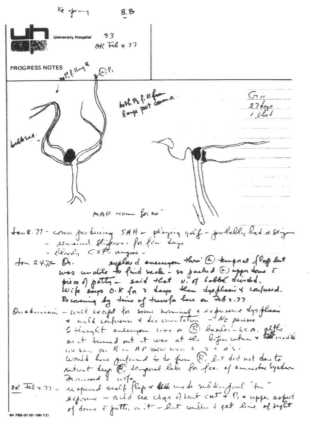

Figure 2.2. A typical track sheet

the World Federation of Neurosurgical Societies. Only 14.5% of patients with non-giant aneurysms were operated upon within 7 days of SAH, most in recent years (cf. Chapter 22). Surgery on days 7 to 10, formerly thought to be ideal timing, has been shown to carry a higher morbidity for ruptured anterior aneurysms, presumably because the peak incidence of vasospasm occurs at this time. Our outcome in this period was not significantly different.

Because of the various sites, sizes and complexity of this series of aneurysms, the results of treatment, including patient outcome and obliteration of the aneurysm, will be discussed under the various aneurysm origins from the vertebrobasilar tree.

In the tables to follow, the data are derived from track sheets on which were traced the pertinent angiograms followed by a written description of the history, the operative procedure and progress during the hospital stay (Fig. 2.2). All patients were analyzed. The data collected included surgeon, age, sex, mode and dates of clinical presentation, pre- and postoperative neurological condition and grade, location, type and size of the aneurysm and its relation to landmarks of the skull base, associated vascular lesions, type and date of surgery, intra- and postoperative complications. These factors were related to clinical outcome. Only in 11 cases, were track sheets not found so that exact site, size and projection of those aneurysms and some other information is unknown, and so listed in the tables.

Surviving patients' outcome was categorized first at the time of discharge and then in follow-up at variable time intervals often amounting to years. Patients in poor condition at the time of discharge often expired after discharge from intercurrent disease. All deaths within three months of surgery were counted as surgical deaths. A significant number of patients improved from poor to good or good to excellent in the month(s) following surgery. We do not have systematic records of long term outcome. However, regular contacts with the referring neurosurgeons kept information on improvements and declines accurate, e.g rebleedings as late as eight years after surgery are included in statistics. In those few cases without follow-up we have recorded the condition at discharge as outcome.

Table 2.1. Location and aneurysm size in 1767 patients with VBAAs

Location	Small	Large	Giant	Total	Percent
Basilar bifurcation	493 55.1	265 29.6	137 15.3	895	50.7
Basilar SCA	153 57.5	57 21.4	56 21.1	266	15.1
Midbasilar	23 16.0	21 14.6	59 41.0	144	8.1
Basilar-AICA	31 21.5	10 6.9			
Vertebro-basilar junction	46 39.7	31 26.7	39 33.6	116	6.6
Vertebral	154 69.7	27 12.2	40 18.1	221	12.5
Posterior cerebral artery	39 31.2	20 16.0	66 52.8	125	7.1
Total	939 53.1	431 24.4	397 22.5	1767	100.0

Table 2.2. Type of aneurysm in 1767 patients with VBAAs

Type of aneurysm	No.	Percent
Saccular	1591	90.0
Fusiform	127	7.2
Dissecting	28	1.6
Atheromatous	10	0.6
Mycotic	3	0.2
Traumatic	3	0.2
Fistulous	4	0.2
No aneurysm found[a]	1	0.1
Total	1767	100.0

[a] As basilar bifurcation aneurysm explored.

12 Clinical Material

Table 2.3. Preoperative Grade (Botterell) and outcome in 1767 patients with VBAAs

Grade	Excellent	Good	Poor	Dead	Total	Percent
0[a]	304	61	61	36	462	26.1
	65.8	13.2	13.2	7.8		
0g	*279*	*36*	*24*	*17*	*356*	*20.1*
	78.4	*10.1*	*6.7*	*4.8*		
0p	*25*	*25*	*37*	*19*	*106*	*6.0*
	23.6	*23.6*	*34.9*	*17.9*		
1	683	88	38	32	841	47.6
	81.2	10.5	4.5	3.8		
2	180	62	27	20	289	16.4
	62.3	21.5	9.3	6.9		
3	42	53	31	13	139	7.8
	30.2	38.1	22.3	9.4		
4	2	6	12	10	30	1.7
	6.7	20.0	40.0	33.3		
5	1			6	7	0.3
	16.7			83.3		
Total	1212	270	169	116	1767	100.0
	68.6	15.3	9.6	6.6		

[a] *0* Unruptured aneurysm or remote hemorrhage (> 1 year). *0g* Good risk without major neurological deficit. *0p* Poor risk patient with major neurological deficit (severe confusion or dementia or stupor or coma, dysarthria or bulbar paralysis, severe dysphasia or severe mono-, hemi-, or tetraparesis).

Table 2.4. Aneurysm size and outcome in 1767 patients with VBAAs

Size	Excellent	Good	Poor	Dead	Total	Percent
Small	736	113	56	34	939	53.1
	78.4	12.0	6.0	3.6		
Large	287	70	44	30	431	24.4
	66.6	16.2	10.2	7.0		
Giant	189	87	69	52	397	22.5
	47.6	21.9	17.4	13.1		
Total	1212	270	169	116	1767	100.0
	68.6	15.3	9.6	6.6		

Table 2.5. Location and outcome in 1767 patients with VBAA

Location	E	G	P	Dead	No.	Percent
Basilar bifurcation	611	140	95	49	895	50.7
	68.3	15.6	10.6	5.5		
Basilar SCA	186	40	23	17	266	15.1
	69.9	15.0	8.6	6.4		
Basilar trunk (AICA and midbasilar)	85	25	14	20	144	8.1
	59.0	17.4	9.7	13.9		
Vertebro-basilar junction	70	19	14	13	116	6.6
	60.3	16.4	12.1	11.2		
Vertebral	171	27	13	10	221	12.5
	77.4	12.2	5.9	4.5		
Posterior cerebral artery	89	19	10	7	125	7.1
	71.2	15.2	8.0	5.6		
Total	1212	270	169	116	1767	100.0
	68.6	15.3	9.6	6.6		

E Excellent, *G* good, *P* poor.

Table 2.6. Location and outcome in 1767 patients with VBAAs

Location	Excellent	Good	Poor	Dead	No.	Percent
Basilar artery						
Bifurcation	611	140	95	49	895	50.7
	68.3	15.6	10.6	5.5		
SCA	179	36	22	16	253	14.3
	70.8	14.2	8.7	6.3		
SCA distal	7	4	1	1	13	0.8
	53.8	30.8	7.7	7.7		
AICA	25	5	2	1	33	1.9
	75.8	15.2	6.1	3.0		
AICA proximal	2		1	1	4	0.2
	50.0		25.0	25.0		
AICA distal	3	1			4	0.2
	75.0	25.0				
Trunk	55	19	11	18	103	5.8
	53.4	18.4	10.7	17.5		
Vertebrobasilar junction						
Junction	69	19	14	13	115	6.5
	60.0	16.5	12.2	11.3		
Hypoglossal artery	1				1	0.1
	100.0					
Vertebral artery						
Proximal	2	1	1		4	0.2
	50.0	25.0	25.0			
PrePICA	8	2	1	3	14	0.8
	57.1	14.3	7.1	21.4		
PostPICA	107	17	6	6	136	7.7
	78.7	12.5	4.4	4.4		
Distal	30	6	5		41	2.3
	73.2	14.6	12.2			
PICA proximal	10				10	0.6
	100.0					
PICA distal	14	1		1	16	0.9
	87.5	6.3		6.3		
Posterior cerebral artery						
P1	29	7	8	2	46	2.6
	63.0	15.2	17.4	4.3		
P1 Mesencephalic branch	1				1	0.1
	100.0					
PCom junction P1-P2	19	2	1	2	24	1.4
	79.2	8.3	4.2	8.3		
P2	27	9	1	3	40	2.3
	67.5	22.5	2.5	7.5		
P3-P4	13	1			14	0.8
	92.9	7.1				
Total	1212	270	169	116	1767	100.0
	68.6	15.3	9.6	6.6		

14 Clinical Material

Table 2.7. Age related to outcome in 1767 patients with VBAAs

Age group (years)	Excellent	Good	Poor	Dead	Total	Percent
0–9	6	1		2	9	0.5
	66.7	11.1		22.2		
10–19	37	4	3		44	2.5
	84.1	9.1	6.8			
20–29	109	15	2	4	130	7.4
	83.8	11.5	1.5	3.1		
30–39	210	43	20	15	288	16.3
	72.9	14.9	6.9	5.2		
40–49	364	66	47	31	508	28.7
	71.7	13.0	9.3	6.1		
50–59	324	88	52	33	497	28.1
	65.2	17.7	10.5	6.6		
60–69	150	47	39	28	264	14.9
	56.8	17.8	14.8	10.6		
70 or more	12	6	6	3	27	1.5
	44.4	22.2	22.2	11.1		
Total	1212	270	169	116	1767	100.0
	68.6	15.3	9.6	6.6		

Table 2.8. Sex and final result of surgery in 1767 patients with VBAAs

Sex	Excellent	Good	Poor	Dead	Total	Percent
Female	781	175	109	75	1140	64.5
	68.5	15.4	9.6	6.6		
Male	431	95	60	41	627	35.5
	68.7	15.2	9.6	6.5		
Total	1212	270	169	116	1767	100.0
	68.6	15.3	9.6	6.6		

Table 2.9. Operative method and outcome in 1767 patients with VBAAs

Operative method	Excel-lent	Good	Poor	Dead	Total	Percent
Clip	974 72.7	194 14.5	112 8.4	60 4.5	1340	75.8
Silk ligature	10 55.6	2 11.1	4 22.2	2 11.1	18	1.0
Hunterian ligation	150 57.5	48 18.4	35 13.4	28 10.7	261	14.8
Trapping	23 51.1	8 17.8	4 8.9	10 22.2	45	2.5
Excision	9 75.0	3 25.0			12	0.7
Wrapping	27 73.0	5 13.5	3 8.1	2 5.4	37	2.1
Endovascular[a]	1 20.0	1 20.0		3 60.0	5	0.3
Transmural injection (horse hair or wire)	1 25.0	1 25.0	1 25.0	1 25.0	4	0.2
Varia[b]	1 25.0		1 25.0	2 50.0	4	0.2
Explored only	16 39.0	8 19.5	9 22.0	8 19.5	41	2.3
Total	1212 68.6	270 15.3	169 9.6	116 6.6	1767	100.0

[a] Cf. Chapter 24, which includes 12 later cases after this series.
[b] Two patients shunted only (PCA aneurysm thrombosed, atherosclerotic basilar trunk giant aneurysm), one induction rebleeding without surgery and one hematoma only removed.

Clinical Material

Table 2.10. Operative method and completeness of aneurysm treatment in 1767 patients with VBAAs

Operative method	Total obliter-ation	Resid-ual neck	Resid-ual fundus	No oblit-eration	Not known	Total
Clip	1211 90.4%	94	33		2	1340
Silk ligature	15 83.3%	1	2			18
Hunterian ligation	170 65.1%	19	61	6	5	261
Trapping	44 97.8%			1		45
Excision	12 100.0%					12
Wrapping	2 5.4%		1	32	2	37
Endo-vascular	2 40.0%		3			5
Transmural injection (horse hair or wire)			2		2	4
Varia	1 25.0%			3		4
Explor-ation only	1 2.4%		2	38		41
Total	1458 82.5%	114	104	80	11	1767

Table 2.11. Timing of surgery after last SAH and outcome in 1305 patients with VBAAs

Timing of surgery	Excel-lent	Good	Poor	Dead	Total
0–1 day	22 50.0	7 15.9	6 13.6	9 20.5	44
2–3 day	34 55.7	10 16.4	9 14.8	8 13.1	61
4–6 day	56 66.7	18 21.4	3 3.6	7 8.3	84
7–10 day	141 75.0	22 11.7	14 7.4	11 5.9	188
11–30 day	465 69.9	108 16.2	55 8.3	37 5.6	665
31–365 day	190 72.2	44 16.7	21 8.0	8 3.0	263
Total	908 69.6	209 16.0	108 8.3	80 6.1	1305

Chapter 3

Small Aneurysms at the Bifurcation of the Basilar Artery
493 Patients

The basilar bifurcation is the most common aneurysm site (50.7%) in the posterior circulation, comprising about 5-6% of all solitary intracranial aneurysms. The majority are saccular, but a few (< 1%) are fusiform in origin. This aneurysm has proved to be the most difficult of all intracranial aneurysms, surgeons having taken a decade longer to reduce its surgical morbidity to near that of any on the anterior circulation.

Clinical Features

Most small saccular aneurysms arising at the basilar bifurcation remain silent, unheralded by specific premonitory signs or symptoms until they rupture. But, in common with all patients who rupture an aneurysm, non-specific symptoms such as headache, dizziness or visual blurring may precede the ictus. Infrequently, transient paresis of upward gaze may be seen after the rupture of basilar bifurcation aneurysms. Third nerve paresis is rare (5% in small and 9% in large aneurysms), but it has occurred after rupture of upward projecting bifurcation aneurysms, whose domes were related to the roots of the nerve, or in those few aneurysms with eccentric lateral projections. In one patient it was bilateral. Fourteen patients had sixth nerve palsy, in six bilaterally. Two patients had fourth nerve palsy, one of which was bilateral. No other cranial nerve palsies were seen. The domes of aneurysms abutting the floor of the hypothalamus may rupture into the third ventricle, flooding the ventricular system with blood. Intra-axial rupture of basilar and vertebral aneurysms is very rare even when much of the dome is embedded in the brain stem, probably because of the pial barrier or that the rupture site at the dome is not buried. The large brain stem and angle cisterns are often packed with clot, but subtemporal subdural collections are unusual, probably because of the barrier of Liljequist's membrane.

Early Surgical Experience

Early on, it was realized that surgical treatment of this aneurysm was extremely hazardous in comparison to sacs of similar size on the anterior circulation. Of the senior author's first eight patients, only three had satisfactory results while three were poor and two died; admittedly, most were in poor grade preoperatively. The sixth and seventh patients with bifurcation aneurysms in this early series made profound impressions. In each, silk ligatures had been passed blindly around the neck with a ligature carrier to occlude the aneurysm. Neither patient awakened from the anesthetic and both remained in deep coma with quadriparesis and fixed dilated pupils, although the postoperative angiograms seemed to show clean, complete occlusion of the necks.

This prompted a review of the anatomy of the region in cadavers. There, under magnifying loupes, were revealed the numerous small thalamoperforating branches arising chiefly from the origins of the P1 segments, but also occasionally from the back of the basilar bifurcation, and entering the posterior perforated substance to irrigate the mid brain. Others ascended more vertically to irrigate the thalami. About that time, Dr. Ian Turnbull of Vancouver kindly sent an intact specimen of a large basilar bifurcation aneurysm in situ, where the relationship of these branches to the sides and back of the neck was seen vividly, forming a sheath around that portion of the neck and waist of the sac embedded in the interpeduncular fossa (Fig. 3.1). It was immediately obvious that injury or occlusion of these branches had been responsible for the persisting coma and paralysis from upper brain stem infarction after these early operations. Since that awareness, most of the effort to improve the surgical results at this site has been concentrated on methods to see, to separate and to preserve the integrity of these vessels, as well as the basilar

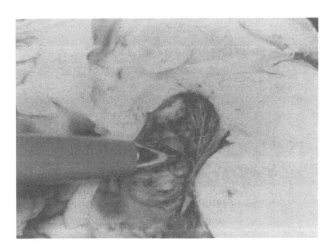

Figure 3.1. Turnbull specimen of basilar bifurcation aneurysm tilted forward of its bed to reveal cluster of thalamoperforating vessels in interpeduncular fossa which arise from P1

bifurcation itself. Although small important ganglionic branches exist at or very near most saccular aneurysm sites, nowhere are they more numerous or more vital than at the basilar artery bifurcation.

Anatomical Features

These aneurysms arise in the crotch of the bifurcation and tend to be half hidden posteriorly in the interpeduncular fossa. Most commonly (73%) they project upward in line with the curve of the basilar artery (Fig. 3.2); less commonly (14%) they project posteriorly into the interpeduncular space (Fig. 3.3). However, for surgical clipping, one must be very certain that the backward projecting sac is not a loculus bending posteriorly from a neck that initially arises vertically. Least common (11%) are those sacs projecting anteriorly with the dome above the dorsum sella or adherent to its posterior surface (Fig. 3.4). Very rarely, this aneurysm may be bilobular with two different projections or project laterally from a bifurcation that has rotated as much as 90 degrees to one side or the other in the coronal plane.

The third nerve is almost never compressed by basilar bifurcation aneurysms except when they are low placed, of giant size or particularly eccentric in their projection.

Associated with the characteristic bulbous features of these aneurysms as they enlarge is a tendency for the basilar bifurcation to become widely ectatic. When viewed from the side at operation, the P1 segment, or even the superior cerebellar artery (SCA), may seem to emerge from the base of the sac itself. There is also a tendency for the neck to bulge anteriorly or more often posteriorly when it forms a "beer belly" buried in the interpeduncular fossa. This can make neck clipping awkward, difficult, even dangerously impossible unless the sac can be made slack so that the "belly" can be displaced out of the interpeduncular fossa.

The host of perforating vessels frequently seen in the angiogram in this region is often interpreted as arising from the aneurysm itself. This is fallacious because a saccular aneurysm originates as a "blow out" of the intimal lining at the distal carina of the bifurcation, through an opening in the media and elastica. Only when the crotch itself expands with the base of a very large saccular aneurysm can branches be said to arise from the sac.

Saeki and Rhoton describe each P1 giving origin to an average of four perforating branches (range 1–13). They arise mainly from the superior and posterior surfaces of P2 near its origin and course superiorly and posteriorly, dividing into numerous branches which terminate in descending order of frequency in the posterior mesencephalon, interpeduncular fossa, cerebral peduncle, posterior perforated substance and mammillary bodies. The posterior and lateral surfaces of the upper centimeter of the basilar artery are also a rich source of perforating arteries. Most end in the pons, but not infrequently one or two arising from the posterior aspect of the bifurcation will cluster with the more lateral thalamoperforating branches on the posterior aspect of the aneurysm. These perforators, which must be preserved, may be adherent to the thin wall of the sac and their separation can be difficult and dangerous. Perforators have been seen crossing from one side to the other, passing usually behind, but rarely in front of the neck and waist of the sac.

The height of the terminal bifurcation of the basilar artery in relation to the dorsum sella varies considerably and is an important consideration in planning and executing the approach to the aneurysm. Ordinarily, the artery bifurcates at the pontomesencephalic junction at the level of the dorsum sella or just above (41% in this series) (Fig. 3.5). However, it may be much higher, at the apex of the interpeduncular space behind the mammillary bodies (31%). Rarely, it may be found even higher

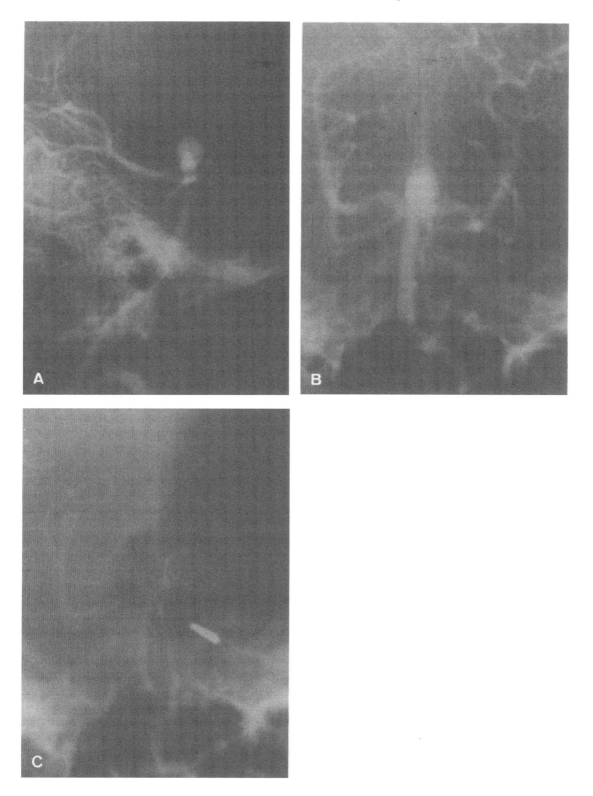

Figure 3.2 A–C. M.A., F, 41, upward pointing basilar bifurcation aneurysm (**A, B**). Ligation with silk in May 1967 12 days after third bleed in Grade 1. Excellent result after removal of a postoperative extradural clot, silver clip on carotid posterior communicating aneurysm (**C**)

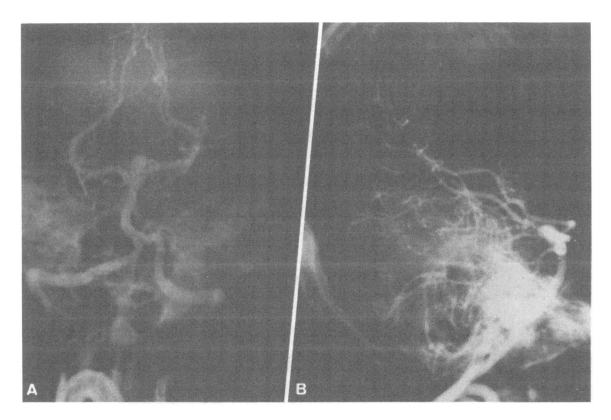

Figure 3.3 A, B. A McM., F, 36, backward pointing basilar bifurcation aneurysm (**A, B**). Ligated with a Mayfield clip in April 1968 13 days after second bleed in Grade 2. Excellent result

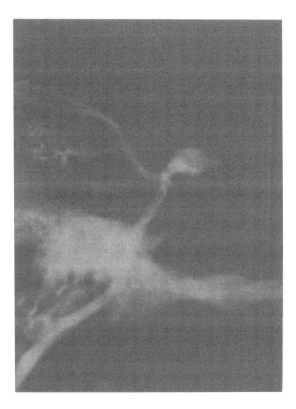

Figure 3.4. J.B-P., F, 32, forward pointing basilar bifurcation aneurysm. Operation in June 1981 8 days after second bleed in Grade 1. Excellent result

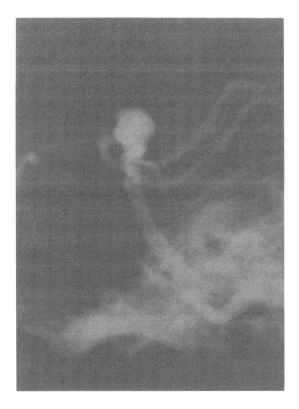

Figure 3.5. W.W., M, 61, high location of basilar bifurcation aneurysm at the apex of the interpeduncular space behind the mammillary bodies. Intact incidental aneurysm operated on in January 1985. Excellent result

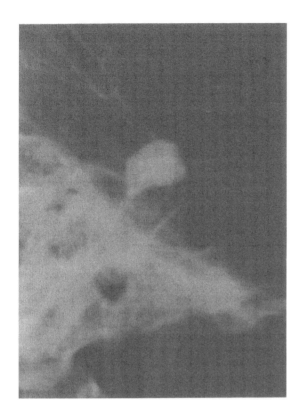

Figure 3.6. S.M., M, 37, low location of basilar bifurcation aneurysm, neck below the level of the floor of the sella. Subtemporal operation with tentorial division in June 1983 22 days after a single bleed in Grade 1 with bilateral oculomotor palsies. Three short applications of a temporary clip with a total occlusion time of 8 minutes. Good result, oculomotor palsies cleared

when the basilar artery is elongated and tortuous with atheroma (dolichocephalic), when it may even be indenting the floor of the hypothalamus and invading the third ventricle. Or, the bifurcation may be low behind the dorsum sellae (28%), even below the level of the floor of the sella (Fig. 3.6). The exposure for a low-placed aneurysm is much more restricted by the bulge of the pons crowded against the clivus and obscured by the edge of the tentorium which often has to be divided. Large basilar bifurcation aneurysms tend to lie lower in relation to the posterior clinoid than the small ones. Then, the fourth nerve will cross the tentorial opening and the fifth nerve may restrict access to the basilar artery below.

Observed in the frontal view, the basilar bifurcation varies from a 'T' configuration to a 'Y' depending on the direction of take off of the P1 segments and the height of the bifurcation. 'T' configurations become more common as the height of the bifurcation rises above the dorsum while 'Y' configurations become the rule with low placed bifurcations, where the P1 segments routinely embrace the aneurysm. Caution must be exercised in the interpretation of the AP angiogram of basilar bifurcation aneurysms in the Towne's projection, where the P1 segments may seem to stand clear from the neck of the aneurysm. It must be remembered that P1 takes a compound curve upward, forward and outward around the peduncle to cross above the third nerve before turning around the edge of the peduncle and becoming hidden under the hippocampal gyrus. The first part of this curve may not be seen in the angiogram, where the artery is often adherent to the base and waist of the sac. Furthermore, even when the neck seems to stand clear for a millimeter or so at its origins in the angiogram, it must be understood that P1 may still be adherent because of the unseen walls of the aneurysm and P1. Therefore, during operation on vertically projecting aneurysms, P1 will usually be applied to the side of the neck with its perforators and may be quite adherent in the larger bulbous sacs. It will seem to arise from the base of the sac itself, although it is really from the common ectatic widening of the basilar artery bifurcation. The ectasia remaining open below a clip placed accurately at the P1 origins has shown no propensity to form a new aneurysm.

The Subtemporal Approach

In 1958, the approaches to various segments of the basilar artery were worked out in the post-mortem room. Subsequently, under the fullness of the living brain at craniotomy, exposure of the same regions was found to be much more limited.

The senior author had been impressed previously with the exposure of the upper basilar artery in the cavity remaining after the subfrontal or transsylvian removal of large suprasellar tumors. However, this exposure on either side of the carotid artery in cadavers seemed narrow and confining. After several dissections, the anterior subtemporal approach across the floor of the middle fossa and tentorial edge into the mouth of the incisura in front of the midbrain seemed to provide the most direct and widest exposure of the interpeduncular region and has been used in more than 80% of small and large basilar bifurcation aneurysms. The main reason for the use of the frontotemporal approach has been multiplicity with another aneurysm(s) on the anterior circulation.

Ordinarily, the right side (86%) is used unless the projection or complexity of the aneurysm, a left oculomotor palsy, a left-sided blindness or a right hemiparesis, demand an approach under the dominant temporal lobe. The left-handed patients were usually operated on by the right-sided approach.

In the lateral decubitus, a small temporal bone flap above and in front of the ear was used for several years and still is appropriate for those beginning or those who prefer wide exposures (Illustration 3.I A–C). It is important to remove the temporal squama with rongeurs – or recently with drill – down to the level of the zygomatic root so that the bony opening is as flush with the floor of the middle fossa as possible.

With experience, a small subtemporal craniectomy through a linear incision, similar to the Frazier-Spiller operation for tic douloureux, has been quite sufficient and is now routine in our unit for most aneurysms in the region of the basilar bifurcation; it can easily be converted to a frontotemporal or posterior temporal bone flap if necessary. The skin incision is perpendicular to the zygoma about 1 cm

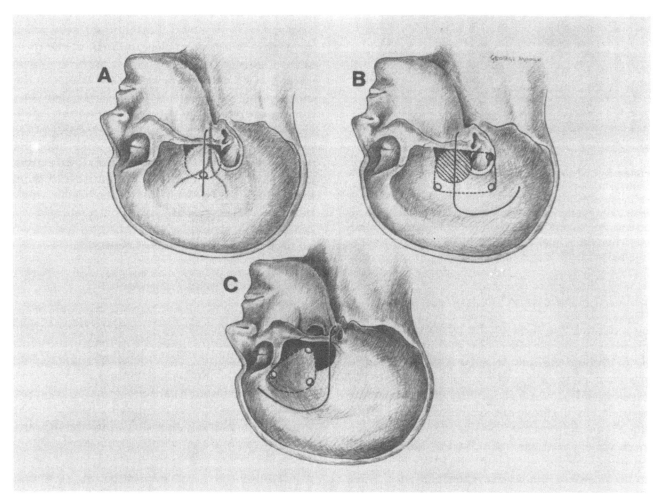

3.I. Subtemporal approach to region basilar artery bifurcation with head flexed slightly downward. **A** A vertical incision in front of the ear with sparing of the trunk and posterior branch of S.T.A. and crossing the zygomatic process of the temporal bone is necessary. The flap is fashioned from a single burr hole and high speed craniotome. Bone must be removed with the drill or rongeurs below the base of the zygoma. **B** The same vertical 'tic' incision can be extended posteriorly to allow the original flap to be extended posteriorly to permit more exposure of the tentorium should it need to be divided to gain access to low lying aneurysms. **C** The pterional transsylvian approach is easily converted to the subtemporal or half and half by removal of the temporal squama in front of the tragus and is carried to the lower border of the zygomatic arch. Here, care must be taken not to injure the frontotemporal branch of the facial nerve. Ordinarily, this branch rises over the zygomatic arch anterior to this incision, in the subcutaneous tissues over the outer lamina of the temporal fascia originating from the lateral border of the arch. After incising the temporal muscle and its fascia vertically to the arch, it is important to remove the muscle with its fascia posteriorly from the temporal root of the zygoma. Anteriorly, both leaves of the temporal fascia are separated from the arch carefully for a centimeter or so usually with blunt dissection so as not to injure the nerve. This allows wider retraction of the temporal muscle so that the temporal squama can be removed down flush with its origin at the lateral floor of the middle fossa for the lowest line of sight under the temporal lobe to the interpeduncular region. The craniotomy should be rongeured to about 4 cm across at the base and 3–4 cm high. Recently we have returned to a small bone flap the same size as the craniectomy with less postoperative discomfort and deformity for better patient acceptance. Quite frankly, the tic craniectomy was used to shorten the operation so that two aneurysm patients could be done in one day, by forestalling cancellation of the second by the anesthesiologist.

For very high bifurcation aneurysms, other authors have used various forms of resection of the zygomatic arch to widen the base of the approach while improving the line of sight into the interpeduncular fossa with lesser temporal lobe retraction. Some middle fossae seem to be deeper than others, but removal of the zygomatic arch, either to lessen temporal lobe pressure or to see higher bifurcations, has not seemed necessary in this series. Anterior temporal lobe resection has not been considered necessary and has never been utilized, except when rupture occurred before exposure of the aneurysm. With modern neuroanesthesia, using Mannitol and lumbar drainage of the spinal fluid as the dura is being opened, the brain will be very slack, even early after bleeding in good grade patients. The retraction can be slowly increased over a large sheet of moist gelfoam used to cover the brain which, if irrigated, does not adhere and prevents sharp angulation of the brain over the edge of the retractor. A second retractor placed at an obtuse angle beside and in front of the first assists in

holding the temporal pole anteriorly out of the field while preventing acute angulations over the edge of the first retractor which may tear the cortex. Retractor pressure has been measured in several cases and has almost never exceeded 10 torr. The angle of the subtemporal approach ordinarily is nearly perpendicular to the sagittal plane. However, an opposite P1 hidden behind a large sac with its perforators can usually be seen by angling the retractor forward a few degrees under the temporal pole and then displacing the waist of the sac posteriorly. This maneuver is particularly appropriate when a temporal bone flap has been used. Associated ipsilateral intact carotid aneurysms are easily exposed for clipping by moving the retractor tip forward a few centimeters under the temporal pole, but for associated middle cerebral, carotid bifurcation and anterior communicating aneurysms, the subtemporal exposure usually must be abandoned for the transsylvian approach.

Occasionally, a temporal vein crossing to the floor of the middle fossa in the line of approach must be divided, but usually other veins on either side can be spared, although put on the stretch for an hour or more. The junction of the vein of Labbé with the lateral sinus ordinarily is well posterior and not in jeopardy in this approach. It is critical that this vein not be injured for fear of major temporal lobe venous infarction (Illustration 3.II A).

The exposure to this point may be done with magnifying loupes, but then the microscope should be brought into position. As the edge of the tentorium comes into view, the uncus will disengage from its position inside the edge of the tentorium (Illustration 3.II B). The uncus is the landmark for this retraction, as its elevation by the retractor tip exposes the opening to the interpeduncular cistern, which will be covered by Liljequists's membrane and crossed by the third nerve. A medial temporal vein may join the dura of the tentorial edge or even pass inside it, and has been divided safely on many occasions before the final retractor placement on the temporal lobe mesially at the base or under the tip of the uncus.

The tentorial edge and the arachnoid sheath of the interpeduncular fossa (Liljequist's membrane) is exposed with a filmy septum covering or surrounding the third nerve which is usually adherent to the tip of the uncus (Illustration 3.II). In early cases, the third nerve was freed from this attachment but was a nuisance crossing the field and the manipulation usually caused complete palsies. Then it was found that as the uncus is raised with the tip of the retractor, the third nerve is elevated with it, ordinarily without placing disturbing angular tension on it (Illustration 3.II C). It is usually possible to work underneath the nerve to clip the aneurysm except in the case of a high basilar bifurcation or a giant sac, when it may be necessary to separate the third nerve from the uncus. The lessening of the third nerve manipulation by this simple expedient of its retraction by the uncus has resulted in fewer (67%) and clearly less complete postoperative third nerve palsies with better tendency for recovery from 81% to 92%. If the nerve appears to be critically angled by the retraction, it may be relaxed by dividing the arachnoid bands holding it near its exit into the triangular ligament anteriorly, or, if necessary, by completing its separation from the uncal adherence. Even though this nerve toler-

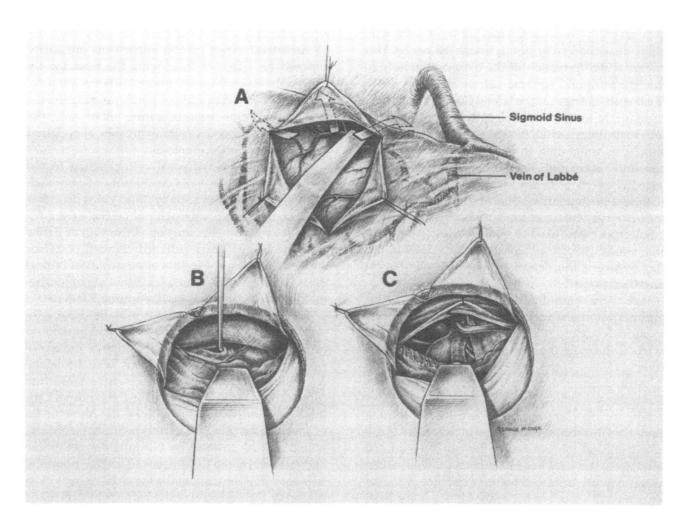

3.II. A After the brain slackens off with lumbar CSF drainage, the undersurface of the temporal lobe is inspected for draining veins to the dura of the middle fossa. The vein of Labbé ordinarily is well posterior to this relatively small craniotomy. B Initial view of entrance to interpeduncular cistern over tentorial edge. – The arachnoid covering the opening into the interpeduncular cistern is revealed by finding and placing the retractor tip at the base of the uncus. The uncus is the landmark which, as it is elevated and disengaged from its position inside the tentorial edge, will uncover the opening, whose arachnoid may now be opened with a hook and microscissors taking great care to avoid the superior cerebellar artery which may loop anterolaterally. C The entrance can be greatly enlarged by two maneuvers: 1. the third nerve is elevated to the superior margin of the exposure and out of harm's way by its natural adherence to the uncus which is placed under the tip of the retractor. 2. the edge of the tentorium can be reflected downward by a cm or more by tethering with a suture placed lateral to or behind the insertion of the fourth nerve and then to the dura of the floor of the middle fossa

ates little manipulation, its potential for recovery is remarkable even when complete paralysis exists postoperatively. After a few weeks or months, recovery becomes complete in virtually all (91%) cases where no paresis existed before. Any persistent residua are usually not disabling and limited to mydriasis and impairment of upward movement of the globe. Missed regenerative changes (synkinesis) may follow when the nerve must be manipulated more vigorously, particularly at its root when freeing perforators from the base of larger aneurysms. Angling of the nerve by the clip handle does not seem to be a factor in either postoperative paresis or its recovery.

Even with the uncal retraction of the third nerve, the opening into the interpeduncular cistern is narrow. However, it can be widened significantly by the simple maneuver of placing a suture in the edge of the tent just in front of, but free of, the insertion and intradural course of the fourth nerve (Illustration 3.II C). After passing it through the dura of the floor of the middle fossa, below the position of the Gasserian ganglion, it can be tied tightly or held so with a clip, thus reflecting the edge of the tentorium downward for 1 cm or more. Any arachnoid tethering the fourth nerve needs to be divided before tension is placed on the nerve by this maneuver. Then the fourth nerve can be tucked below the tentorial edge for safety. Introduction of this simple but effective maneuver in 1969 to open the entrance into the interpeduncular cistern has obviated the necessity of dividing the tentorium for most aneurysms at the basilar bifurcation including those arising at the origin of the SCA. However, in one-third of the cases with low-lying basilar bifurcation aneurysms tentorium division remains necessary.

At this stage, the membrane of Liljequist is widely opened beginning just above the fourth nerve and the SCA on the side of the midbrain and extending forward below the third nerve to the clivus, taking great care not to injure the SCA or a low positioned posterior communicating artery (PComA).

The size of the interpeduncular cistern is quite variable. Ordinarily, a centimeter or so of space exists between the peduncle and the dorsum sellae laterally, although the peduncle tends to angle forward medially in the interpeduncular fossa. Occasionally, the brain stem can be crowded against the clivus, hiding the interpeduncular fossa; however, the peduncle seems to withstand considerable retraction without causing hemiparesis in order to see the basilar artery and the base of the aneurysm. It has never been necessary to remove the posterior clinoid.

Depending upon the extent of bleeding and the interval, the interpeduncular fossa may alternatively be filled with clear cerebrospinal fluid (CSF), packed with fresh or disintegrating clot, or occasionally in long delayed cases, obliterated with a dense arachnoiditis.

To avoid heavier retractor pressure to see the posterior cerebral artery above CNIII, it is convenient to follow the SCA back under CNIII to the basilar artery, sucking away clot to expose its origin just below that of P1. The lower aspect of P1 then followed outward will disappear underneath the third nerve. Even though still covered in clot, the position of the lateral aspect of the neck and waist of the aneurysm is now known as being just medial to P1 and usually partially covered laterally and posteriorly by the P1 perforators. Only twice was it necessary to divide the PComA; in fact, it should be carefully preserved in case some injury to P1 occurs or if it becomes necessary to include P1 in the clip (rarely). Furthermore, the communicating artery gives rise to important diencephalic branches (anterior thalamoperforating arteries) the integrity of which might be compromised by its occlusion.

P1 and the SCA can be identified by their relation to the third nerve. P1 is above the nerve and the PComA joins it; the SCA is below. The same relationship can be used to identify these vessels on the opposite side.

At this stage, a segment of the basilar artery below the SCA and free of perforators for two or three millimeters should be exposed for placement of a temporary clip. Of all the measures to solve the technical problems with this aneurysm, temporary basilar clipping has been most important (Illustration 3.III B).

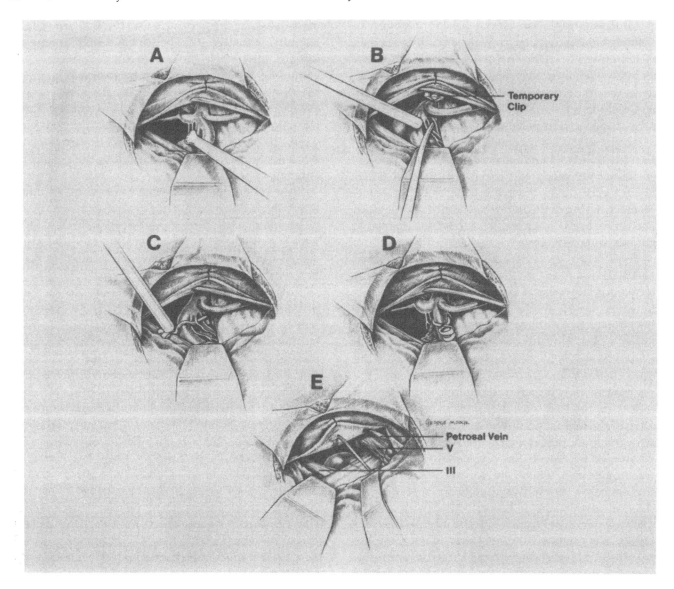

3.III. A Compression of waist of aneurysm to see opposite P1, often its medial perforators and the opposite posterior communicating artery. **B** Anterior displacement of sac with sucker tip or dissector to see and separate thalamoperforating vessels not only ipsilaterally, but behind and on the far side of the neck. There is often a glimpse of the root of the opposite third nerve. The temporary Kleinert-Kurtz clip on the basilar artery below softens the aneurysm for these maneuvers. **C** A fenestrated clip has been placed, but on immediate inspection posteriorly, by tilting the clip handle forward with an instrument, a perforator is found caught under the blade. **D** After immediate removal and further separation of the perforator(s), during temporary basilar artery clipping, the fenestrated clip is replaced as many times as necessary for certainty that no perforator is caught under the blade, or on the far side, or is safe in the clip aperture. **E** Division of inner third of tentorium for low lying basilar bifurcation or superior cerebellar aneurysms. Their exposure is usually between CNIII and the slender CNIV which crosses the field and is easily torn by inadvertent movement of a sucker tip or blunt hook. This approach can be used also for clipping midbasilar trunk aneurysms by working above CNV and above and below CNIV. The petrosal vein may be left intact

Induced Intraoperative Hypotension

Since tension in the aneurysm wall is related in almost linear fashion to systemic blood pressure (Ferguson), surgeons have attempted to induce hypotension by various means since the beginning of direct aneurysm surgery (Table 3.1). Undoubtedly, this has contributed to the safety and surety of aneurysm surgery with minimal risk of ischemia.

Systemic hypotension, down to a mean arterial pressure (MAP) for 40–50 torr has been widely recognized to reduce the tension and fragility of the aneurysm wall. There has been a lingering concern about its use in patients with vasospasm and reduced cerebral blood flow. In the last decade, Isoflurane has been our agent of choice providing rapid, precise control.

Recently, local or regional hypotension induced by temporary occlusion of the parent artery is replacing systemic hypotension on our unit. In fact, only one-fifth of the patients were operated on under hypotension (below 70 torr) in the last ten years. For over 35 years, the anesthesiologist's finger has been used for intermittent compression of the carotid artery in the neck for carotid aneurysms during critical phases of the dissection, coagulation or clipping. It is simple, safe and very effective in reducing tension in the aneurysm, but not appropriate to use in vertebrobasilar aneurysms.

Temporary intracranial arterial clipping had a brief vogue after 1959 when Pool reintroduced the concept using the early Mayfield spring clip. While a few surgeons continued to use temporary clipping our initial experience with a fatal anterior cerebral artery thrombosis from the clip site made us abandon its use immediately. Pool subsequently stated that he had as well because of local thrombogenic intimal injury (personal communication).

After occasional use in the 1970's our unit returned to the use of temporary clipping in 1981, especially on the basilar artery, using the modern, gentle temporary clips. They had been in routine use at our institution during extracranial to intracranial (EC-IC) bypass procedures. The 98% patency rate in over 400 cases implied no significant intimal injury at the clip sites, even on these small M1 branches. Elsewhere, Suzuki in Japan was using a temporary clip on virtually all cases, including arteriovenous malformations (AVMs), for several minutes, even up to an hour or more with AVMs.

He claimed no local arterial thrombosis or significant ischemia. To prevent ischemia, the "Sendai cocktail", consisting of 20% Mannitol 500 ml, vitamin E 500 mg, and steroid 50 mg (later phenytoin) was used during the period of temporary clipping.

On our unit gentle temporary clips with very low closing pressures (Kleinert, Kutz, Sugita, Drake) have been used in more than 400 cases of posterior circulation aneurysms in most of which postoperative angiography has been done. In none was neurological deficit attributed to the clip, and the only evidence of injury at the temporary clip site has been a napkin ring-like narrowing of the upper basilar artery in two cases, in spite of re-application many times at the same clip site for difficult aneurysms (Fig. 3.7). There have been no arterial occlusions. However, in one case a rent in the basilar bifurcation occurred inexplicably during preparation of the artery for a temporary clip. A Sundt clip graft had to be used around the bifurcation and the patient had a bad outcome from branch and perforator occlusion.

We are convinced of the safety and usefulness of temporary clipping when very low tension in the aneurysm deemed essential for dissection, coagulation or clipping. What is not known is the safe time for their application at normothermia; our experience indicates that three to four minute intervals are safe for any artery, and much dissection can be done in that time. Mean total occlusion time in small and large basilar bifurcation aneurysms has been 11 minutes with 3 to 4 applications of the temporary clip. There were no undue side-effects in the cases with a total application time of less than 30 minutes. The highly variable collateral circulation will be a major factor in the time element for each artery. Under Mannitol protection only (1–2 gms/kilo), up to 10 minutes of single total occlusion times seems to be safe; between 10 and 15 minutes in small and large basilar bifurcation aneurysms the mortality and morbidity rises implying more technically difficult aneurysms.

The argument that repeated applications are more likely to cause ischemia in perforator territory seems tenuous in view of the large number of temporary upper basilar artery occlusions in this series (mean 3.1 per operation, range 1–14). Up to five applications seem to be safe and there is no difference in the results. With more than five appli-

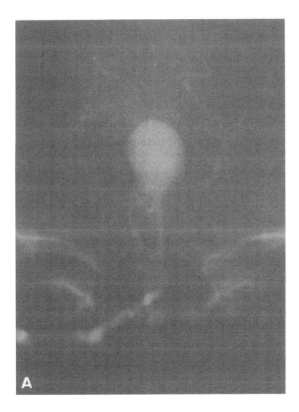 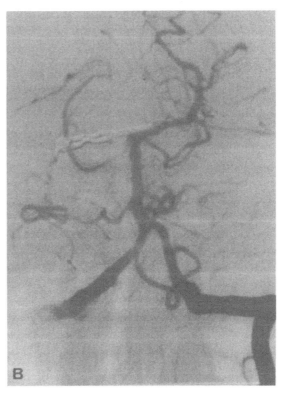

Figure 3.7 A, B. Illustrating an effect, benign, of repeated temporary occlusion of basilar artery. R.H., M, 42, giant basilar bifurcation aneurysm explored elsewhere (**A**). Two operations in August 1986 12 days after a single bleed in Grade 1. In the first operation clip slipped down over atheromatous neck; three days later the slipped clip was left in place and the sac aspirated, then another clip could stay on the neck. The slipped clip was removed. Angiogram after clipping shows "napkin ring" stenosis (arrow) at site of 8 temporary clip placements (4 in each operation) (**B**). Excellent result

cations the mortality and morbidity increases again implying technical difficulty. Perforator ischemia has always seemed due to the vessel's injury during dissection and/or clipping. Remarkably the frequency of perforator infarction has not increased or decreased with temporary clipping.

Recently, for difficult aneurysms, especially large ones at the basilar bifurcation, particularly when one or both PComAs are large, temporary trapping has been used by occluding one or both PComAs during the basilar artery occlusion. The opposite PComA is usually easily seen unless the aneurysm fills the space. It is more convenient to leave the temporary basilar clip in place while removing and replacing the clip on a large PComA to provide the intervals for reflow. Analogously temporary bilateral vertebral occlusion has been used for demanding aneurysms at the vertebrobasilar junction.

Recently W. Schucart (personal communication) has used temporary endovascular balloon occlusion of the basilar as well as the carotid arteries with aspiration to partially empty the sac. This method has been published by the Sendai group both in anterior and posterior circulation.

The Transsylvian (Pterional) Approach

Many surgeons prefer the transsylvian approach because of familiarity with its use for anterior aneurysms, as well as providing less temporal lobe retraction and third nerve paresis. After splitting the anterior limb of the Sylvian fissure, the approach is on one or the other side of the carotid, between it and the chiasm medially or the third nerve and uncus laterally. It gives excellent, though narrow, visualization of the anterior aspect of most basilar bifurcation aneurysms and particularly the opposite P1 origin and its perforators. H. Batjer (personal communication) has found it necessary often to remove the uncus, even the anterior hippocampus.

On this unit, trials of the transsylvian exposure since 1967 have not been persuasive, and in fact it has been used in only nine cases of small and large basilar bifurcation aneurysms without associated aneurysms. It has usually been found to be narrow and confining, with less visualization of the aneurysm, especially posteriorly in the interpeduncular fossa. The present clip applicators are often too large for this narrow space, and the route itself has lead to carotid injuries. It is most suitable for aneurysms with small necks lying in an ideal position near the level of the dorsum sellae and pointing upward or forward. The height of the basilar bifurcation, and therefore of the aneurysm neck, varies considerably from 1–2 cm above or below the dorsum sellae. High necks may not be seen transsylvian unless the approach is above the carotid bifurcation, with the danger to its perforators; low necks are hidden by the dorsum sellae and tentorial edge. Most importantly, the Sylvian approach does not allow nearly the same visualization behind the aneurysm, where most of the trouble lurks with the perforating vessels. The necks of posteriorly projecting aneurysms are also poorly seen.

The neck of an aneurysm is most completely obliterated when the clip blades fall across the neck in parallel with the parent bifurcation and there is less risk of kinking P1, particularly with large necks. This ideal placement is more likely to occur with the subtemporal exposure. Clips placed more perpendicular to this crotch often leave tags of neck in front and behind ("dog ears"), as the sides of the neck are approximated and the bifurcation crimped. "Dog ears" of residual neck have been shown to grow into new aneurysms on the carotid artery in several cases and probably do so at the basilar bifurcation as well. Further, basilar bifurcation aneurysms can be visualized subtemporally regardless of their size, height, direction or multilocularity. The inner third of the tent can be divided easily for very low necks and placement of a temporary basilar artery clip, and there is no necessity to remove the posterior clinoid or inner petrous apex. Finally, control of vigorous hemorrhage from premature or inadvertent rupture of the aneurysm is far easier through the subtemporal rather than a transsylvian exposure. These concerns have tended to outweigh the minor risk factors associated with

temporal lobe retraction and the more frequent temporary CNIII paresis.

The Sylvian approach has been utilized mostly for appropriately placed intact aneurysms in the basilar bifurcation region, after clipping a ruptured anterior circulation aneurysm. The two approaches have been used frequently in complementary fashion, for the Sylvian approach can be modified quickly to the subtemporal by removing the temporal squama.

A "half and half" combination of the two approaches is useful where the Sylvian exposure does not allow visualization of the back of the neck of the larger aneurysms, or where the neck has a more horizontal takeoff posteriorly. A mobile temporal pole may be readily displaced backward, but we do not divide large temporal-sphenoidal veins, for severe temporal edema or hemorrhage may occur. If it were not for these usually large veins tethering the temporal pole to the sphenoid ridge, the half and half approach would be the ideal, for it combines the good features of each while minimizing their drawbacks, but it has been used only on four occasions. If tethered by veins, the pole may be elevated so as to provide a more anterior subtemporal approach. With these more anterior exposures the clip may be applied from in front, over or beside the dorsum, with all vessels in view. Much of the merit of an approach is a matter of continued use and familiarity with the anatomy.

Delay in conversion of a transsylvian to a subtemporal approach undoubtedly resulted in one of the fatal intraoperative ruptures – a transsylvian approach to obliterate a ruptured basilar bifurcation and intact left pointing SCA aneurysm. The latter was clipped uneventfully, but the basilar aneurysm projected posteriorly and had a large perforator crossing the neck obliquely *anteriorly*. Persistence in attempting to work a clip blade under the perforator and across the neck ultimately resulted in rupture of the poorly seen posterior part of the neck with a fatal outcome. A subtemporal lateral approach, which had been postponed for one more try, would have allowed easier placement of the clip blade under the perforator.

Other Approaches

Several modifications of the pterional approach have been proposed to improve the angle and width of exposure, with less brain retraction. These include mobilization or removal of the zygomatic arch, part of the orbital roof laterally, and the outer two-thirds of the sphenoid ridge. Heros has divided the temporalis muscle from its origin to displace its bulk posteriorly. The temporopolar approach of Sano is similar to the half and half approach described earlier when the transsylvian is not satisfactory. A few surgeons have found it necessary to divide the PComA or even an atrophic A1 to provide more exposure beside or over the carotid artery.

For extremely high basilar bifurcation aneurysms on dolicho-ectatic basilar arteries, where the aneurysm lies subependymally in the wall of or even within the third ventricle, two approaches into the ventricle have been used, either through the lamina terminalis or interfornicial through the corpus callosum. In this series, six cases of highly located small or large basilar bifurcation aneurysms had to be treated with basilar occlusion (three with tourniquet), and two operations remained explorative.

Upward Projecting Basilar Bifurcation Aneurysms

After identifying the basilar artery and the origins of the SCA and P1 segments, it is wise to clear a short segment of the basilar artery below, which is free of perforators, for placement of a temporary clip. For some protection from ischemia, Mannitol, 1–2 gm/kg, has been injected into the circulation by this time. If one or both PComAs are large, then one or both may have to be temporarily clipped as well as the basilar artery to soften the aneurysm significantly. Ordinarily, the opposite PComA can be found easily and verified by its connection to the opposite P1 segment. However, it may be difficult to see with large or low-placed sacs.

The front of the basilar artery is cleared of clot gently upward across the ipsilateral P1 origin where the bulging of the anterior aspect of the neck of the aneurysm is first seen. If the clot sucks or is teased away easily, the whole of the front of the neck and waist of the aneurysm can be exposed quickly. Occasionally, it is tough and adherent to a thin neck; then, only enough neck is cleared to accept the width of the clip blade. Depending on the bulge of the neck and the projection of the aneurysm, the opposite P1 can usually be seen, if need be, by displacing the waist of the sac posteriorly with a dissector (Illustration 3.III A). This will confirm the angle the clip blades must take during application, and further, will often help to visualize the perforators arising from the opposite P1, as well as the opposite third nerve. Sometimes, it will be necessary to clear arachnoid with blunt or sharp dissection on the other side of the neck to see the opposite P1 origin clearly with its perforators.

The major difficulties with this aneurysm lie behind the sac. Rarely, it will stand free in the interpeduncular space; usually, it will be half buried in the interpeduncular fossa.

Clearing the base of P1 behind will prepare the way for the all important task of finding and separating the perforators (Illustration 3.III B). Gentle retraction of the crus is well tolerated and will expose the posterolateral aspect of the neck and waist of the sac, sucking or teasing away old clot if need be. Most of the perforators arise from P1 near its origin and course obliquely upward and backward on the side and back of the neck and waist of the sac. They are often free or only lightly adherent to small sacs, but are usually adherent, sometimes densely, to large aneurysms. Not infrequently, one or more perforators arising from the upper basilar artery course upward on the back of the neck. Large perforators have been seen crossing the back, even the front, of a neck. Getting behind the neck usually requires gentle retraction forward of the waist of the sac with the sucker tip, while using the small curved dissector to clear and separate any perforators clinging to the back of the neck. Usually, the perforators can be teased off, but occasionally one or more can be quite adherent to a thin-walled neck. More forceful dissection to free them is made less dangerous by temporary basilar artery occlusion, used in nearly half of the cases of small aneurysms since 1981. Ordinarily, the neck can be displaced forward enough to see across the interpeduncular fossa to the opposite peduncle, the origin of the opposite P1 and the root of the opposite third nerve. The perforators most difficult to see and separate are those that cling to the opposite side of the neck, posterolaterally. Adherent perforators must be separated upward far enough so that the posterior clip blade can slip inside them without kinking or tearing their origin.

The upward curve of P1 only stands free beside small aneurysms, but is usually adherent to larger sacs, often densely. In many early cases, when only straight spring clips were available, P1 with its perforators had to be freed carefully from this adherence so that one blade could be slipped beneath P1 from either in front or behind to cross the neck. This is quite reasonable where P1 is slanted either toward the front or back of the sac. However, it is most commonly placed mid way on the side of the sac and it can be awkward and dangerous to try to free a firm P1 adherence from a very thin-walled sac and then to slide one blade underneath P1 nearly at right angles to the surgeon. It was frustration with this situation that resulted in the design of the fenestrated clip in 1969 (cf. Chapter 2, p. 8 and Illustration 3.IV). With this clip, P1 can be left adherent to the sac, but open in the aperture while the blades fall across the neck of the aneurysm. Some perforators too may be included safely in the aperture. The use of a fenestrated clip alone demands that the clip blades be exactly the width of the flattened aneurysm neck, which is about one and a half times its diameter. The blades of the clip must be selected or trimmed and polished with a diamond burr or whetstone so that they just cross the compressed neck leaving the opposite P1 and its perforators free of the tips. To obscure vision least during clip application, the lowest profile clip applier should be used. We now use the Sugita modification of the Drake-Mayfield fenestrated clip.

There are three concerns when using the fenestrated clip; first, the fenestrating ring beyond the applier tips tends to obscure vision in the narrow confines, especially behind the aneurysm. Second, the clip blades must be no longer than the flattened, occluded neck or else the P1 origin(s) and its perforators may be stenosed or occluded. Two common errors are to use blades longer than necessary, which may occlude the opposite P1 or its perforators, or to place the clip too far out on the neck. It is remarkable how short the blades need to be when placed down at the very origin of the neck at the P1 roots. It must be certain too, that the origin of the SCA is not mistaken for P1, else inadvertent occlusion of the basilar bifurcation will occur (cf. Chapter 4, p. 42). The third concern is that not uncommonly a bit of the neck is left open in the aperture just medial to the P1 root (Illustration 3.IV B). This is usually the cause of an aneurysm that still pulsates or bleeds on needling, although it must be certain that the clip tips cross to the far side of the neck (Illustration 3.IV A). Repositioning of the clip a little lower or with slightly longer blades may suffice to occlude the remaining neck. Otherwise, a straight tandem clip can be added (vide infra). As the posterior blade is passed behind the neck, one must be certain that it is inside the perforators while using temporary basilar occlusion to soften a dangerously thin neck. As the blades are allowed to close and narrow the neck, the opposite P1 will come into view so that final alignment, flush with the neck at the upper origins of P1 on each side, can be made before final closure. The posterior blade must not be put too far across, for the root of the opposite third nerve courses up just behind the opposite P1 and can be brushed or actually injured by this blade. As for any aneurysm, immediate inspection is done in front of and behind the neck to determine that each P1 is open and no perforators are caught or kinked by the blades. Rotating the clip handle forward usually exposes the posterior blade and looking just above the blade will determine whether or not any perforators emerge from underneath it. If so the clip must be removed, retrimmed if necessary and reapplied as many times as is necessary for perfect placement (Illustration 3.III D). Not infrequently with the first placement, the blades will be too high or too low on the opposite side and it is sobering how often, when surely all the perforators have been seen and separated, one or more are found caught under the blade (Illustration 3.III C). Adherent ipsilateral perforating vessels, even CNIII, may be left in the aperture of the clip with P1. Quick *advantage* may be taken of a *malpositioned clip* either to separate adherent perforators, even P1, from a slack sac or to separate the sac itself from the higher reaches of the interpeduncular fossa. It is remarkable that inadvertent temporary perforator occlusion with the strong blades, even for several minutes, has not usually produced infarction. After final position, if enough of the sac can be seen, it should be pierced first with the stylet of the lumbar puncture needle then, if no bleeding occurs, the sac usually can be needled and collapsed. This will provide an even better view of the position of the clip. If imperfect still, the bleeding from a needle hole will always stop with a little suction and pressure on a pattie so that a dry field will be available for repositioning

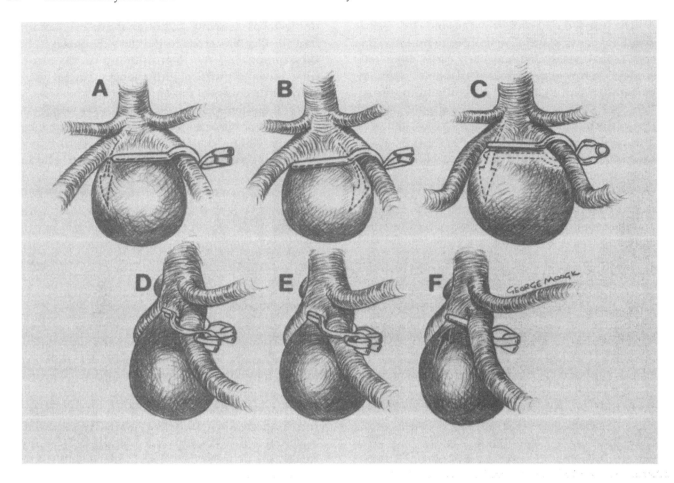

3.IV. Illustrated are three ways when fenestrated clipping may be incomplete and the use of tandem clipping for completion. **A** Clip tips not reaching far side of neck. **B** Blades a little short leaving small portion of neck open in clip aperture. **C** The tips of clip blades closing on a thick atheromatous neck can be held far enough apart to allow a narrow arterial stream between them. **D** Tandem clipping using short straight clip to close the bit of neck left open in the aperture. **E** In recent years, to avoid incomplete clipping, a long straight clip is placed in tandem instead and **F** then after removal of the initial fenestrated clip, is replaced down accurately, across the full neck of the aneurysm

the clip. It must be made as certain as possible that the aneurysm is occluded, for there is no greater calamity than rebleeding during closure or early in the postoperative period. Rupture during closure may cause such rapid bursting temporal lobe swelling that irreversible brain stem injury occurs before urgent temporal lobe removal allows even a chance to control the bleeding. In small basilar bifurcation aneurysms a rupture during closure happened three times, but luckily, in all three after clip replacement the final outcome was good.

If single fenestrated clip blades cannot be positioned perfectly without concern for the P1 origins or perforators, then shorter, fenestrated blades should be placed so as to occlude accurately the far two-thirds of the neck, leaving the near neck and P1 and perforators open in the fenestration (Illustration 3.IV D). Usually then it is simple to separate this open but narrowed portion of the neck from P1 and the perforators, and occlude it by adding a tandem straight clip. This short clip may be applied in front of or behind P1 and the perforators while being certain that it crosses all the neck remaining open in the aperture of the first clip. More often now, instead of using short blades for the tandem clip just to occlude the remaining neck in the fenestration, longer straight blades are used and worked across the *whole* of the neck, just beyond the fenestrated clip, which then can be removed (Illustration 3.IV E, F and Fig. 3.8). The straight clip blades then

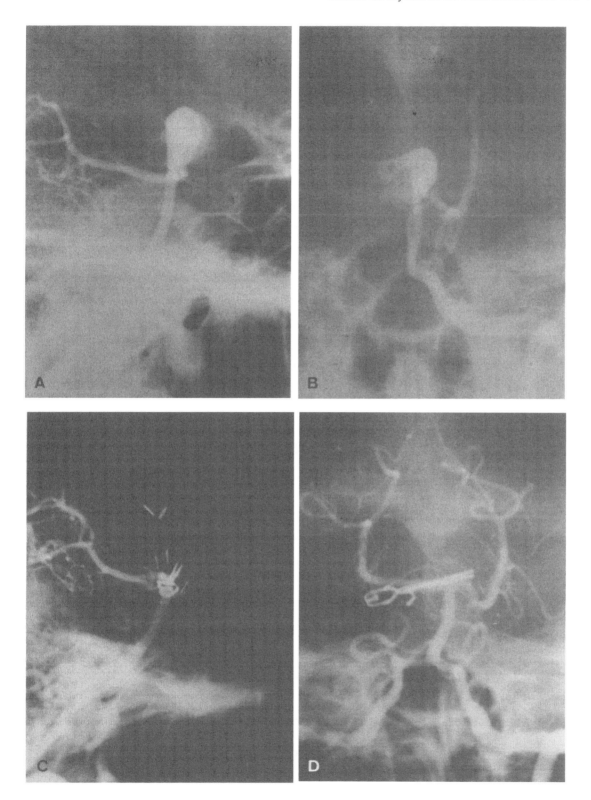

Figure 3.8 A–D. L.A., M, 55, partially thrombosed giant basilar bifurcation aneurysm operated on in April 1981 19 days after a single bleed in Grade 1 (**A, B**). The single straight clip was applied in tandem to an incompletely occluding fenestrated clip and then repositioned more accurately across the neck after removal of the fenestrated clip (**C, D**). Excellent outcome

can be repositioned lower on the neck if necessary. This is of particular value if the fenestrated clip has slid down to stenose the P1(s) or if the fenestrated blades cannot be positioned so as to occlude both sides of the neck. Providing they do not kink P1, straight blades are more satisfactory; there is no worry about any open near neck and without the obscuration of the fenestrating rings, the tips can be positioned very accurately on the far side of the neck. If the neck is thick at the fulcrum, it may keep the blades of a long clip open on the far side to allow continued filling of the aneurysm (Illustration 3.IV C). Then a tandem, fenestrated clip will close the far side of the neck. Although sometimes difficult to see because of the clip handles, an effort should still be made to needle and collapse the sac to prove completed clipping.

In six cases where it seemed dangerous to complete the occlusion on the far side because of encroachment on P1 or perforators, or where postoperative angiography revealed that side still to be open, a second craniotomy was done on the oppo-

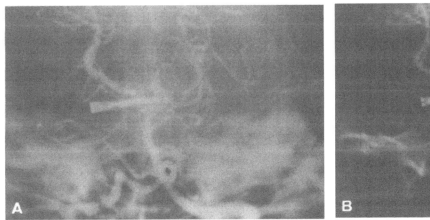
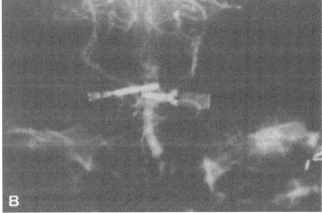

Figure 3.9 A, B. J.G., F, 41, small basilar bifurcation aneurysm was operated on initially in October 1982 21 days after a single bleed in Grade 1. Clip blades are placed too short in avoiding perforators on the left side (**A**). Residual neck was clipped from left approach 10 days later (**B**). Excellent result

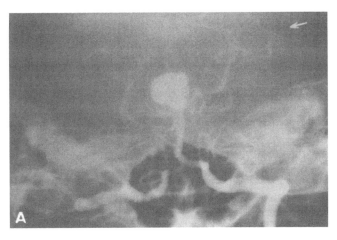
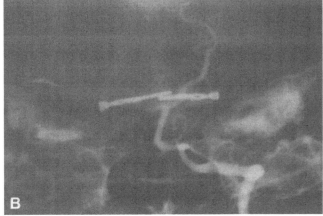

Figure 3.10 A, B. R.H., M, 46, large basilar bifurcation aneurysm (**A**) was operated on in November 1982 23 days after a second bleed in Grade 2. An intact right middle cerebral artery aneurysm was clipped simultaneously. Opposite neck of the basilar bifurcation aneurysm was thick with atheroma, postoperative angiogram showed the clip blades to be held open. Residual neck was clipped from left approach 6 weeks later (**B**). Excellent result

site side within a few days. In each, the neck remaining was easily occluded with a straight clip and in none was there any evidence of injury to the memory mechanisms from bilateral hippocampal retraction (Figs. 3.9 and 3.10).

Where P1 rises either toward the front or back of the aneurysm, and is free of or can be freed from the sac, a straight clip (non-fenestrated) is preferred if one blade can be slipped under P1 from one side of it or the other. The reason is that the length of the blades is not a consideration and the tips can be positioned accurately so as to cross the neck without encroaching on the opposite P1 origin with its perforators, but without concern for the ipsilateral P1 and its perforators, provided there is no kinking of P1. There is then no worry about the sac remaining open in the aperture requiring a second tandem clip. When P1 rises near the front of the neck, the tips of the clip can be spread so that the anterior blade goes under P1 and the posterior blade under the perforators. Both tips have to be watched carefully to be sure not to puncture the aneurysm and that the posterior blade is under the perforators. For P1 rising up the back of the aneurysm, the posterior blade must be in front of both the origin of P1 and the perforators. The sac softened by temporary clipping makes this maneuver much simpler and safer.

Inadvertent rupture of the sac (12.2%) during dissection or clip placement in these narrow confines can be harrowing, and may be controlled better with temporary clipping. Inadvertent rupture has added 8% to the mortality overall. Remarkably, temporary clipping has not reduced its incidence but this may imply more bold dissection or use of temporary clipping after rupture. In fact, scrutiny of small basilar bifurcation aneurysms showed that if those cases where temporary clipping was used after rupture were excluded, the frequency of inadvertent rupture was only 4.7% as compared to 11.3% in patients without temporary clipping.

These aneurysms ordinarily are partially buried in the interpeduncular fossa on the posterior perforated substance, with the domes above and behind the mammillary bodies. Small tears from separation of a perforator or tentative clip application were not uncommon before more routine use of a temporary basilar artery clip, but this bleeding usually stopped spontaneously by the tamponade effect when the sac was allowed to re-expand, or by suction on a small cottonoid. The tamponade effect with re-expansion is also helpful when the seal over the ruptured dome is torn, as when an unsatisfactory clip application retracts the sac from an adherence to the hypothalamic floor or dorsum sellae. Although a major rupture can be calamitous, panic and frantic selection and application of a clip must be avoided. Suction to clear the field must be used carefully to prevent injury to the brain stem and third and fourth nerves during reapplication of the temporary clip or even trapping, at which point the bleeding will slow down so that the site and size of a larger rent can be seen and dealt with. First the dissection of the neck must be completed with the perforators freed and the origins of P1 seen. Seldom is it possible to put the rent into the sucker tip so as to collapse the sac for quickly finishing the dissection and clip application, as with anterior aneurysms. Tearing just above the neck must be controlled by exquisitely accurate clip placement. Rents at the origin may require clip blade placement that compromises the origin of a P1, hopefully one that has a reasonable PComA for collateral to P2 as well as the P1 perforators retrogradely. Permanent trapping of the basilar bifurcation in this circumstance is almost certain to be ruinous or fatal where clip application is not successful in controlling the bleeding, but another maneuver using a small pack is usually successful. This entails stuffing the orifice of the rent with surgicel or a piece of patty under temporary basilar occlusion and then allowing the blades of the clip to fall upon the pack which plugs the rent. The clip blades may have to be trimmed quite short, for the pack itself tends to close the neck on either side of the rent. Only rarely has the basilar artery had to be left occluded with a clip below a torn neck to control bleeding through a surgicel or muscle pack, and only if at least one of the PComAs is of reasonable calibre.

Anatomical rotation of the basilar bifurcation and hence, the neck of the aneurysm, in the coronal plane deserves some comment. Often this is considerable, and, if down and away from the surgeon, makes it awkward for clip application since not enough temporal lobe retraction can be safely achieved to get a line of sight along the neck. Except in the rare circumstance of a laterally directed basilar bifurcation, this is not enough of a problem to warrant approach under the dominant temporal lobe. Usually, it is possible to rotate the clip and/or its applier or to retract P1 downward enough to orient the neck properly for accurate placement. In the same way those aneurysms slightly or more off the midline to the left (10% of all small basilar bifurcation aneurysms) should be approached from the right side.

When can a perforator be taken? Ideally never, although a tiny, very adherent one on the back of a very thin neck has been occluded on occasion without demonstrable deficit. Rarely, small mid brain or thalamic infarcts have been seen in CT scan of patients without complaints. Altogether, in 14 of 62 verified perforator injuries in small aneurysms there was no deterioration in the postoperative clinical state and the ultimate outcome was excellent. Most perforators can be dissected free with a tiny dissector under temporary basilar artery occlusion or trapping. If one or more of a large size cannot be freed, then it is best to use other means to occlude the aneurysm. Tandem clipping, with the beginning of the clip fenestration just beyond the perforators and then a tandem clip just short of the perforator, may suffice. The Sylvian approach may allow blades to be placed so as to close on the very edge of the sac just short of an adherent large posterior perforator. Sometimes, thickening of the wall of the sac with bipolar coagulation beside the perforator will make it possible to dissect it free without rupturing the aneurysm.

While coagulation is occasionally useful to shrink and firm up bulbous or otherwise awkward necks of aneurysms at other sites, it has rarely been used at the basilar bifurcation. It is not only that forcep blades usually cannot be placed across the neck in the lateral approach without including P1, but the fear that an unseen perforator(s) might be coagulated too.

High Basilar Bifurcation

The greater the height above the dorsum sella, the greater must be the retraction of the mesial temporal parahippocampal region. If the neck of the sac reaches the apex of the interpeduncular space, it and the perforators are more effectively hidden by the mammillary bodies in front, and the peduncle laterally and behind. In only two early cases was it necessary to abandon clipping for incomplete gauze packing because of its obscuration by the

height of the bifurcation. In another later case with a high buried aneurysm, the basilar artery was occluded by the tourniquet. Although the thrombosis was incomplete she has remained well for over 10 years. It is here that mobilization of the zygoma by dividing each end might be helpful. A very high bifurcation indeed, may be preferentially approached from the frontotemporal exposure after splitting of the Sylvian fissure. It may be necessary to work above the carotid bifurcation where its perforators must carefully be avoided. A hypoplastic A1 could be divided to provide more room. Gentle retraction of the mammillary bodies or crus has not had any serious consequences.

Low Basilar Bifurcations

At the other extreme, the bifurcation may be quite low, at the level of the floor of the sella or even lower down the clivus (Illustration 3.III E). Rhoton describes low bifurcations in 10% of cadavers. In this series of small aneurysms one-fourth of the cases had low basilar bifurcations (large aneurysms 38%) – which might be due to the referral policy. However the number of redo aneurysms was not higher in this than other groups. This position of the neck is confining to the surgeon because the edge of the tentorium cannot be reflected downward far enough by the "tenting" suture and it hides the base of the sac which is wedged between the pontomesencephalic junction and the clivus. With a little more retraction applied under the lateral temporal lobe, and more upper squamal removal (if the tic opening is used) to increase the angle of vision over the depressed tentorial edge, it may be possible to place a temporary basilar clip and clear the neck for clipping without dividing the tentorium. The waist of a larger sac may have to be separated from adherence to the dorsum or clivus carefully under high magnification and temporary clipping. However, if the neck is obscured or the basilar artery cannot be adequately seen for temporary clipping, the inner third of the tentorium should be divided (in 30% in low necks) beginning behind the insertion of the fourth nerve. The anterior leaflet is sewn back into the floor of the middle fossa to give more line of sight down behind the clivus. The fourth nerve should be freed of any arachnoid attachment so that undue tension is not put upon it. N. Martin (personal communication) has described freeing the nerve from its channel in the tentorial edge to the back of the cavernous sinus so that more forcible retraction of this corner of the leaflet will increase the exposure behind the clivus without placing undue tension on the nerve. For these low aneurysms, it is always wise to have the scalp marked for a posterior temporal flap for further division of the tentorium laterally which was necessary in 10%. The transmastoid-transpetrosal sinus approach, through a completely divided tentorium, has been used once for a difficult, large, low placed neck. After the tentorium is divided, the dissection of the neck is usually done medial to the fifth nerve and on either side of the fourth nerve. This slender, fragile nerve is a nuisance in this exposure and great care must be taken to avoid tearing it with an inadvertent movement of a blunt hook or sucker. This has occurred four times in small aneurysms, usually in a trying circumstance, such as bleeding. Single suture repair of the nerve or use of Tisseal® has not resulted in functional reinnervation and diplopia on downward gaze has persisted.

Forward Projecting Aneurysms

Forward projecting aneurysms, unfortunately rare, are the most straightforward for clipping except those located very low. They project anteriorly from the front of the basilar bifurcation, free in the interpeduncular space, often above the dorsum sella and free of perforators, since none arise from the anterior aspect of the artery. When the basilar bifurcation is low, caution is needed, for the dome of this aneurysm is often adherent to the dorsum or clivus and may be torn loose with manipulation or clipping. The perforators often have a longer adherence to the sac because of the 'Y' configuration of the bifurcation. Actually, this specific subgroup had the worst operative results (Table 5.8). The clip blades should be gently pressed back against the bifurcation so that no vestige of the neck remains behind at the crotch. Another hazard to avoid is that the clip blades do not encroach on the base of the opposite P1 or its perforators. These sacs are easily seen for needle aspiration to verify perforator preservation and complete clipping.

Backward Projecting Aneurysms

Backward projecting aneurysms, half of them located at the posterior clinoid level, are buried in the interpeduncular fossa and may have perforators on either sides, as well as beneath the neck. A few have been seen crossing above the neck, even from one side to the other, and prevented safe clipping in one case. The third nerve is more in the way because of its downward slope from above and behind in the interpeduncular fossa, and it may cross the neck. Only a glimpse of the upper neck is seen from in front, although the opposite P1 is seen clearly. Because of the rise of P1 from its origin, it will be necessary to work behind and below it, and either above or below the third nerve, depending on its position and easiest displacement. The neck can be brought into view by gentle displacement of the crus posteriorly, sometimes in combination with a little pressure forward on P1 with a sucker tip. Strangely, these perforators often seem less adherent and separate easily from the neck after this maneuver. As the blades of the clip, placed above and below the neck behind P1 and inside the perforators, are allowed to close slowly, the narrowing of the neck will reveal the origin of the opposite P1 and its perforators. The opposite P1 will not ordinarily be in the way of the blades, and as long as the blades close only across the far side of the neck, an unseen perforator will not be caught. More reassurance can be gained by needling and collapsing the sac, although it may be difficult to see behind the clip because of the crus. One or two small perforators have been seen free between the tips of the blades on the far sides, which were held just far enough apart by the bulk of the neck to accommodate them, although this is not a circumstance to rely upon.

Particular caution should be exercised to ensure that what appears to be a backward pointing aneurysm is not really a saccule coming off at a right angle from a neck that initially is projecting upward. With modern subtraction films, it would be unlikely for this portion of the neck to be hidden in control angiograms but this mistake has resulted in four deaths several years after clipping when the original base of the sac, in front of the clip, enlarged and ruptured (Fig. 3.11).

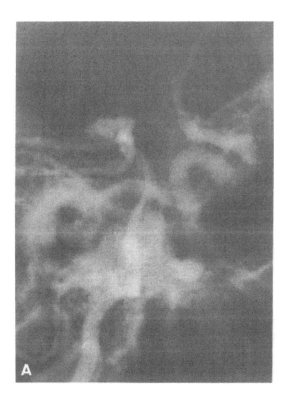
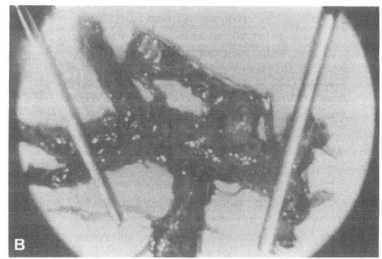

Figure 3.11 A, B. P.V., F, 33, basilar bifurcation aneurysm (**A**) interpreted as backward pointing in operation in January 1972 12 days after a second bleed in Grade 1. Excellent result, but she rebled to death in 1975. Autopsy specimen shows clip occluding posterior loculus. Upward portion of neck remaining had enlarged and ruptured (**B**)

Results

The results can be seen in Tables 3.2 to 3.11.

The small aneurysms are further subdivided as to their projection from the basilar bifurcation, forward, backward or upward, since the surgical problems with the perforating vessels vary significantly (cf. Chapter 5). In spite of this, the surgical results were not remarkably different.

None of the patients with unruptured aneurysms died, but three had poor results from perforator injury: two patients with remote bleeds (one of which was a redo operation for complete occlusion of the aneurysm), and the third had an ischemic brain lesion prior to operation. Curiously no deaths occurred in the seven patients operated on in Grade 4 or in the seven patients aged 70 years or more (Tables 3.2 and 3.3).

All but a few of the small bifurcation aneurysms were treated by clipping (95%). Other methods of treatment are summarized in Table 3.4. Nine small aneurysms were wrapped, one with hammered muscle, eight with gauze. Muscle was used in 1965 because a large perforator could not be separated from the side and dome of a small aneurysm. Remarkably, this woman, then 51, remains well without sequelae. Two small intact aneurysms would not hold a clip and each was shrunk to complete obliteration with coagulation and the coagulum was packed in gauze. A ruptured aneurysm at the apex of a dolichocephalic artery was packed incompletely in gauze when it could not be seen well enough for clipping, Five further aneurysms were unsuitable for clipping. Surprisingly none of these wrapped aneurysms has become symptomatic even though the shortest follow-up is eight years.

Proximal basilar artery clip occlusion was used in two small aneurysms, one located very high, the other very low in relation to the posterior clinoid, both with excellent results.

In seven patients the subtemporal approach remained exploratory, three of them died: in all of these deaths an early intraoperative aneurysm rupture occurred; all these aneurysms were located very low. Three of the other four patients with good outcomes had a very high basilar bifurcation making safe clipping seem impossible at the time; additionally, one had severe basal arachnoiditis after several SAHs and four earlier operations and one had a dense hard calcification of the aneurysm. It was felt then that other methods were not warranted for these patients, e.g. basilar occlusion.

During induction of anesthesia nine days after the initial hemorrhage, a 45 year old male in Grade 1 had severe rebleeding. Operation was abandoned and he remained deeply unconscious with both pupils maximally dilated and died the next day (Table 3.5).

Forward projecting aneurysms are clear of the perforator clusters and no perforator infarction occurred. However among the various heights of the bifurcation the low lying aneurysms projecting forward produced the highest mortality and morbidity (for further analysis see Chapter 5 with Table 5.7). One of the deaths occurred on day 3 from rupture of a previously intact left middle cerebral aneurysm. Three of four poor results resulted from ischemia with vasospasm. One occurred postoperatively, and two patients had hemiplegias preoperatively, but desired repair of their aneurysms.

Table 3.1. Methods for induced hypotension

1) Systemic:	Controlled transvenous blood volume reduction
	Ganglionic blockade
	Nitroprusside
	Anesthetic agents – Isoflurane
2) Local:	Temporary carotid occlusion in neck
	– anesthesiologist's finger
	– cutdown and clamp
	Temporary clip(s) intracranially

Table 3.2. Preoperative Grade (Botterell) and outcome in 493 patient with small basilar bifurcation aneurysms

Grade	Excellent	Good	Poor	Dead	Total
0	78	2	3		83
1	213	32	12	7	264
2	70	17	8	8	103
3	13	12	8	3	36
4	2	2	3		7
Total	376	65	34	18	493
	76.3%	13.2%	6.9%	3.7%	100.0%

Table 3.3. Age related to outcome in 493 patients with small basilar bifurcation aneurysms

Age group (years)	Excellent	Good	Poor	Dead	Total
10–19	2				2
20–29	29	1			30
30–39	69	15	5	4	93
40–49	130	22	12	6	170
50–59	95	18	8	4	125
60–69	47	7	8	4	66
70 or more	4	2	1		7
Total	376	65	34	18	493

40 Small Aneurysms at the Bifurcation of the Basilar Artery

Table 3.4. Operative method and outcome in 493 patients with small basilar bifurcation aneurysms

Operative method	Excel-lent	Good	Poor	Dead	Total
Neck clipping	361	64	30	14	469
Wrapping	8	1			9
Silk ligature	1		4		5
Basilar occlusion	2				2
Explorative	4			3[a]	7
Rebleed during induction, no operation				1	1
Total	376	65	34	18	493

[a] Craniotomies remained explorative due to rebleedings.

Table 3.5. Operative method and completeness of aneurysm treatment in 493 patients with small basilar bifurcation aneurysms

Operative method	Total obliter-ation	Resid-ual neck	Resid-ual fundus	No oblit-eration	Not known	Total
Neck clipping	428	33	7		1	469
Silk ligature	5					5
Wrapping	2		1	5	1	9
Basilar occlusion			2			2
Exploration only				7		7
Rebleed during induction, no operation				1		1
Total	435	33	10	13	2	493

Table 3.6. Timing of surgery and outcome in 410 patients with small basilar bifurcation aneurysms

Timing of surgery	Excel-lent	Good	Poor	Dead	Total
0–1 day	6	2	2	1	11
2–3 day	14	3	5	3	25
4–6 day	16	6	2		24
7–10 day	46	6	6	4	62
11–30 day	168	36	13	9	226
31–365 day	48	10	3	1	62
Total	298	63	31	18	410

Table 3.7. Basilar aneurysm projection and outcome in 493 patient with small basilar bifurcation aneurysms

Basilar projection	Excel-lent	Good	Poor	Dead	Total
Forward	48	6	4	3	61
Upward	272	50	28	12	362[a]
Backward	48	9	2	3	62
Bilobed	8				8
Total	376	65	34	18	493

[a] Includes one patient with no aneurysm (as basilar bifurcation aneurysm explored).

Table 3.8. Preoperative Grade (Botterell) and outcome in 362 patients with small and upward projecting basilar bifurcation aneurysms

Grade	Excellent	Good	Poor	Dead	Total
0	62	2	2		66
1	150	24	11	6	191
2	49	13	8	3	73
3	9	9	4	3	25
4	2	2	3		7
Total	272	50	28	12	362

Table 3. 9. Preoperative Grade (Botterell) and outcome in 61 patients with small anterior projecting basilar bifurcation aneurysms

Grade	Excellent	Good	Poor	Dead	Total
0	7				7
1	27	2	1	1	31
2	12	1		2	15
3	2	3	3		8
Total	48	6	4	3	61

Table 3. 10. Preoperative Grade (Botterell) and outcome in 62 patients with small and posterior projecting basilar bifurcation aneurysms

Grade	Excellent	Good	Poor	Dead	Total
0	7		1		8
1	30	6			36
2	9	3		3	15
3	2		1		3
Total	48	9	2	3	62

Table 3.11. Relation of basilar aneurysm to clinoid and outcome in 493 patients with small basilar bifurcation aneurysms

Basilar-clinoid	Excellent	Good	Poor	Dead	Total
Above	105	23	9	1	138
At clinoid	144	21	11	7	183
Below	91	18	9	6	124
Not known[a]	36	3	5	4	48
Total	376	65	34	18	493

[a] Posterior clinoid not seen in angiogram tracings.

Chapter 4

Large (or Bulbous) Basilar Bifurcation Aneurysms (12.5–25 mm)
265 Patients

Clinical Features

Two patients with remote bleeds 15 months and 4 years ago were classified with the 40 unruptured aneurysms (Table 4.1). In the remaining, besides the usual clinical symptoms of subarachnoid hemorrhage (SAH), 23 had CNIII palsy, one of them bilaterally. Trochlear nerve palsy was seen in four, one bilaterally, and sixth nerve palsy in seven patients, three times bilaterally.

Three-quarters of these aneurysms projected vertically and had broad bulbous necks whose girths increased proportionately the difficulties of exposure and clipping. Additionally, these necks are more often (38%) low lying in relation to the posterior clinoid. Part of the problem is that the basilar bifurcation is often ectatic and seemingly a part of the neck. As a consequence, the P1 segments seem to arise from the side of the neck and rise vertically in close approximation to the neck and waist of the aneurysm along with the thalamoperforating vessels. The ectasia often includes the origins of the superior cerebellar arteries (SCAs). However, the ectatic arterial wall must be reasonably normal, for it has never been known to form another aneurysm later, provided that a clip has been properly placed between the medial portions of the P1 origins. The sheer bulk of the neck makes it more difficult to see to the other side, particularly behind the aneurysm. The necks of these larger aneurysms tend to be thicker and often yellow with atheromata.

If there is any doubt about the probability of clipping a large basilar bifurcation aneurysm, the alternative of basilar artery occlusion just below the SCA origins should be investigated preoperatively. The size and potential collateral function of the posterior communicating arteries (PComAs) must be known. If not visualized on the carotid injections, they can be opacified by vertebral artery injection while one, then the other, carotid is temporarily manually occluded in the neck (Allcock's test). If one or both PComAs are obviously large enough to carry the basilar circulation, then the basilar artery can be clip occluded at the appropriate site. If they are marginal in calibre, then the Drake tourniquet can be applied for subsequent basilar artery occlusion after the patient is awake (vide infra). Fourteen non-giant basilar bifurcation aneurysms were treated by basilar occlusion, in five instances with the tourniquet. Because of the proximity of the origins of SCA and P1, only once was it possible to occlude the terminal basilar artery safely between their origins with a clip (Fig. 4.1).

The subtemporal approach was used in 90% of the cases. The main reason for using the frontotemporal approach were associated anterior circulation aneurysms. After initial exposure and with temporary basilar clipping if necessary, it is best to firmly indent the neck of the sac anteriorly with a small dissector so as to see across to the origin of the opposite P1 and its perforators. Identification of the opposite P1 is vital to clip placement in all basilar bifurcation aneurysms. To mistake its origin for that of the opposite SCA means that the clip will occlude the origin of the opposite P1 and probably its perforators and a portion of the basilar bifurcation (Fig. 4.2). The opposite P1 may be identified by confirming that the oculomotor nerve passes beneath it, and that the opposite PComA joins it. Further identification of the PComA is confirmed by thalamic perforators arising from its upper aspect.

These large aneurysms tend to bulge far back into the interpeduncular space, or may have a "beer belly" projecting anteriorly or more often posteriorly from the neck and waist of the sac. Fairly firm retraction of the peduncle is necessary to expose the back of the neck. However, it is remarkable how much retraction the peduncle will take without producing any deficit. The surgeon may get a "feel" of the curve and extent of the neck by blindly, but gently, working a small curved dissector backward

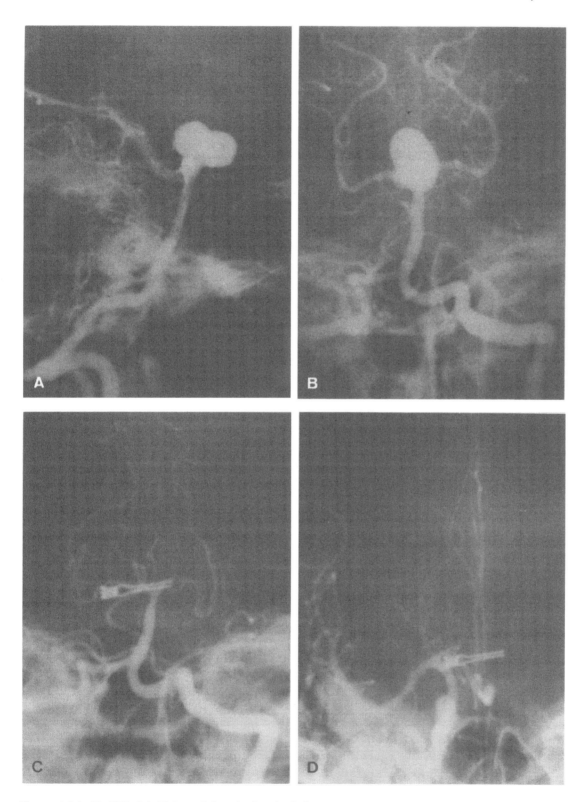

Figure 4.1 A–D. T.D., M, 15, large bilocular basilar bifurcation aneurysm (A, B) was operated on using hypothermia (27°C) in May 1976 10 days after fourth bleed in Grade 1. The neck of the aneurysm had expanded to include basilar bifurcation with P1s emerging from the sac (C). This expansion allowed placement of Scoville clip on basilar artery *between* the origins of P1s and superior cerebellar arteries. Large posterior communication arteries filled posterior cerebral arteries (D). Outcome excellent

44 Large (or Bulbous) Basilar Bifurcation Aneurysms (12.5–25 mm)

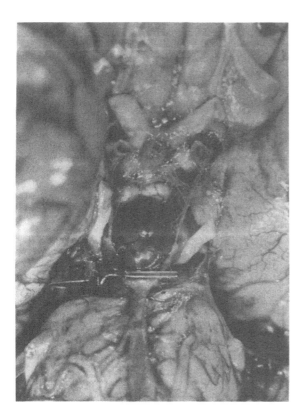

Figure 4.2. B.L., F, 61, large basilar bifurcation aneurysm was operated on in deep hypotension (21 minutes 40 mm HG) in September 1974 39 days after single bleed in Grade 1 with a subtemporal approach. Clip blades placed across left P1 when SCA mistaken for P1. Extensive infarction of left thalamus, midbrain and occipital lobe after death 11 days later. Furthermore, the 10 mm blades are far too long. A 6 mm clip would have sufficed. (Reprinted from Clin Neurosurg 26, 1979, p. 123 by courtesy of Williams and Wilkins)

beside then behind the neck inside the medial aspect of the peduncle.

Finally, it will be necessary to work either the sucker tip or the dissector gradually behind displacing the waist forward as the instrument advances and separating perforators until reaching the apex of the curve. Temporary basilar artery occlusion is very appropriate here to make the sac soft and more easily displaceable, and was used in two-thirds of the cases since its more routine use in vertebrobasilar aneurysms from 1981. If the communicating arteries are large enough that slackening does not take place, then temporary occlusion of one or both posterior communicating artery will collapse the sac. More forward displacement of the waist of the sac will disclose the contents of the interpeduncular fossa, the opposite perforators and often the opposite P1. If the origin of the opposite P1 is seen, its position should be noted carefully in order to get a line for the angle that the clip blades must take.

If the neck is not too broad, the fenestrated clip blades can usually be worked across gradually with a rocking motion inside the perforators, and slowly allowed to close (Fig. 4.3). Because of the breadth of the neck, it may be necessary to use a sucker tip to indent the waist of the sac behind to expose the base of the neck and the perforators in the interpeduncular fossa for initiating clip application. As the neck is narrowed by slow closure of the blades, the origin of the opposite P1 should come into view either in front or behind, so that the tips of the blades can be accurately positioned just across the neck at the upper aspect of P1, but not beyond so that no perforators are inadvertently taken. It is just as important with this aneurysm that the blades be fashioned so as to close only the width of the flattened neck. Also, on these steeply sloping necks, clip blades tend to slip down and occlude one or both P1 origins. In this event, the clip blades should be positioned a little further up on the neck in the hope that "slippage" will be less. If the sac can be needled and collapsed, the position of the clip may be retained by the arterial pressure below.

With very large bulbous necks buried in the interpeduncular fossa or those with a "beer belly" behind, it may be dangerous or impossible to utilize the above technique (Fig. 4.4). Then the clip blades must be slipped up onto the neck from below after initial placement just below the ballooning base but inside any perforators. With the sac softened by a temporary basilar clip or trapping, the blades may be worked up with a rocking motion, gathering in the neck of the aneurysm between the blades while displacing the sac out of the interpeduncular fossa. Quite firm upward pressure may have to be applied for this maneuver. The blades must be placed high enough so that they just clear each P1 after closing. As the blades close, the opposite P1 will be seen so that an adjustment of their angle can be made. The root of the opposite third nerve is more in jeopardy during application of a clip on these large aneurysms, for it may be thinned and flattened on the far side and apt to be brushed by the widely opened posterior blade. Rare large bilocular aneurysms with the neck emerging at right angles from in front

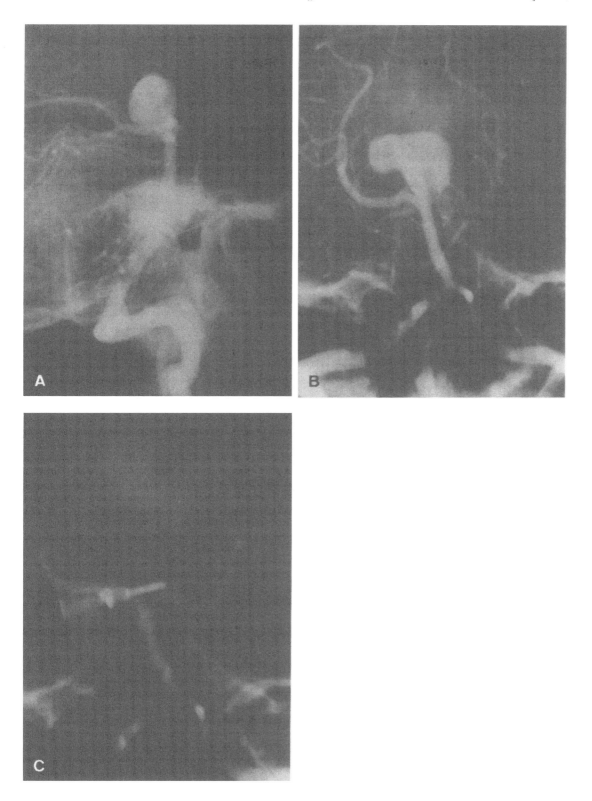

Figure 4.3 A–C. J.W., M, 59, large basilar bifurcation aneurysm (**A, B**) was clipped with a single fenestrated Drake clip in February 1977, 7 weeks after third bleed in Grade 1 (**C**). Outcome excellent

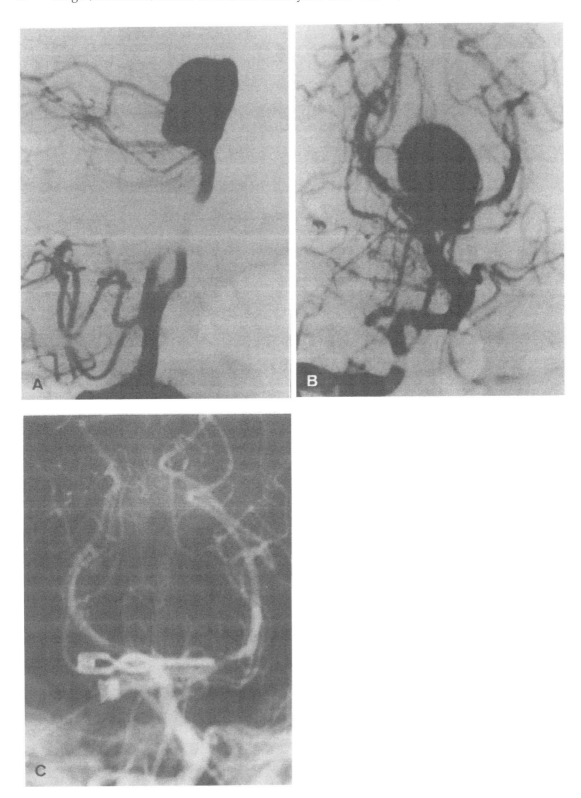

Figure 4.4 A–C. J.O., M, 34, "Beer belly" on posterior neck of large basilar bifurcation aneurysm (**A, B**) could be "gathered in" by clip blades after two previous attempts elsewhere in August 1978 21 days after single bleed in Grade 2 (**C**). Lower Heifetz clip is on an intact anterior communicating aneurysm. Outcome excellent

Large (or Bulbous) Basilar Bifurcation Aneurysms (12.5–25 mm) 47

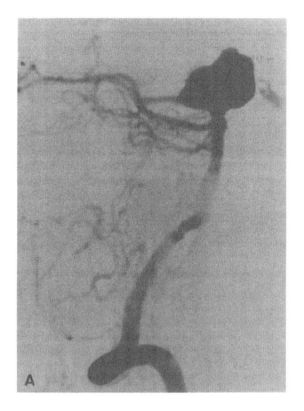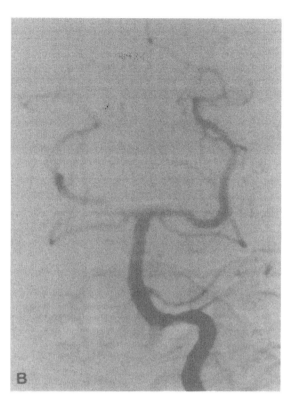

Figure 4.5 A–B. L.W., M, 47, large basilar bifurcation aneurysm with neck expanding horizontally 180° forward and backward (**A**) was operated on in February 1983 11 days after single bleed in Grade 1. Neck could be "gathered in" between clip blades after 11 short temporary basilar clippings (total occlusion time 21 minutes) (**B**). Excellent outcome

and behind the bifurcation in the sagittal plane can usually be managed similarly with the "gathering" method (Fig. 4.5). If not, each loculus may be clipped separately, the posterior loculus first, then the anterior, so that the clip blades lie side by side in front of and behind the bifurcation; this was done in two of the six cases (Fig. 4.6).

A continuing difficulty with a firm atherosclerotic neck is that, although the open blades may be initially in the correct position, they slide down to occlude the bifurcation as they are allowed to close. Sometimes, the anterior blade can be held up on the far side of the neck with the sucker tip as the blades are allowed to close. Repeated trials sometimes soften the neck so that the blades will stay in position, but often it requires drastic narrowing of the waist of the sac with forceps or with the sucker tip to produce a slope on which they will close and remain. Adding clips in parallel beyond the first malpositioned clip may produce a stable clip so that those slipped proximally can be removed. It may be necessary to place the blades deliberately up on the waist and then try to get another set of blades below, or vice versa. In this situation, the tandem clip principle may be of great value and was used in one-fifth of the large aneurysms (Fig. 4.7). A shorter pair of fenestrated blades may stay up on the far side of the neck while the near side of the neck remains open in the aperture. Then another tandem clip can be applied a little higher on the near side to close off the portion of the neck remaining open in the fenestration. This tandem clip principle usually solves the problem when the tips of a well positioned long clip are held open by the bulk of the neck in the fulcrum, thus allowing flow into the aneurysm, which will pulsate or bleed on needling.

Large bulbous sacs can be associated with another dangerous anomaly. The ectasia of the bifurcation may develop in such a manner that the P1 segments emerge *downward* from the base of the sac (Figs. 4.8, 4.9). Here, it may be impossible to prevent the blades of the clip from slipping down and stenosing or occluding the P1 orifices. Providing there is a good PComA, then an ipsilateral P1 can be

48   Large (or Bulbous) Basilar Bifurcation Aneurysms (12.5–25 mm)

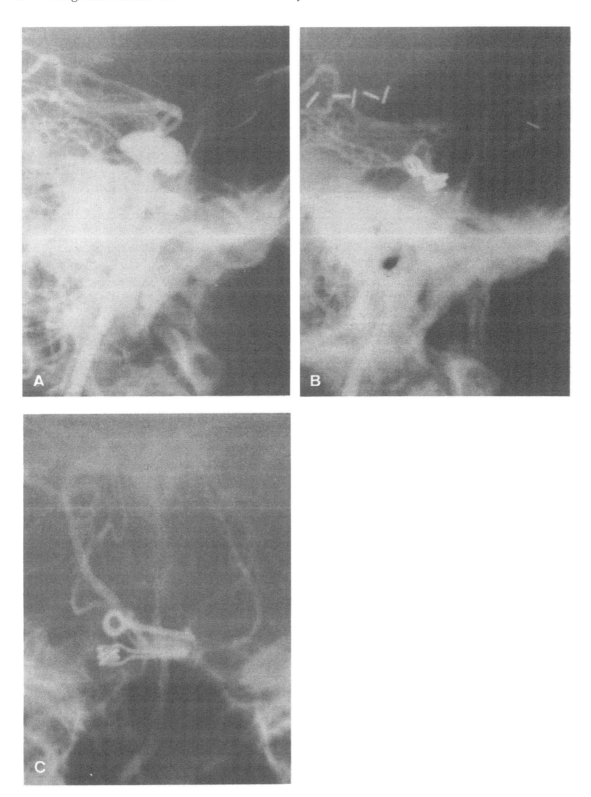

Figure 4.6 A–C. W.McA., M, 25, very low bilobed large basilar bifurcation aneurysm (**A**) was operated on in June 1974 2 months after single bleed in Grade 1. Clip blades placed side by side on each locule (**B**). In spite of residual neck between blades (**C**), patient has remained well for over 20 years

Large (or Bulbous) Basilar Bifurcation Aneurysms (12.5–25 mm)   49

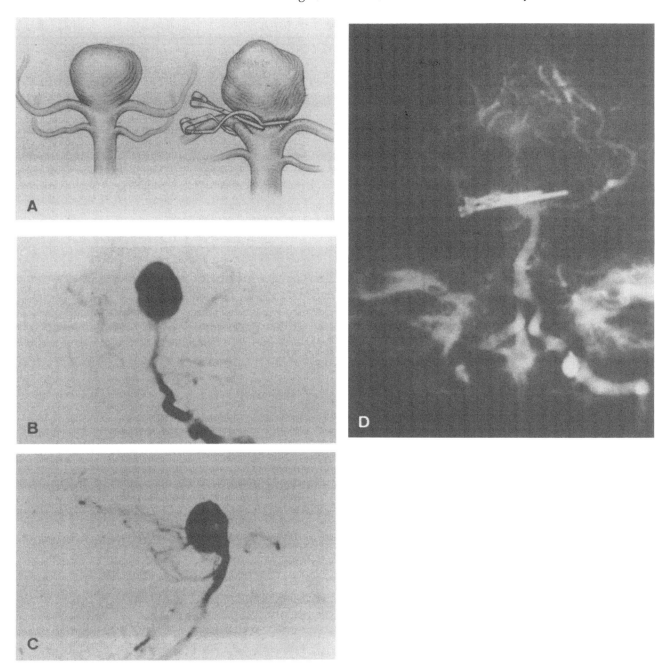

Figure 4.7 A–D. Principle of tandem clipping (**A**) as seen in the case of a large basilar bifurcation aneurysm (**B–D**). Ectasia of bifurcation seen below clip blades

50   Large (or Bulbous) Basilar Bifurcation Aneurysms (12.5–25 mm)

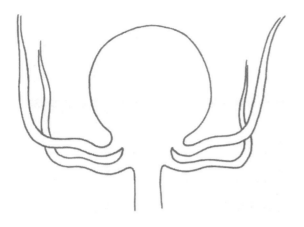

Figure 4.8. When P1s emerge downward from neck of large aneurysm, clip blades should be placed higher on neck to avoid stenosis or occlusion of the orifices of these vessels and perforators. (Reprinted from Clin Neurosurg 26, 1979, p. 64 by courtesy of Williams and Wilkins)

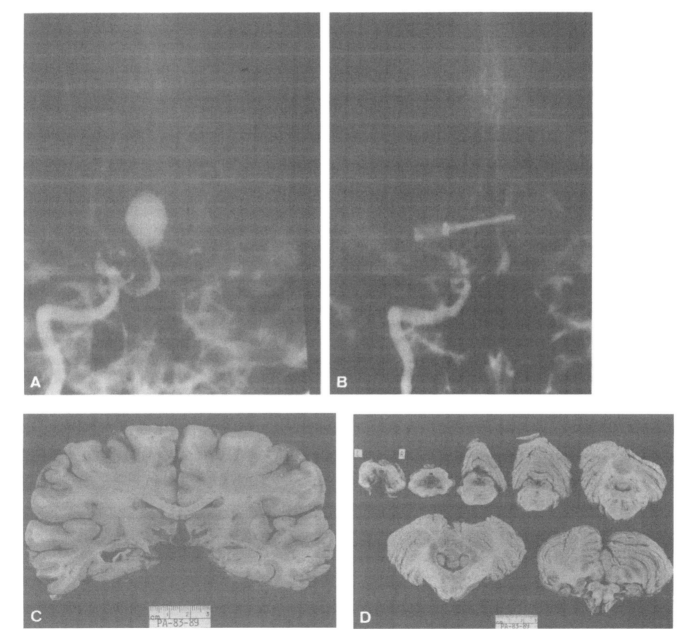

Fig. 4.9

taken cautiously in the clip, if there is no alternative and no perforators are included. This was done five times in large aneurysms with one death and four excellent results. Another maneuver that has been successful is to apply shorter fenestrated clip blades *obliquely* from below upwards placing the ipsilateral P1, even SCA, in the aperture. The clip blades then close from the center of the ectatic basilar bifurcation across the far side of the neck at the level of the origin of the opposite P1. With this narrowing of the neck, another tandem clip can usually be placed above the ipsilateral P1 with the tips closing flush with the blades of the first clip. Rarely, it has been possible to use very short blades and allow them to fall in the center of a widened thick basilar bifurcation, just at the base of the neck, leaving a current on either side to irrigate the P2 segments.

When thrombus extends down around the neck of a larger aneurysm, shortened fenestrated blades can be used to close the open neck centrally and leave the thrombosed near neck in the aperture while the tips close flush with the thrombus on the other side (Fig. 4.10).

Results

The results are seen in Tables 4.1 to 4.10.

Three of four patients with poor results in unruptured aneurysms had perforator injuries, one had Hunterian ligation with tourniquet(vide infra). A 38 year old female remained one month in Grade 4 after her fourth SAH and had her aneurysm repaired. A shunting procedure was done and she made a surprising recovery being self-sufficient 10 years later (Table 4.1).

All patients aged 70 or more made good recoveries: three patients aged 70, 72 and 75 years had excellent results and all had early surgery in Grade 2, 3–5 days after bleeding; the one with good recovery had transient postoperative hemiparesis (Table 4.2). The poor result in a 12 year old boy is explained below.

All but a few of the large bifurcation aneurysms were treated by clipping (91.4%). Other methods of

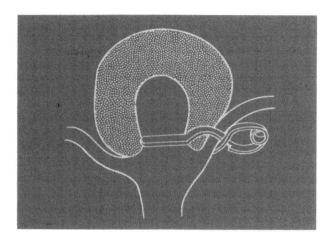

Figure 4.10. The clip blades close the open neck between masses of thrombus extending into neck of aneurysm

treatment are summarized in Table 4.3. A female aged 33 in Grade 3 in 1967 had a silk ligature of the aneurysmal neck, she died two months later due to perforator injury and inadvertent major vessel occlusion. Four large aneurysms were wrapped in gauze, probably incompletely. Three were done early in the series; one is known to have survived for three years, but the others died of rebleeding within a few months. The last one in 1980 was a high posteriorly projecting unruptured aneurysm in a lady, 67, who remains in excellent condition 12 years later.

Proximal basilar artery occlusion was used in 12 large aneurysms, using a clip in 7 and the tourniquet in 5. One large aneurysm was not suitable for clipping because of its fusiform nature, the remainder had wide bulbous thick stiff necks which would not hold a clip or were additionally highly located (5). Two patients died. A 62 year old man in Grade 2 had good clip occlusion 33 days after SAH, but died 3 weeks later from staphylococcal meningitis. The other was a female, 57, in Grade 1 but five days after bleed when the tourniquet was applied – she died one week after operation from massive temporo-occipital infarction from feeble filling of the right posterior cerebral artery (PCA). Two patients died more than three months after operation and are

Figure 4.9 A–D. T.N., F, 48, large basilar bifurcation aneurysm (A) was operated on in January 1977 6 months after single bleed in Grade 1. Postoperatively she remained quadriplegic in coma, and died more than 6 years later in 1983. Clip blades have slipped down to occlude orifices of P1s emerging downward from thick bulbous neck of large bifurcation aneurysm (B) resulting in extensive infarction thalamus, midbrain, pons and medial temporal and occipital lobes (C, D)

classified in the Tables as poor surgical results: a 12 year old boy with a highly located aneurysm in Grade 1 remained in poor condition after clip occlusion on the 11th day after bleeding and died five months later. A 55 year old female had a tourniquet occlusion for her unruptured aneurysm located high above the posterior clinoid level, remained in rather poor condition and died 10 months later from rupture when a patent PComA prevented thrombosis in the sac.

In two recent unruptured aneurysms it was felt that clipping carried high risk and the craniotomies remained exploratory: the one was a 45 year old and after prolonged dissection, the fusiform nature of the aneurysm was detected, the other was a 69 year old with a low posterior projecting partially fusiform calcified aneurysm. In both a yellow fusiform enlargement of the basilar bifurcation was found giving rise to smaller saccules but as well to P1s and SCAs. Finally one young female aged 37 deeply unconscious in Grade 5 had her temporal hematoma removed on the day of bleeding (Day 0) and died.

Endovascular coils were used in two patients. The first had suffered a myocardial infarction on the day after hemorrhage and the bulk of the sac was occluded with coils soon after the hemorrhage as the patient still was in Grade 4–5. She recovered but six months later the coils had been compacted into the periphery of the sac which was slightly larger. One end of a coil projected near the orifice of the left P1 and application of a clip was felt to be too dangerous. The residual sac was repacked nearly completely with GDCs and she will be followed for recurrence when basilar artery occlusion may be necessary. The other patient was in Grade 4 condition but rapidly deteriorated after the catheter was seen projecting through the dome of the aneurysm, although post mortem angiography revealed complete occlusion of the aneurysm (Table 4.3).

One death occurred in a patient with a forward projecting aneurysm with a neck lying far below the posterior clinoid: this 54 year old male in Grade 3 and 7 days after bleeding had inadvertent PCA occlusion and died 10 days later. The poor result was due to perforator injury in an aneurysm with the same low location. The other death in this group was due to perioperative aneurysm rupture in a female aged 48 in Grade 1 who remained deeply unconscious and died one week later, the aneurysmal neck was located at the clinoid. The only poor result in non-giant bilobed aneurysms was in a 46 year old female in Grade 1 with a low lying aneurysm (Tables 4.5 to 4.10).

Table 4.1. Preoperative Grade and outcome in 265 patients with large basilar bifurcation aneurysms

Grade	Excellent	Good	Poor	Dead	Total
0	33	3	4		40
1	99	16	10	7	132
2	37	16	7	2	62
3	8	8	7	3	26
4		1	1	1	3
5	1			1	2
Total	178	44	29	14	265
	67.2%	16.6%	10.9%	5.3%	100.0%

Table 4.2. Age related to outcome in 265 patients with large basilar bifurcation aneurysms

Age group (years)	Excellent	Good	Poor	Dead	Total
0–9	1				1
10–19	2		1		3
20–29	7	2			9
30–39	42	7	2	3	54
40–49	60	12	8	2	82
50–59	48	16	13	6	83
60–69	15	6	5	3	29
70 or more	3	1			4
Total	178	44	29	14	265

Table 4.3. Operative method and outcome in 265 patients with large basilar bifurcation aneurysms

Operative method	Excellent	Good	Poor	Dead	Total
Neck clipping	166	41	27	9	243
Silk ligature				1	1
Wrapping	3	1			4
Basilar occlusion	6	2	2	2	12
Endovascular	1			1	2
Only hematoma removed				1	1
Explored only	2				2
Total	178	44	29	14	265

Table 4.4. Operative method and completeness of aneurysm treatment in 265 patients with large basilar bifurcation aneurysms

Operative method	Total obliteration	Residual neck	Residual fundus	No obliteration	Total
Neck clipping	219	15	9		243
Silk ligature		1			1
Wrapping				4	4
Basilar occlusion	6		6		12
Endovascular			2		2
Only hematoma removed				1	1
Exploration only				2	2
Total	225	16	17	7	265

Table 4.5. Outcome as related to timing of surgery in 225 patients with large basilar bifurcation aneurysms

Timing of surgery	Excel-lent	Good	Poor	Dead	Total
0–1 day	6	1		1	8
2–3 day	7	1	1	2	11
4–6 day	12	3		1	16
7–10 day	25	8	3	2	38
11–30 day	77	24	11	5	117
31–365 day	18	4	10	3	35
Total	145	41	25	14	225

Table 4.6. Basilar aneurysm projection and outcome in 265 patients with large basilar bifurcation aneurysms

Basilar projection	Excel-lent	Good	Poor	Dead	Total
Forward	14	4	1	2	21
Upward	131	33	23	10	197
Backward	30	5	4	2	41
Bilobed	3	2	1		6
Total	178	44	29	14	265

Table 4.7. Relation of basilar aneurysm to clinoid and outcome in 265 patients with large basilar bifurcation aneurysms

Basilar-clinoid	Excel-lent	Good	Poor	Dead	Total
Above	36	6	3		45
At clinoid	71	21	11	10	113
Below	66	16	14	4	100
Not known	5	1	1		7
Total	178	44	29	14	265

Table 4.8. Preoperative Grade (Botterell) and outcome in 197 patients with large and upward projecting basilar bifurcation aneurysms

Grade	Excellent	Good	Poor	Dead	Total
0	22	2	2		26
1	74	10	7	4	95
2	28	14	6	2	50
3	6	7	7	2	22
4		1		1	2
5	1			1	2
Total	131	33	23	10	197

Table 4.9. Preoperative Grade (Botterell) and outcome in 21 patients with large and anterior projecting basilar bifurcation aneurysms

Grade	Excellent	Good	Poor	Dead	Total
0	5	1			6
1	3	2		1	6
2	5		1		6
3	1	1		1	3
Total	14	4	1	2	21

Table 4.10. Preoperative Grade (Botterell) and outcome in 41 patients with large and posterior projecting basilar bifurcation aneurysms

Grade	Excellent	Good	Poor	Dead	Total
0	6		2		8
1	20	4	2	2	28
2	3	1			4
3	1				1
Total	30	5	4	2	41

Chapter 5

Analysis of Operative Morbidity in Basilar Bifurcation Aneurysms: Small and Large (Non-Giant)

758 Patients

Operative complications specific for non-giant basilar bifurcation aneurysms were chiefly midbrain and/or thalamic infarction from perforator injury or occlusion, inadvertent intraoperative rupture, imperfect clipping with early rerupture, and frequent but nearly always transient third cranial nerve paresis (Tables 5.1 to 5.8).

The most catastrophic complication of operation in this region is a major operative tear of the aneurysm or incomplete clipping of the aneurysm with the potential for rebleeding during closure or early in the postoperative period. Prior to 1983, four deaths and two poor results resulted from major intraoperative ruptures that were difficult to control.

Early rebleeding from incomplete clipping occurred 13 times with 7 deaths and 1 poor result (cf. Table 5.2). In most, the blades of a fenestrated clip were thought to occlude the neck completely while trying to avoid perforators on the far side (Fig. 5.1) or accommodate them in the aperture on the near side with P1 (Fig. 5.2). Even though the refilling of the aneurysm was through a tiny portion of the neck remaining in the fenestration or just beyond the clip tips, catastrophic rebleeding occurred in an hour to three days. The frequency of early postoperative rebleedings although low has remained about the same in the recent years inspite of increasing experience and sophisticated methods: temporary clipping, careful inspection to be certain the clip is in as perfect a position as possible and proving complete clipping by needling. These figures are higher than in anterior circulation reflecting the special difficulties in the treatment of these aneurysms, and also more follow-up of the patients (as half of the rebleedings occurred late). One early fatal rebleeding occurred from two millimetres of *intact* neck remaining *below* a clip that had occluded the aneurysm beyond. The last fatality occurred from a small tear in the front of the basilar bifurcation below a completely clipped aneurysm. This proved to be a ruptured dissection presumably related to the clipping although there was no known misapplication of the clip before final placement. Another similar tear is described under temporary clipping. One patient died on day 3 from rupture of a previously intact middle cerebral aneurysm.

Thirty-two postoperative, *coma-producing* extracerebral clots occurred in 1089 subtemporal approaches for aneurysms on the upper two-thirds of the basilar artery; 11 were extradural and 21 were subdural. Recovery was complete after removal of eight extradural clots, one was poor, but two died; one was the only death in the small superior cerebellar aneurysms. Acute subdural hematoma carried a much worse prognosis; only seven patients had good outcomes, seven were poor and seven died.

Brain stem or cerebral ischemia with vasospasm alone caused 11 poor outcomes and 9 deaths in nongiant basilar bifurcation aneurysms (cf. Fig. 9.10). Recently, higher levels of artificial hypertension after volume expansion and more recently angioplasty have undoubtedly saved several patients from this fate. Two men, with large ruptured bifurcation aneurysms developed early postoperative hemiplegias with vasospasm. Neither responded to volume expansion and moderate hypertension. It was not until the hypertension was raised to systolic pressures of 230–240 in the first and 210–220 in the second that recovery began rapidly, even though the younger man had been solidly hemiplegic for 36 hours. Systolic pressures over 200 had to be maintained for 10 days before either could be weaned without recurrence. Both made complete recoveries.

Perforator Injury or Occlusion

The most common, serious complication was brain stem infarction from perforator injury and occlu-

56 Analysis of Operative Morbidity in Basilar Bifurcation Aneurysms

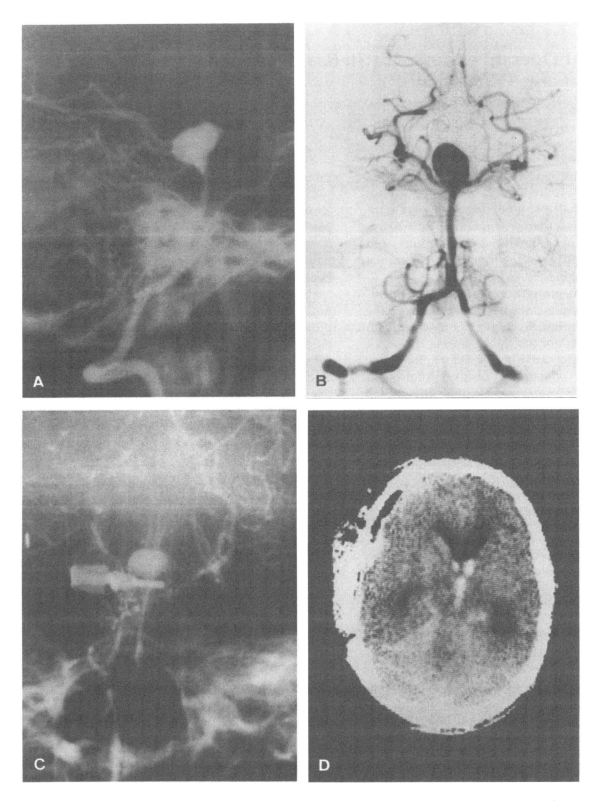

Figure 5.1 A–D. B.P., F, 48, small basilar bifurcation aneurysm (**A, B**), operation in deep hypotension(45mm Hg 30 minutes) in July 1978 22 days after single bleed in Grade 1. Clip tips just short allowing filling through tiny opening on left side of neck (**C**). Fatal rebleeding after awakening intact in recovery room (**D**)

Analysis of Operative Morbidity in Basilar Bifurcation Aneurysms 57

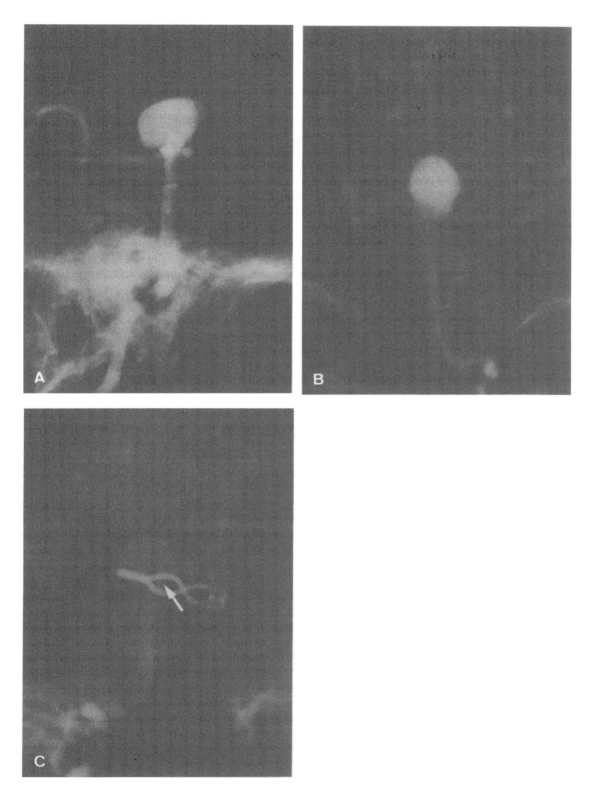

Figure 5.2 A–C. B.B., F, 69, large basilar bifurcation aneurysm (**A, B**), operation in August 1982 18 days after single bleed in Grade 2. Postoperatively well for 10 hours then fatal rebleeding from rerupture of sac still filling through small portion of neck remaining open in fenestration (**C**)

sion. This accounted for about two-fifths of the poor results in small aneurysms and nearly three-fifths in the large aneurysms (Tables 5.3, 5.4, and 5.8). Interestingly, perforator injuries were only slightly, not significantly more common in patients with intraoperative aneurysm rupture than in patients without rupture (21% versus 15%). Even after the early catastrophes with massive multiple perforator infarction, it took some time to recognize the features of smaller infarctions, e.g. that a contralateral postoperative third nerve paresis usually was evidence of perforator infarction and not due to injury of the nerve with a clip blade. CT and MR scanning finally revealed the site and size of the midbrain and thalamic perforator infarctions (Figs. 5.3, 5.4, 5.5, and 5.6).

The projection and size of the aneurysms were important for both the incidence and outcome of perforator injury (Tables 5.3, 5.4, and 5.8).

Understandably, no perforator injury occurred in the forward projecting *small* aneurysms, since the course of the perforators is upward and backward, away from the necks of these aneurysms, which usually lie free in the interpeduncular space at the front of the basilar artery bifurcation.

Perforators commonly lie under and on either side of *backward* projecting sacs and although their injury rate (20.4%) was only slightly higher as for upward projecting sacs (16.4%), only in large aneurysms did a perforator infarction alone contribute to a poor result. However, and as seen in the upward projecting aneurysms, isolated perforator injury does contribute to more cases being classed as good rather than excellent results because of residual oculomotor paresis and/or non-disabling slurred speech and unsteadiness, albeit with clear intellect (Table 5.4).

For *upward* projecting small aneurysms, perforator injury occurred in 14%, but contributed to 53% of the poor results (Table 5.3). The outcome of perforator infarction was related to the size and position of the infarction as seen in later cases with CT or MR scanning. In review of the outcome, it became apparent that most who recovered completely, or nearly so, had minor degrees of gaze palsy, often only a medial rectus and/or an upward gaze palsy. One of these patients had a perforator occluded deliberately. The recovery of these pareses often takes place while in hospital. Major degrees of ophthalmoparesis, especially if bilateral

(although it was often difficult to be sure of the contribution of ipsilateral third cranial nerve manipulation) signalled either a poor outcome, or that the patient might recover to a good but seldom an excellent outcome. The prognosis was worse when ophthalmoparesis was associated with one or a combination of pseudobulbar slurring dysarthria, ataxia, rubral tremor, hemiparesis or coma. However, it was remarkable how, over many months, significant and satisfactory recovery occurred in a few of these patients (Tables 5.3 and 5.4).

In spite of the frequency of perforator infarction with small aneurysms, the majority of these patients (72.5%) ultimately have a satisfactory outcome, although about one-third of these are classed as good rather than excellent results.

For *large* basilar bifurcation aneurysms, perforator injury was of even greater significance; the incidence was 21% and it accounted for nearly two-thirds of the poor results (59%) (Table 5.3). The problem is twofold. First is the bulbous nature of the neck with its expansion into the ectasia of the basilar bifurcation, from which perforators may arise. Second is the difficulty in preventing the clip blades from slipping down and kinking the orifices of the P1 origins, particularly when they emerge downwards from the neck. However, there has been a significant decline in major perforator infarction since 1988 even though the more routine use of temporary basilar artery clipping, with or without trapping, began earlier. Even so, the surgeon should be cautious because prolonged temporary occlusion of a perforator, as by tentative aneurysm clipping, with a temporary clip in place or during systemic hypotension, may sufficiently impair its meager collateral flow to produce an infarction. In the total series of non-giant basilar bifurcation aneurysms, the frequency of perforator injuries was not influenced by temporary clipping (cf. Table 5.7).

Although inadvertent P1 occlusion carried high morbidity in large aneurysms, its occurrence ipsilaterally in nine *small* aneurysms was uneventful in eight; one patient remained poor. P1 was deliberately occluded in three patients with a good posterior communicating artery (PComA), also without effect. The PComA was divided in two cases without consequences. In 265 *large* aneurysms, inadvertent P1 occlusion occurred 14 times, 6 times bilaterally and was usually associated with larger

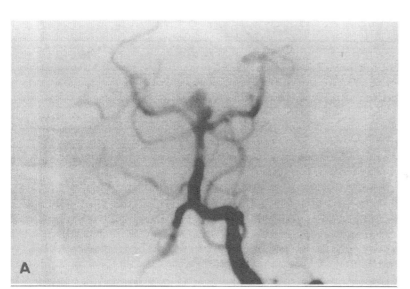
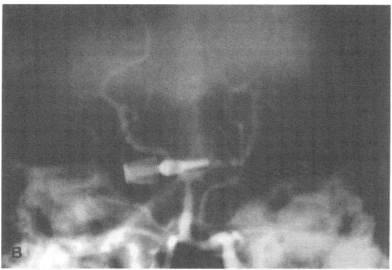
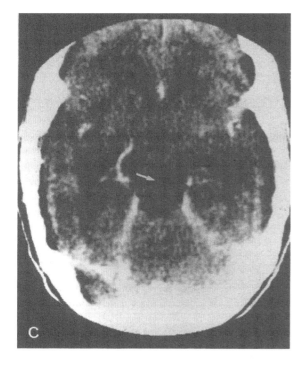

Figure 5.3 A–C. E.W., F, 58, small basilar bifurcation aneurysm (**A**), operation in December 1979 5 days after second bleed in Grade 2. Postoperatively EOM paresis and rubral tremor. Fenestrated clip blades too long and occlude left side P1 perforators. Central and posterior midbrain infarcts (arrow) (**C**). Poor outcome

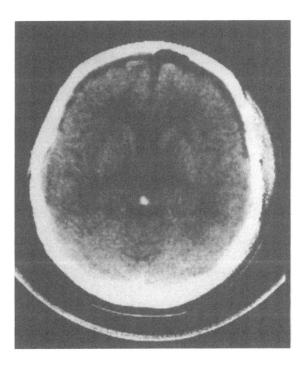

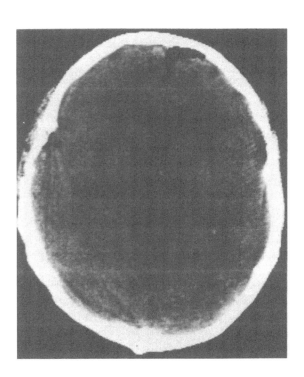

Figure 5.4. F.S., F, 44, small basilar bifurcation aneurysm, had a rebleeding during opening of the skull. Before operation in September 1985, 16 days after the first bleed she was in Grade 1. Postoperatively she was amnestic with upward gaze paresis and dysarthria but with good ultimate recovery. CT reveals 1.5 cm lower left thalamic infarct

Figure 5.5. F.R., M, 39, large intact basilar bifurcation aneurysm, headache, operation in January 1982. Postoperatively she was well except for paresis of upward gaze and partial left ptosis. CT reveals small preaqueductal midbrain infarct. Later excellent recovery

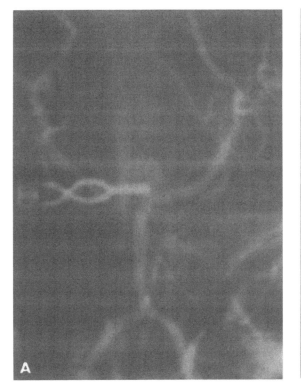

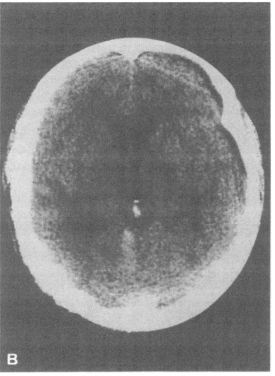

Figure 5.6 A, B. E.P., M, 51, small basilar bifurcation aneurysm. Operation in June 1982 in Grade 1 11 days after single bleed. Incomplete fenestrated clip trying to avoid left side perforators (**A**). Postoperatively drowsy with bilateral vertical ophthalmoplegia. CT reveals bilateral thalamic and small midbrain infarcts, then fatal rebleeding on day 8 (**B**)

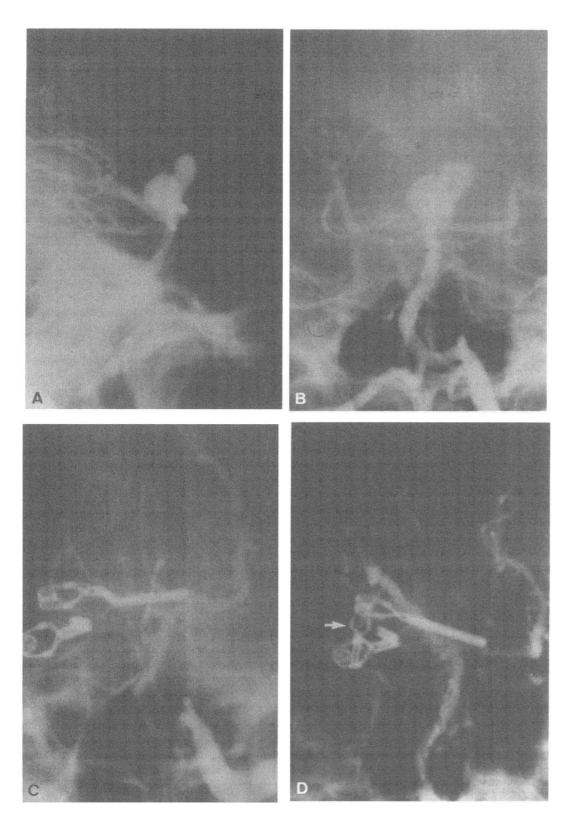

Figure 5.7 A–D. G.G., M, 58, large basilar bifurcation aneurysm (**A, B**), operation 8 days after single bleed in Grade 1 in July 1987. Postoperative occlusion of right P1 causing stupor and hemiparesis (**C**). The lower clip is on a carotid aneurysm. At reoperation clip blades were in good position on the aneurysmal neck but the descent of the temporal lobe on the clip handle after retraction had torqued the blades so as to occlude P1. Maintenance of the correct clip angle by propping the handle up with another clip attached to the tentorium (arrow) was followed by restoration of P1 flow and complete recovery (**D**)

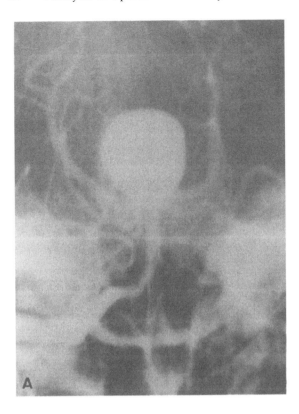 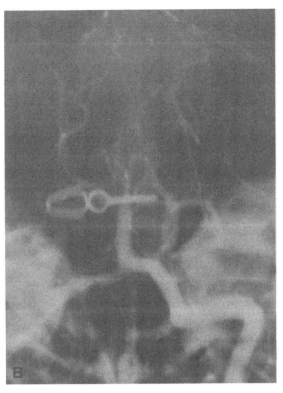

Figure 5.8 A, B. J.D., F, 56, large basilar bifurcation aneurysm (**A**), using deep hypotension (28 minutes 35 mmHG) she was operated on 13 days after single bleed in Grade 1 in July 1977. Postoperatively she was well for 24 hours, then confused with right hemiparesis and upward gaze paresis. Clip blades had stayed up on neck only on third application but must have slipped down again to occlude basilar bifurcation and stenose origins of SCA (**B**). Good outcome after recovery using hypertension. Good leptomeningeal collateral to both posterior cerebral arteries

midbrain and thalamic infarctions resulting in 6 poor results and 3 deaths. P1 was deliberately occluded in five cases with one death. In two patients severe P1 stenosis resulted in minor infarction. One of these was in coma postoperatively, and urgent reposition of the clip, which had been rotated by the temporal lobe descent, resulted in immediate dramatic recovery (Fig. 5.7). In two patients, bilateral P1 occlusion was well tolerated (Fig. 5.8), one of which included the origin of the left superior cerebellar artery (SCA)!

Altogether, inadvertent arterial occlusion occurred in 27 patients with small and large basilar bifurcation aneurysms. The basilar bifurcation was inadvertently occluded with P1 or SCA uni- or bilaterally in 7 patients, P1 alone in 14 patients, P1 associated with SCA in 1 patient and both P1s in 1 patient, SCA alone in 1 patient and PComA in 1 patient. Two patients had mysterious thromboembolic occlusions in distal middle cerebral artery (MCA) and distal pericallosal artery (Tables 5.9 and 25.6).

In several patients in the total series of large aneurysms, the occlusion of a major branching was thought to be due to apposition of thick atheromatous walls *proximal* to the clip blades (Fig. 5.9). If this is suspected at operation, the clip blades should be repositioned a little further out on the neck so that the apposition of the walls proximally takes place only to the beginning of the neck.

Medical complications have seemed no different in this group of aneurysms (Table 5.6). There were two deaths from massive pulmonary embolism, five patients survived this complication. Myocardial infarctions accounted for a poor result with anoxic encephalopathy on day 1, and a sudden death on day 3. Two other patients with cardiac complications made good recoveries. One man, aged 64, operated on day 4, with occlusion of a ruptured basilar bifurcation and intact left MCA aneurysms, was found comatose and pulseless in hemorrhagic shock on day 8. Retroperitoneal and duodenal bleeding were identified and angiogra-

Analysis of Operative Morbidity in Basilar Bifurcation Aneurysms 63

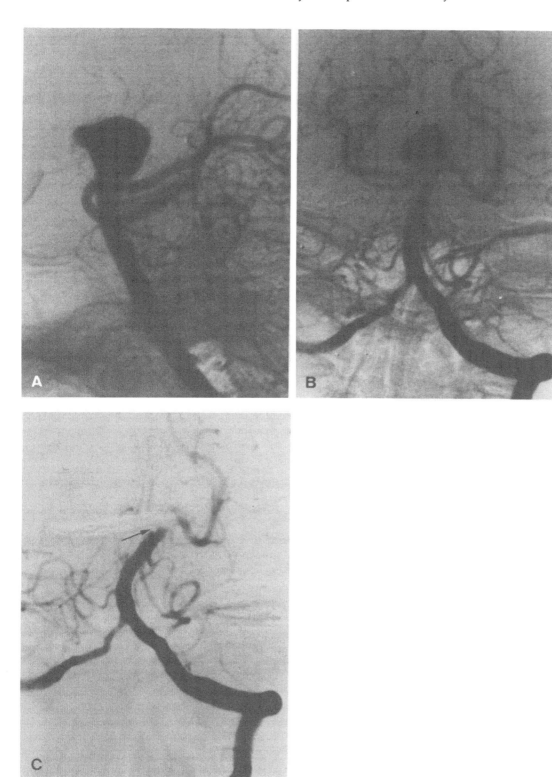

Figure 5.9 A–C. S.Z., F, 62, large basilar bifurcation aneurysm explored elsewhere (**A, B**), operation 7 weeks after single bleed in Grade 1 in January 1983. Tandem clip seemed to stay in position on neck but a complete Weber's syndrome followed. The right P1 and SCA occlusion felt to be due to apposition of thick atheromatous walls *proximal* to clip blades (**C,** arrow). Poor outcome

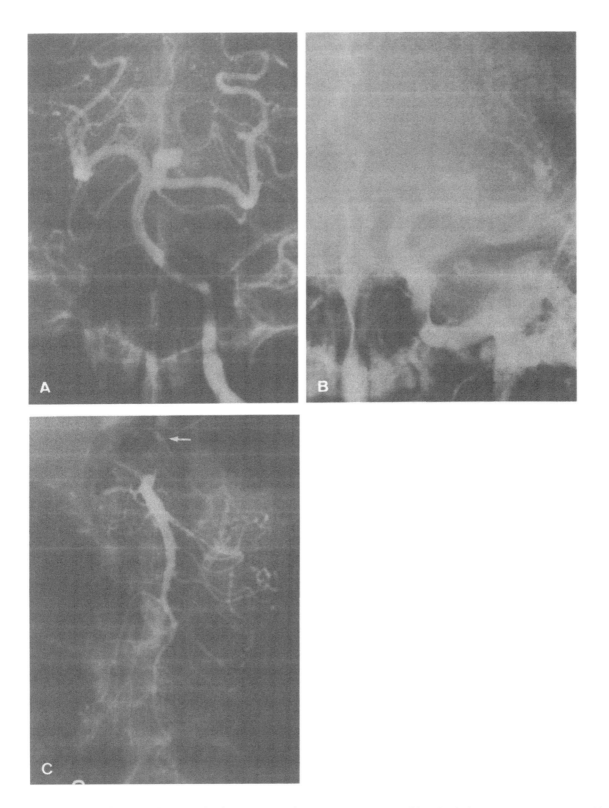

Figure 5.10 A–C. D.J., M, 62, multiple intracranial aneurysms, ruptured basilar bifurcation aneurysm and bilateral middle cerebral artery aneurysms (**A, B**), operation 4 days after single bleed in Grade 2 in April 1988. Postoperatively on day 4 found ashen and pulseless and on resuscitation was hemiplegic and aphasic. A distended abdomen led to the discovery of massive retroperitoneal hemorrhage. Angiography revealed innumerable aneurysms on the celiac vessels (**C**). The largest of the multiple celiac artery aneurysms (arrow) was embolized but the hemiplegia persisted but with good speech recovery. A tiny low density in the external capsule seen on day 1 had expanded to infarction of the corpus striatum and corona radiata above. Poor outcome

phy revealed innumerable aneurysms on the celiac vessels (Fig. 5.10). After embolic occlusion of the gastroduodenal artery giving rise to the larger aneurysm, he survived, but with a right hemiplegia and expressive aphasia related to hemodynamic infarction of striatum and corona.

Final Comments on Non-Giant Basilar Bifurcation Aneurysms

The major technical problem in the clipping of basilar bifurcation aneurysms in distinction from most others has been preserving the integrity of all the intimately associated perforating arteries in the confines of the interpeduncular space. Outcome has improved over the 34 years of this series beginning with the recognition of the perforator problem, the introduction of the spring clip and the use of loupe magnification after 1958. Soon after, ever deepening levels of systemic hypotension for bolder dissection were used and microtechniques after 1970. The fenestrated clip eased the situation further, particularly for larger aneurysms. Finally, increasing experience undoubtedly was a factor as well as significant alteration of ischemia with vasospasm using volume expansion and hypertension. In non-giant basilar bifurcation aneurysms operated on in the microsurgical era since 1970 by the senior authors, the operative mortality within 90 days was in the first half 5.7% and in the last half 2.7% in nearly identical number of cases (all grades included, cf. with Table 5.7 with good risk patients).

For no other aneurysm has induced hypotension (used in 58.6%) been more important and the authors believe that the increasing use of temporary clipping since 1981 (in 54% of non-giant basilar bifurcation aneurysms), with its even more profound softening of the aneurysm, has had another significant effect over the last decade. The benefit of temporary clipping is difficult to prove statistically, because of its most frequent use in the difficult aneurysms which, in the notes, could not always be separated from those less dangerous where its use was less common. Even so, its use gives some comfort to the surgeon in lessening anxiety over inadvertent rupture while being more bold with difficult dissection, even making the experience a pleasant one.

In order to compare these two periods, the results in good condition patients only, in the microsurgical era before and after 1981, when temporary clipping was used, are matched in Table 5.7. The exclusion of poor condition patients removes most of the morbidity from subarachnoid hemorrhage (SAH) allowing the morbidity from technical surgical problems to be seen more clearly. Breaking down the figures in Table 5.7 further, an improvement in results is seen as follows. For small bifurcation aneurysms, the combined operative morbidity and mortality was reduced from 10.3% (mortality 4.8%) down to 6.5% (mortality 2.2%); for the large aneurysms the reduction was from 16.7% (mortality 6.0%) down to 10.4% (mortality 2.1%). Correspondingly, good outcome was raised to 93.5% and 89.6% respectively. The causes of the surgical morbidity in this selected recent good risk group of small aneurysms differ significantly; only 9.6% perforator injury in the small aneurysm group as compared to 16.8% in the first period (in large aneurysms the decrease was from 26.2% to 19.4%). Four poor results were due to vasospasm reflecting the increasing use of early operation. The unexplained postoperative spontaneous rupture of the upper basilar artery proximal to the clip and the massive retroperitoneal bleeding from one of multiple coeliac aneurysms accounted for two others and a man, 80, made no recovery from a Grade 2 confusional state. There were still three perforator infarctions in the large aneurysms and one P1 occlusion. Vasospasm, operative tear of the aneurysm and an airway-induced postoperative cardiac arrest with anoxic encephalopathy accounted for the remainder.

Analysis of Operative Morbidity in Basilar Bifurcation Aneurysms

Table 5.1. Operative complications in 493 patients with small basilar bifurcation aneurysms

Complication	No.	Percent
Intraoperative aneurysm rupture	68	13.8
Perforator injury	62	12.6
Inadvertent major vessel occlusion	11	2.2
Brain injury	3	0.6
Cranial nerve injury	5	1.0
Postoperative significant spasm	34	6.9
Postoperative hematoma removed	12	2.4

Table 5.2. Death from rebleeding in 758 non-giant basilar bifurcation aneurysms. Six patients survived recurrent bleed and five had subsequent operations

Time of rebleeding	Neck clipping	Other methods than neck clipping	Total
< 1 month	7	5	12
1 month–1 year	0	4	4
> 1 year	6	0	6
Total	13	9	22

Table 5.3. Influence of perforator injury on outcome in 758 patients with non-giant basilar bifurcation aneurysms. Number of perforator injuries / Number of patients in each outcome group

Aneurysm size	Excellent	Good	Poor	Dead	Total
Basilar projection					
Small	27/377	18/65	14/33	3/18	62/493
Forward	0/48	0/6	0/4	0/3	0/61
Upward	22/273	12/50	14/27	2/12	50/362
Backward	5/48	6/9	0/2	1/3	12/62
Bilobed	0/8				0/8
Large	20/178	16/44	17/29	2/14	55/265
Forward	2/14	1/4	1/1	0/2	4/21
Upward	16/131	12/33	13/23	1/10	42/197
Backward	2/30	3/5	3/4	1/2	9/41
Bilobed	0/3	0/2	0/1		0/6

Table 5.4. Outcome (%) in 758 non-giant basilar bifurcation aneurysms as related to perforator injury

Perforator injury	Excellent	Good	Poor	Dead
No	78.9	11.6	5.0	4.5
Yes	40.2	29.1	26.5	4.3
Total	73.0	14.3	8.3	4.5

Table 5.5. Cranial nerve deficits (%) in 493 patients with small basilar bifurcation aneurysms

Cranial nerves paralyzed	Pre-operative %	Post-operative %	Follow-up %
CNIII unilateral	5.3	70.2	7.5
CNIII bilateral	0.2	4.9	2.0
Other cranial nerves	3.4	7.7	1.6

Table 5.6. Medical complications in 493 patients with small basilar bifurcation aneurysms

Nature	No.	Percent
Electrolyte disturbances	3	0.6
Cardiac	2	0.4
Respiratory	9	1.8
Gastrointestinal	6	1.2
Genitourinary	1	0.2
Pulmonary embolus/DVT	4	0.8
Combined medical	13	2.7

Table 5.7. Outcome of surgery in 666 good risk patients with small and large basilar bifurcation aneurysms in two different time periods (microsurgical era)

Timing period	Excellent	Good	Poor	Dead	Total
1970–1980	213 72.9	44 15.1	20 6.8	15 5.1	292
1981–1992	302 80.7	42 11.2	22 5.9	8 2.1	374
Total	515 77.3	86 12.9	42 6.3	23 3.5	666 100.0

Table 5.8. Direction of aneurysm fundus (forward, upward, backward) and relation of the neck to the posterior clinoid (above, at clinoid, below) in 683 patients with small or large basilar bifurcation aneurysms. Excluded were patients without known aneurysm projection or without known height of the aneurysmal neck in relation to posterior clinoid or patients with endovascular surgery (14 patients with bilobular aneurysms were also excluded[a])

Aneurysm projection Relation to posterior clinoid process	No. of patients	Poor + dead %
Anterior projection		
above clinoid	28	0
at clinoid	28	11
below clinoid	20	35
Superior projection		
above clinoid	128	9
at clinoid	207	13
below clinoid	177	12
Posterior projection		
above clinoid	23	4
at clinoid	51	14
below clinoid	21	14
Total	683	12

[a] The only poor result in 14 bilobular aneurysms occurred in one of the five aneurysms located below clinoid.

Table 5.9. Major vessel occlusion in 758 small and large basilar bifurcation aneurysms. Excluded are 14 patients with planned basilar artery occlusion

Vessel occlusion	Excellent	Good	Poor	Dead
Planned (other than basilar artery)	8	0	1	1
Inadvertent	10	6	8	3
Total	18	6	9	4

Chapter 6
Giant Basilar Artery Bifurcation Aneurysms
137 Cases

Our early experience with giant intracranial aneurysms, based on 174 patients, was published in 1979. That report included 76 on the carotid and 98 on the vertebral-basilar circulations, whose characteristics, methods of treatment and outcome were described in some detail. The series now number 732 cases, with the addition of 259 anterior and 299 posterior giant aneurysms.

The origin, size and shape of giant aneurysms and the extent of their mural thrombosis were described and illustrated by tracings in the early experience (Fig. 6.1). There have been no significant changes since, except for the recognition of a significant number of non-atherosclerotic fusiform aneurysms in more than one-fifth (21%) of the series, mainly in the vicinity of the union of vertebral and basilar arteries: at basilar trunk, vertebrobasilar junction and distal vertebral artery in diminishing frequency. Finally they were common in the posterior cerebral artery (PCA), especially its more distal part. Fusiform giant aneurysms occurred in 14 year younger age group and while some may have arisen from the expansion of the base of saccular aneurysms, most were presumed to have their origin in an arterial wall disorder of unknown nature.

The series will be brought up to date with the addition of the salient features of presentation, management and outcome in the additional patients.

Anatomical Features of Giant Basilar Bifurcation Aneurysms

As this aneurysm reaches a large size, the ectasia of the basilar artery bifurcation usually expands concomitantly so that both P1s and the superior cerebellar arteries (SCAs) arise from the base of the sac which makes that portion of the sac between the P1 origins (the neck) much wider and clipping more difficult. Rarely, the expansion tends to spare the neck so that clipping is reasonably straightforward and safe, but this usually occurs in aneurysms projecting forwards or backwards from the bifurcation. However, 42% of the aneurysms could be clipped (Table 6.1).

Large necks tend to be bulbous and thickened with fibrous and collagenous tissues, atheroma and mural thrombus, so that even strong clips will slide down to occlude the basilar bifurcation and one or more of its branches. The perforators are usually attenuated and more adherent, although the thicker neck allows more bold dissection to free them.

Clinical Features

About half of these giant aneurysms presented with recent subarachnoid hemorrhage (SAH) (62/137), most of them Grades 1 to 3 (Botterell), but 6 were Grade 4 at operation. Eight patients had a history of remote bleeding $2^{1}/_{2}$ to 22 years previously, presumably when their aneurysms were smaller; several had been told at the time that their aneurysms were "inoperable." These aneurysms with a remote bleeding more than one year back have been classified in this series (and also at other sites of the total series of vertebrobasilar aneurysms) as unruptured. The remaining 67 patients presented with mass effect causing headache and various combinations of oculomotor paresis and rostral brain stem compression signs. Sixteen patients had severe and 41 a mild limb paresis. Severe quadriparesis was rare, usually one hemiparesis dominated, often associated with ataxia and pseudobulbar dysarthria, emotional lability, or even pathological laughter in one patient. Recent memory was frequently impaired in one-third, often profoundly, and two patients had rubral tremor. Only one had hallucinations. Upward gaze paresis was common, and unilateral oculomotor nerve involvement was present in 26%. A fully developed Weber's syndrome was much less common (eight patients) than with the giant basilar-superior cerebellar aneurysms.

Unilateral CNIII paresis occurred in 35 patients. Bilateral CNIII paresis was seen in four patients with aneurysms arising from a low bifurcation or with unusually large sacs embedded deeply in the midbrain. In five patients, the sac had enough forward projection under the hypothalamus and optic tracts to produce declining vision with field defects (Fig. 6.2). Four patients had sixth nerve palsy, two of them bilaterally. Hydrocephalus requiring a shunt during admission occurred only once, but 17 additional patients were shunted later in other centers.

The future for a patient harboring an untreated giant intracranial aneurysm is bleak. In a follow-up of 31 personal cases not operated upon for various reasons, 68% were dead within 2 years and after 5 years all but one were dead or disabled.

Treatment

Giant intracranial aneurysms are quite individualistic in their presentation and requirements for treatment. All known methods of treatment have been used alone or in combination (one-fifth of the cases) in attempting to manage these dangerous lesions (Table 6.8).

Explored Only

Half of this group of aneurysms were explored early in the series in an attempt at neck clipping, before modern clip development, the use of the tourniquet and the routine use of temporary clipping. Even so, those early views of huge sacs buried in the interpeduncular fossa and brain stem, with the P1 origins and even the SCAs emerging from the base of the bulbous neck, were discouraging. None of the clips of the day would stay up on the neck or were even long enough to reach the other side.

Treatment in the later cases was abandoned for other reasons: one man refused to consider extracranial-intracranial (EC-IC) bypass to P2 for basilar artery occlusion; in two others, no space for the tourniquet could be found between numerous perforators (one was treated later with balloon detachment in the aneurysm); one basilar artery, rock hard with atheroma, could not even be stenosed with the tourniquet; temporary basilar clip occlusion in another produced severe hypertension (270/110).

The results for exploration in Table 6.8 only reflect the condition at discharge or short term follow-up (less than 90 days). Only 2 of the 14 patients are known to have had long survival; one for 14 years to die of myocardial infarction, although he had become confused and nearly blind preterminally. The last patient continues to farm after four years although the balloon detached in the base of the massively thrombosed aneurysm worked its way up into the mural thrombus within three months. Three patients were lost to follow-up, but two were in poor condition at discharge. Five patients died from presumed rupture of the aneurysm from the early postoperative period to 2.5 years.

Intra-Aneurysmal Occlusion

Attempts to occlude the lumen of systemic arterial aneurysms with transfixing sutures or intraluminal wire date back to the turn of the century. The method was revived by Gallagher for intracranial aneurysms in 1963 using animal hair injected into the wall of the aneurysm. Mullan in the late 1960's began to inject long lengths of fine copper-beryllium wire through a needle. Alksne developed a stereotactic technique to inject iron filings into the interior of aneurysms while holding them in place with a magnet. These methods have had limited use not only because of the risks, but because the neck of the aneurysm left open often enlarged into another dangerous sac under the thrombosed dome, as occurred in our three cases.

Over 40 horsehairs were injected into each of two basilar bifurcation aneurysms with extensive but incomplete thrombosis, leaving the neck open. The first giant intact sac, causing loss of vision, ruptured fatally at the neck 3.5 months later. The second patient remained well for seven years before rebleeding three times from aneurysmal enlargement of the open neck, and remained in poor condition. In a third patient, about 18 feet of thrombogenic wire was injected using the Mullan technique. Complete thrombosis of the aneurysm occurred and no discernible neck remained open (Fig. 6.3). Nine months later, she declined rapidly into irreversible coma with clear cerebrospinal fluid (CSF). The neck had blown out into a new aneurysm under the unchanged wire mesh thrombus, pushing the dome further into the hypothalamus.

Giant Basilar Artery Bifurcation Aneurysms

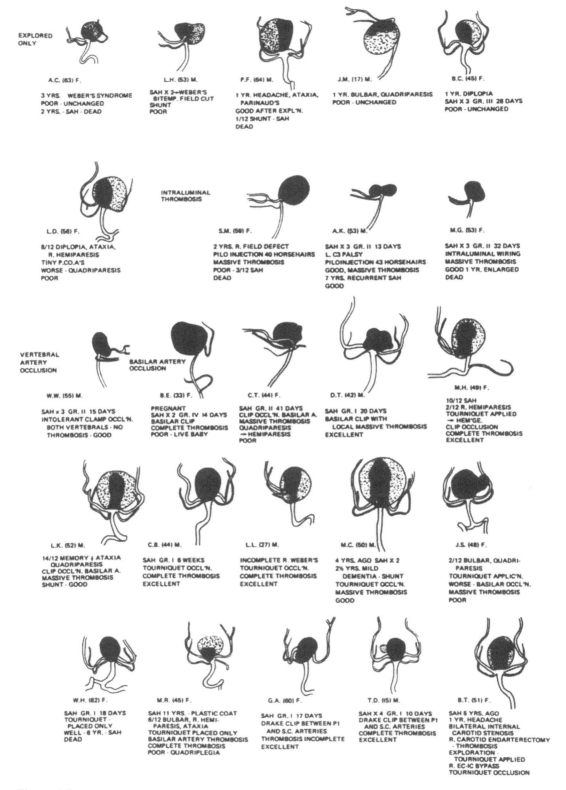

Figure 6.1

Giant Basilar Artery Bifurcation Aneurysms 71

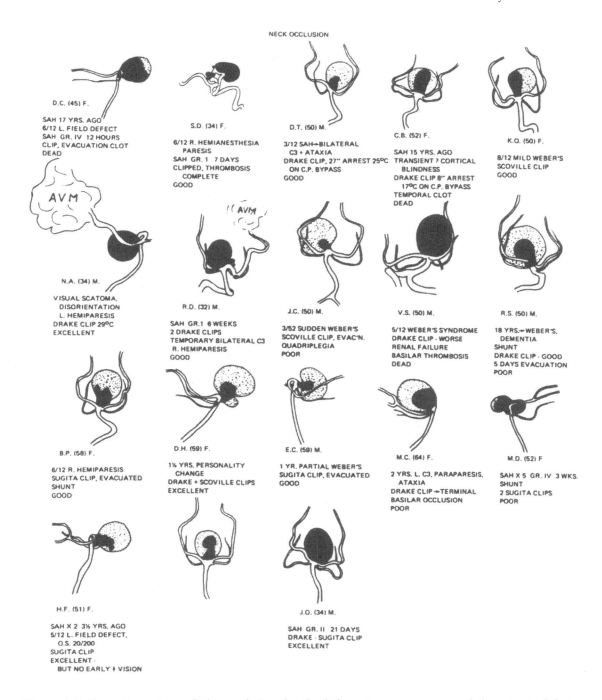

Figure 6.1. The origin, size and shape of giant basilar bifurcation aneurysms and the extent of their mural thrombosis described and illustrated by tracings in the early experience. (Reprinted from Clin Neurosurg 26, 1979, pp. 62–63 by courtesy of Williams and Wilkins)

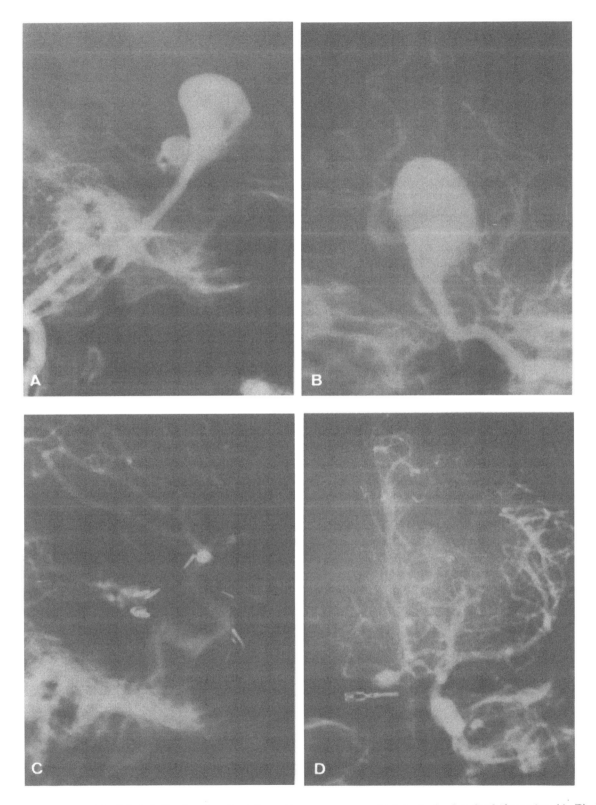

Figure 6.2 A–D. S.S., M, 11, giant basilar bifurcation aneurysm which includes basilar bifurcation (**A, B**), declining vision (O.D. 20/200, O.S. 20/60) with inferior bitemporal field cuts and right inferior altitudinal central scotoma. After clip occlusion of basilar artery there is virtual complete *thrombotic* occlusion of aneurysm with filling only of ectatic bifurcation (**C, D**). Outcome excellent with recovery of vision

In a fourth patient, five feet of wire was injected into a huge bifurcation aneurysm. She was poor thereafter and died one week later.

Two giant basilar bifurcation aneurysms have had their lumens reduced by transfemoral endovascular techniques. In one man, 42, in whom no perforator-free space could be found on the upper basilar artery for a clip, a balloon was detached in the residual base of a ruptured but largely thrombosed giant aneurysm. He returned to work, but follow-up angiograms four months later revealed that the balloon had worked its way up into the clot, reopening the neck and waist of the aneurysm. Recently, the residual sac was largely obliterated using coils (GDC) under the balloon. He may need basilar artery occlusion if further recanalization occurs.

Recently, a 47 year old woman suffered a myocardial infarction shortly after rupturing a giant bifurcation aneurysm. Because of the high cardiac operative risk, and in order to give some protection against rebleeding, the aneurysm was treated by endovascular detachment of platinum wire coils within it (Fig. 6.4). This resulted in thrombosis of the bulk of the sac, but the neck was left open. Follow-up angiography at six months revealed massive enlargement of the aneurysm with recanal-ization and radial impact dispersion of the wire coils. She was treated with tourniquet occlusion of the upper basilar artery which was uneventful except for a brief hemiparesis. Massive thrombosis occurred in the sac although a centimetre of the neck remained open.

This experience with induced intraluminal thrombosis by hair and wire had not as yet been satisfactory, for the neck left open has merely expanded into another dangerous aneurysm beneath the thrombosed dome. Detachable balloons also have been disappointing on our unit, burrowing their way into the thrombus and even through the wall of the aneurysm in one carotid case. Detachment of platinum coils may have a temporary use for prevention of early rebleeding in medically unfit or poor grade patients, so that definitive treatment by clipping can be deferred to a better time. It may be that upper basilar occlusion *after* endovascular wiring will be more successful in delaying or preventing neck enlargement by removing the pounding axial stream. In two patients (vide infra), Mullan wiring has been introduced into the residual base of partially thrombosed aneurysms *after* basilar artery occlusion, although in neither was the neck completely obliterated.

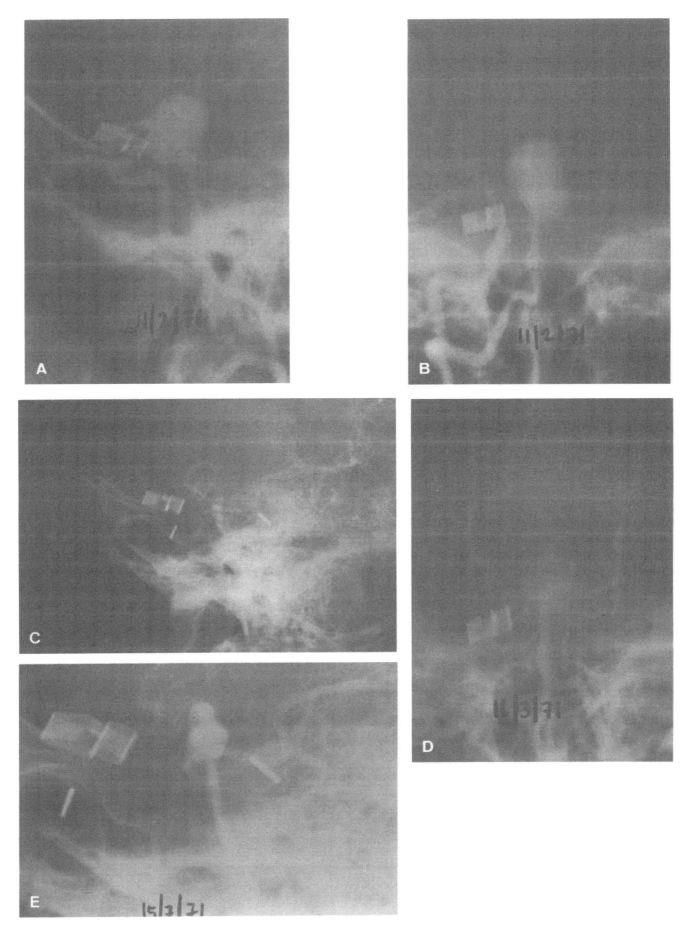

Figure 6.3

Neck Clipping

In less than half the cases (58/137), was the aneurysm clipped. The ratio of clipping to basilar artery occlusion did not increase after 1979 (Table 6.1).

In one-third, the neck remained reasonably small for a centimeter or so, usually in sacs that had more of a forward or backward projection (Fig. 6.5). These necks then stood out in front or behind the basilar bifurcation so that a straight clip could be applied easily across the neck in front or behind the P1s, occasionally reinforced with a tandem clip (Table 6.2).

In most others (i.e. those projecting vertically), a fenestrated clip was placed so that the ipsilateral P1, occasionally with its perforators, remained free in the aperture. After 1978, the addition of tandem clipping led to higher success rates for larger necks that would hold two sets of blades beside each other (Fig. 6.6). Thin-walled necks have been the best for clipping, especially when softened during temporary basilar artery occlusion (19 cases). When indented with a narrow dissector, the opposite P1 could be seen in front, while behind, the neck could be displaced from the interpeduncular fossa to see and separate the perforators and then allow the blades to be placed under them and hold their position on the neck.

Thick-walled necks, whether from fibrous collagenous tissue, atheroma or mural thrombus, have remained a problem. As clip blades were allowed to close they merely slid down the rigid slopes of the neck to close on the P1 origins or the basilar bifurcation, even with temporary clipping or trapping. Occasionally, with repeated attempts, a neck would "soften up" enough to hold the blades precariously, just above the P1 origins. Rarely could tandem clipping be used although the second or third clip might stay in position out on the neck when the proximal clips were removed. Occasionally, the very shortened blades of a Drake-Sugita clip placed out a few millimeters on the neck would hold and narrow it enough for placement of longer clip blades beside.

Three giant basilar bifurcation aneurysms were done during circulatory arrest under deep hypothermia on cardiopulmonary bypass. Then the sac could be opened, thrombus removed if necessary, and the neck collapsed for clipping. One patient had an excellent result (Fig. 6.7), but two died; one from a massive recurrent temporal lobe clot from the retractor bruising and heparin. The recent patient was little different and declined from her preoperative quadriplegic coma. The technique probably deserves further trial.

That the results were not significantly better after 1979, with the addition of temporary and tandem clipping, is partly because more attempts were made on large bulbous rigid necks. Clearly, patients in good condition had far better outcomes, 75% as compared to 45% for those already in poor condition from hemorrhage or mass effect (Table 6.6).

The reasons for new postoperative deficits seemed independent of preoperative condition, except for four patients who declined from Grade 2 and Grade 4 post-SAH states.

The reasons for postoperative morbidity and mortality can be seen in Table 6.3. In half (29) of the patients, significant complications occurred; many patients had several serious complications contributing to poor result or death. In three patients, poor preoperative grade was thought to be the only reason for poor postoperative result.

Perforator injury was inferred in those with poor outcome from upper brain stem signs and with CT evidence of low density in the midbrain and/or thalamus but intact major vessels angiographically. It was in most cases unanticipated, for the surgeon was certain that perforators were free and uninjured. Unseen perforator injury, kinking by a nearby clip or clip slippage may have occurred.

Similarly, none of the major vessel(s) occlusions were deliberate. Clip slippage was a possibility.

Figure 6.3 A–E. M.G., F, 53, giant basilar bifurcation aneurysm, clip graft placed on carotid aneurysm 6 months before (**A, B**). Operation was done 34 days after third bleed in Grade 2 in March 1971: about 18 feet (6 meter) of copper-beryllium wire were inserted transmurally into aneurysm, producing complete occlusion of the aneurysm (**C, D**). Nine months later she became rapidly unresponsive with clear CSF and died. An earlier angiogram shows enlargement of aneurysm under the wire thrombosis projecting the mass further into the hypothalamus (**E**)

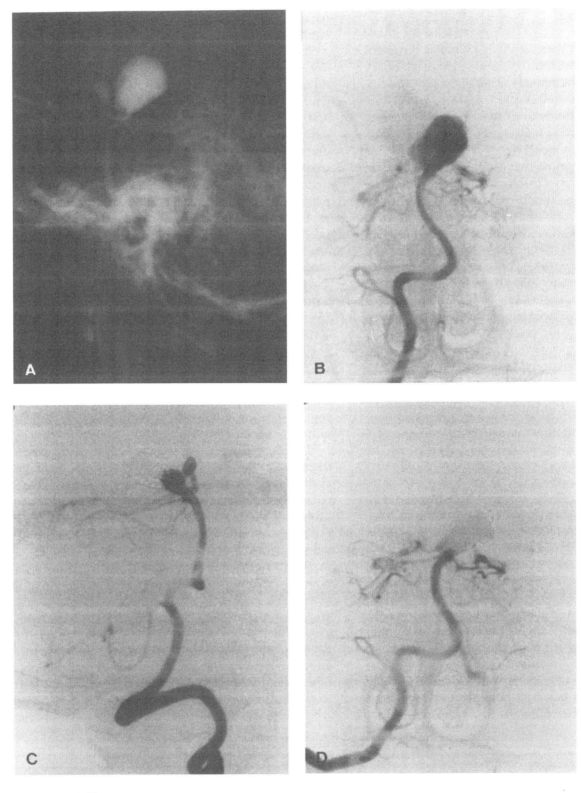

Figure 6.4 A–D

Giant Basilar Artery Bifurcation Aneurysms 77

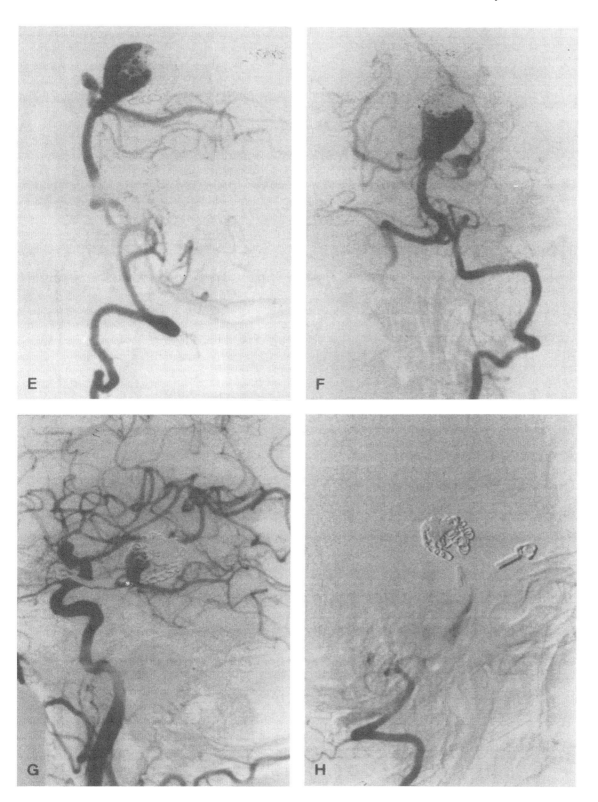

Figure 6.4 E–H

Figure 6.4 A–H. M.W., F, 57, giant basilar bifurcation aneurysm (**A, B**), one bleed with acute myocardial infarction. Endovascular wire coil embolization was done 3 days after third bleed in Grade 3 in February 1990. Three months later angiogram shows main part of the aneurysm thrombosed (**C, D**), but at seven months coils are radially displaced and impacted, aneurysm is enlarged (**E, F**). After tourniquet occlusion of basilar artery, angiograms show aneurysm has massively thrombosed except for a small portion above the neck (**G, H**). Outcome excellent

78 Giant Basilar Artery Bifurcation Aneurysms

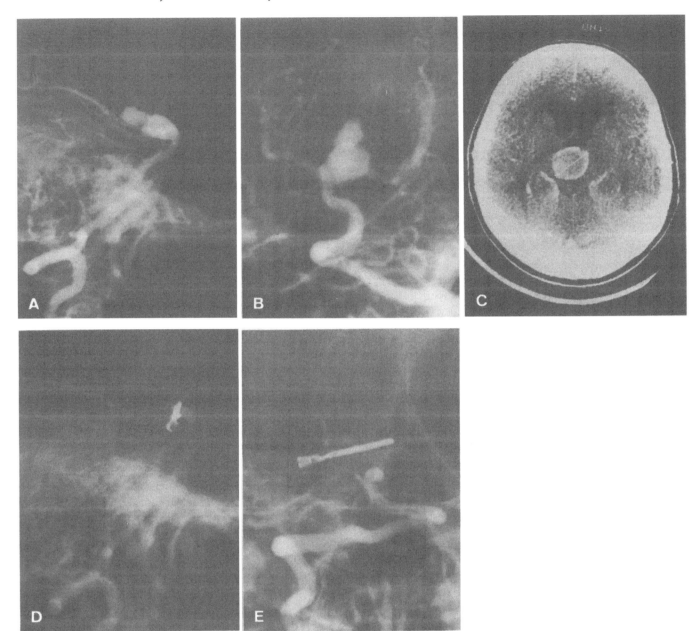

Figure 6.5 A–E. M.S., F, 63, unruptured posterior projecting giant basilar bifurcation aneurysm (**A–C**), mass effect with mild hemiparesis and severe ataxia. Single clip occlusion of neck was done in March 1984 (**D, E**). Outcome excellent

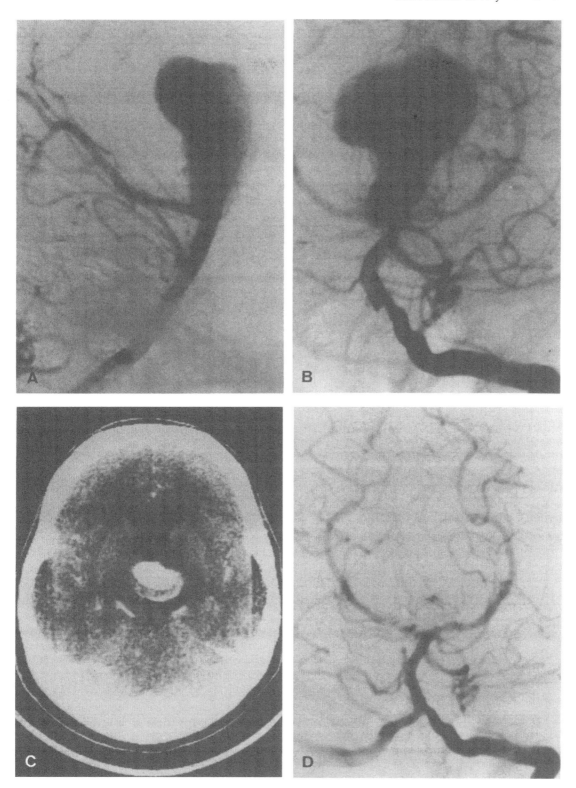

Figure 6.6 A–D. P.D., F, 48, unruptured upward projecting giant basilar bifurcation aneurysm (**A–C**), headache and memory decline. Complete occlusion of neck by tandem clipping in August 1983 (**D**). Outcome excellent

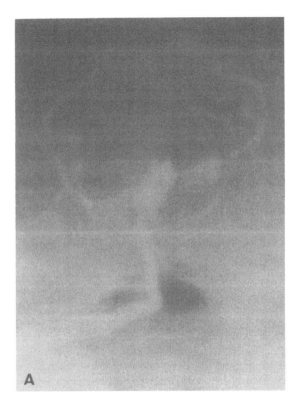 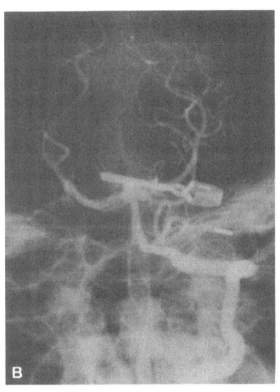

Figure 6.7 A, B. L.M., F, 60, unruptured huge basilar bifurcation aneurysm (A), severe Weber's syndrome. After clipping under deep hypothermia to 14°C and arrest on cardiopulmonary bypass in December 1973 she had a good recovery in spite of large postoperative left sided temporal hematoma (B reprinted from Clin Neurosurg 26, 1979, p. 80 by courtesy of Williams and Wilkins)

More likely, precarious placement allowed kinking or stenosis to occur. The approximation of thick neck walls proximal to the clip blades could have stenosed or occluded the P1 orifices and their perforators (Fig. 5.9). If there was any doubt about P1 patency, it was better to place the clip further out, and leave a little neck below which would likely be occluded by approximation of its thick walls. Both clip occlusions of the terminal basilar artery occurred in thick-walled necks; one artery was severely atherosclerotic and the occlusion extended 1 cm below the clip.

Altogether in 11 giant basilar bifurcation aneurysms, the basilar bifurcation was inadvertently occluded with P1 or SCA uni- or bilaterally in three patients, P1 alone in four patients, P1 associated with SCA in two patients and SCA alone in one patient. Retrograde thrombosis of a dilated atherosclerotic upper end of basilar artery for at least a centimeter with SCA and P1 occurred in one patient with subsequent death.

Slavish devotion to and persistence in trying to clip the neck of the aneurysm may lead to calamity when the final placement is going to be precarious in preserving the crotch of origin and its branches. In these circumstances, it may be wise to abandon clipping for Hunterian proximal occlusion of the parent artery if it can be tolerated.

Vertebral Artery Occlusion (1 Case)

In one patient, in 1973 after explorative surgery, bilateral occlusion of the vertebral arteries in the vertebral triangle in the neck was attempted using Selverstone clamps. After uneventful occlusion on the left, the right was occluded three months later. Thirty hours later, decerebrate coma occurred suddenly, but subsided after the clamp was opened within 30 minutes. He rebled and died eight months later.

Basilar Artery Occlusion (60 Cases)

Hunterian occlusion is still a mainstay for treatment of certain giant carotid circulation aneurysms, and more recently has been shown to be effective for non-clippable giant saccular and a few fusiform aneurysms on the posterior circulation. In fact, every major artery in the vertebral-basilar system has now been occluded on our unit for unclippable aneurysms arising from them. Admittedly, most of the few occlusions of posterior-inferior cerebellar artery (PICA) and anterior-inferior cerebellar artery (AICA) have been proximal to non-giant aneurysms arising on the artery feeding an arteriovenous malformation (AVM), where it is very safe because of the generous collateral flow.

The success in promoting complete thrombosis within a saccular aneurysm varies with the potential for significant collateral flow to continue to fill the aneurysm, e.g. occlusion of the upper basilar requires enough flow from the posterior communicating arteries (PComAs) into the P1s to irrigate the basilar bifurcation and SCAs; some of this flow will also enter the aneurysm. Thrombotic occlusion of a saccular aneurysm filling retrogradely, but isolated from the pounding parental axial stream, depends on the backwater effect generating enough stasis to promote thrombosis. On the other hand, occlusion of an artery proximal to an aneurysm arising from a *peripheral* branch (i.g. A2, P2, SCA, AICA, PICA) where the only collateral is retrograde through many small leptomeningeal circuits, is virtually always successful in promoting complete thrombosis.

The authors were encouraged to attempt deliberate basilar artery occlusion after experiences with clipping the necks of large basilar trunk aneurysms, in which inadvertent occlusion of the artery was without sequalae. Experience has been gained with attempts to occlude the upper basilar in 60 patients with giant bifurcation aneurysms. Clip occlusion is used when there seems little doubt that one or both of the PComAs are of sufficient size to irrigate the upper basilar territory (Fig. 6.2). The microtourniquet, first used in 1975 (Figs. 1.4, 6.8), is used when the PComAs are small, single or not visible angiographically (Figs. 6.9, 6.10). Either or both PComAs larger than 1 mm correlates with good outcome but no size of PComA has been identified as a minimum. In fact, it is remarkable how even tiny PComAs are sufficient immediately, although, in some of these, leptomeningeal collateral from PICA and AICA has been seen by filling the SCAs retrogradely (Figs. 6.11, 6.12).

The results of basilar artery occlusion in Table 6.4 indicate that 73% of patients with completed basilar artery occlusion had good outcomes. Surprisingly, patients assessed as good risk patients preoperatively did not do better than those patients with neurological deficits. All patients with incomplete basilar artery occlusion did badly.

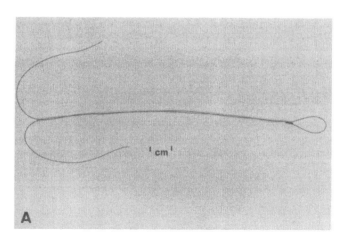 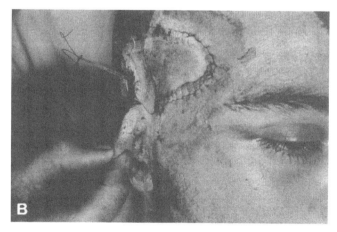

Figure 6.8 A, B. L.L., M, 27, giant basilar bifurcation aneurysm. Tourniquet October 1975, 3 o plastic suture inside PE 190 tubing with marker clip (**A**). Tourniquet clipped closed for 24 hours. Patient had bilateral partial oculomotor nerve palsies. Outcome excellent with complete thrombosis of aneurysm (**B**). (Reprinted from Clin Neurosurg 26, 1979, p. 17 by courtesy of Williams and Wilkins)

82 Giant Basilar Artery Bifurcation Aneurysms

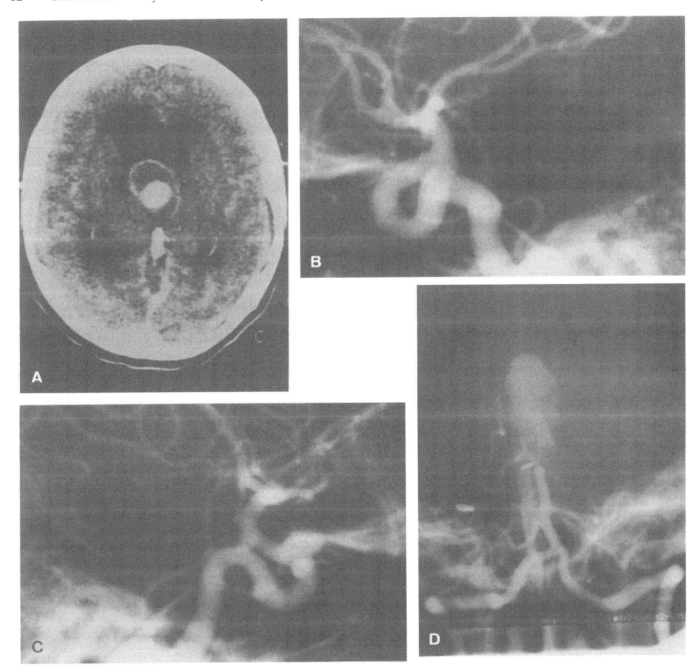

Figure 6.9 A–D

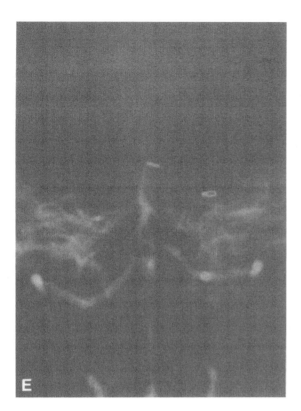
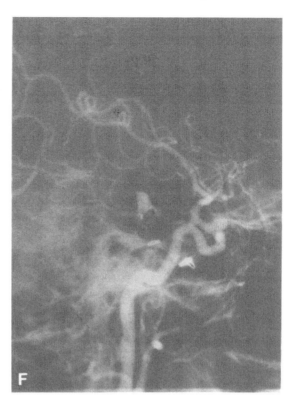

Figure 6.9 E, F

Figure 6.9 A–F. J.S., F, 43, unruptured giant basilar bifurcation, headache and ataxia. CT shows partial thrombosis (**A**). Right and left carotid studies show tiny posterior communicating arteries (**B, C**). Inadvertent severe tourniquet stenosis after application (December 1984) probably from bending of polyethylene tubing (**D**). The following day the basilar artery is spontaneously completely occluded (**E**). The aneurysm is virtually completely thrombosed and the small posterior communicating artery fills the upper basilar circulation without sequelae (**F**). Outcome excellent

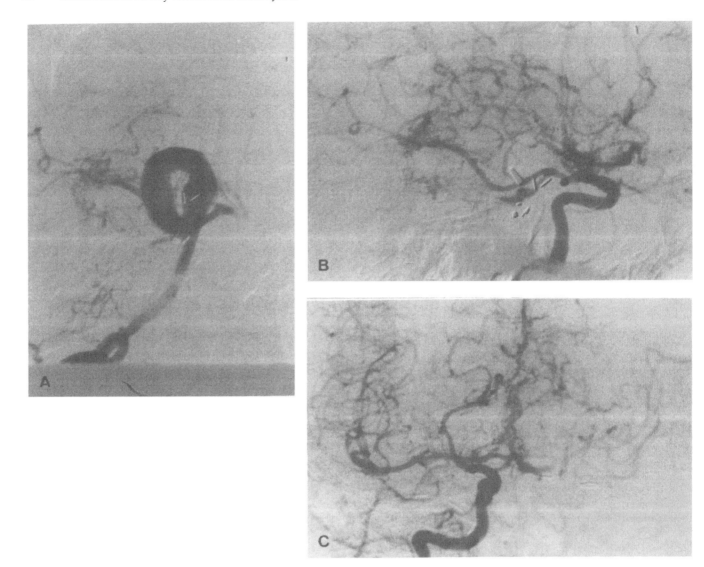

Figure 6.10 A–C. M.H., F, 58, unruptured giant basilar bifurcation aneurysm (**A**) with old left carotid artery thrombosis, partial Weber's syndrome. After tourniquet occlusion of the basilar artery in June 1979 the remaining *right* carotid fills the upper basilar circulation through a large posterior communicating artery and there is complete thrombosis of the aneurysm (**B, C**). Outcome excellent

Results of basilar artery occlusion must be considered from two aspects:

(1) early consequences, re. ischemia or rupture;
(2) degree of thrombosis produced in the aneurysm to prevent future growth and/or rupture (Table 6.5).

Calamitous infarction (13) or bleeding (5) occurred in 18 of the 60 patients. All five bleedings died. In two, the aneurysm still filled after basilar clipping through generous PComAs and rebleeding occurred after 4 hours and 34 days, in the latter after recanalization of the sac. In three, the tourniquet was not closed and the results were tragic. One rebled and died the night of tourniquet application before planned closure the next day. In the second, the basilar artery was shown to be occluded at the site of application and the tourniquet was not closed for fear of cutting through a presumed dissection of the artery from practice occlusions at operation the day before (as presumably occurred with a basilar trunk aneurysm). The fatal bleeding occurred on day 4 when the artery and the aneurysm were shown by angiography to have recanalized. Were this to be seen again, it would be best to re-explore and clip the artery under direct vision. The third patient, intolerant of complete occlusion, was left with a 90% stenosis in the hope that the PComAs would enlarge. A CSF leak occurred when the buried tourniquet protruded through the wound after three weeks.[1] After repair, a lumbar drain was left in place; fatal rupture of this previously intact aneurysm occurred 24 hours later, presumably from the change in transmural pressure from the lumbar drain.

Varying degrees of upper brain stem infarction occurred in the other 13 patients who were worse after upper basilar occlusion. Clip occlusion caused infarction in six, even though in five, the bifurcation and its branches were well and quickly filled from one or both PComAs. Blamed were kinking and thrombosis of a perforator just above or below the clip, and in two a short area of thrombosis in the basilar artery below the clip (Fig. 6.13). In one other, the right P1 was part of a fusiform bifurcation aneurysm. It thrombosed as well, cutting off flow from the only large PComA.

Brain stem infarction accounted for 8 of the 15 bad outcomes where the tourniquet was used. In four patients, the tourniquet was not closed when they awakened with major postoperative brain stem infarctions; two were unexplained, although the distribution and shape of the mural thrombus in the aneurysm had changed; but in two, thrombosis of the upper basilar artery below the tourniquet occurred, in one retrogradely to AICA. Presumably, the artery was injured during tourniquet application and practice occlusion. Practice occlusion in the operating room is no longer done.

In two patients, well postoperatively, inadvertent tourniquet stenosis at the site was shown angiographically; one went on to uneventful spontaneous occlusion (Fig. 6.9), the other was closed deliberately resulting in a delayed hemiplegia.

The use of the tourniquet is not without some hazard. Mere application of an open tourniquet has

---

[1] Protrusion and extrusion of the end of the tourniquet into and through the scalp may occur when the operative scalp and muscle swelling subside. When burying the tourniquet after 24 hours of extracranial occlusion, it is most important to reclip and divide the tourniquet as close to the level of the skull or dura as possible.

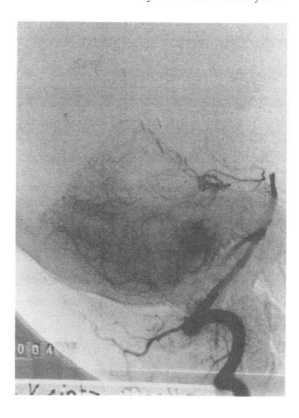

Figure 6.11. M.K., F, 29, unruptured giant basilar bifurcation aneurysm, dysarthria and slight hemiparesis. Tourniquet occlusion of the basilar artery in March 1988. Excellent collateral filling of superior cerebellar vessels from AICA and PICA. Excellent outcome

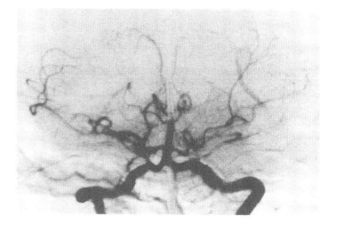

Figure 6.12. P.M., F, 33, giant basilar bifurcation aneurysm. Tourniquet occlusion of basilar artery in Grade 1 $4^{1}/_{2}$ months after fourth bleed in March 1985. Luxuriant leptomeningeal collateral from AICA can be seen filling SCAs back to region of their basilar origin. Excellent outcome

86   Giant Basilar Artery Bifurcation Aneurysms

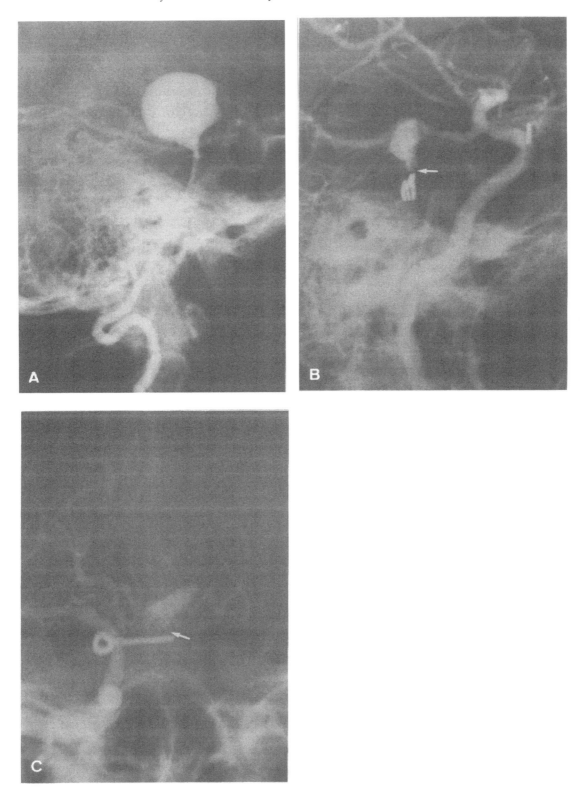

Figure 6.13 A–C. C.T., F, 44, giant basilar bifurcation aneurysm, lateral view (**A**). Clip occlusion of basilar artery in Grade 2 six weeks after single bleed in January 1975. Complete thrombosis of aneurysm except at neck. P1s can be seen emerging downward from neck. Patient was initially in quadriplegic coma from thrombosis of small portion of basilar artery and its perforators just above the clip (**B**, **C**, arrows). In spite of residual left hemiplegia she has remained active for nearly 20 years

caused immediate decline, but this may be due to the preliminary exploration of the giant basilar bifurcation aneurysm which alone can produce more deficit. It did allow early rebleeding in two patients before it could be closed and did not prevent aneurysm rupture in one patient who could tolerate only a severe basilar artery stenosis. It may be difficult to find a segment of the upper basilar artery free of perforators and long enough so that tourniquet closure does not kink and occlude them. Practice occlusion in the operating room is deemed to have produced a dissection of the artery in three or four patients; it was verified in one (Fig. 6.14).

But its ability to test marginal PComA collateral when the patient is awake has allowed many successful basilar occlusions that would not have been undertaken by sudden permanent clip occlusion with any confidence. The tourniquet can also be used to create a severe stenosis of the artery, when occlusion is not tolerated, to reduce the pressure in the aneurysm while promoting an increase in collateral flow. Presumably this occurred in three patients who later tolerated complete occlusion (Fig. 6.15).

Five patients were intolerant of tourniquet occlusion of the upper basilar artery in the operating room (1 cardiorespiratory change) or early after closure when awake (4), developing coma or quadriparesis in 30 seconds, 40 minutes, 1 1/2 hours and 16 hours. Recovery was prompt on opening the tourniquet. One aneurysm ruptured fatally (vide supra); one having rebled in the recovery room became comatose 40 minutes after closure of the tourniquet. She tolerated a severe basilar artery stenosis which later resulted in complete occlusion and a right hemiparesis from which she made a remarkable recovery. Another tolerated a 70% stenosis and remained well for three years before a sudden cerebral demise. Two intolerant patients were discharged and gradually declined to their deaths in a few months to 1 1/2 years. In one, an interposition vein graft to P2 was done, but the graft became thrombosed, as occurred in two other P2 grafts for lower aneurysms. A problem with a vigorous bypass would probably be continued or refilling of the aneurysm.

There were six other bad outcomes when the tourniquet was permanently occluded; three were in poor condition preoperatively. Two had awakened with increased deficits. Closure of the

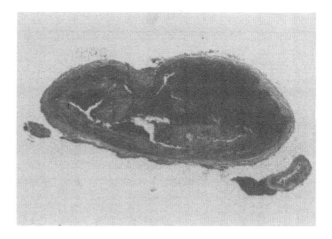

Figure 6.14. L.G., F, 33, giant vertebrobasilar junction aneurysm, 1 1/2 years headache and ataxia. Dissecting aneurysm of vertebral artery from application and practice occlusions of tourniquet in the operating room. (Reprinted from Clin Neurosurg 26, 1979, p. 87 by courtesy of Williams and Wilkins)

tourniquet for control of the aneurysm left them unchanged. Three declined after 12, 36 and 48 hours and it was decided not to open the tourniquet for fear of embolism. None made significant recovery.

Although the overall outcome in good condition patients is similar whether a clip or tourniquet was used, it must be recalled that in 9 of the 33 tourniquet cases, the tourniquet was not closed, in 5 because of early intolerance with ischemia. While use of the tourniquet to test for ischemia with marginal collateral undoubtedly prevented some brain stem infarctions, all nine patients had bad outcomes, three from rebleeding, four from infarction induced by exploration or the application and two, although immediately unchanged, gradually declined from the uncontrolled aneurysm itself.

The poor condition patients, with three exceptions, fared poorly, particularly when the tourniquet was used. The results were surprising in the patients with clip occlusion as there were no deaths and only 2 poor results in 11 poor risk patients (Table 6.4).

The higher incidence of complete thrombosis beyond a tourniquet as opposed to clip occlusion is surely due to the smaller PComAs, whose lower volume flow would allow more stasis in the aneurysm.

88   Giant Basilar Artery Bifurcation Aneurysms

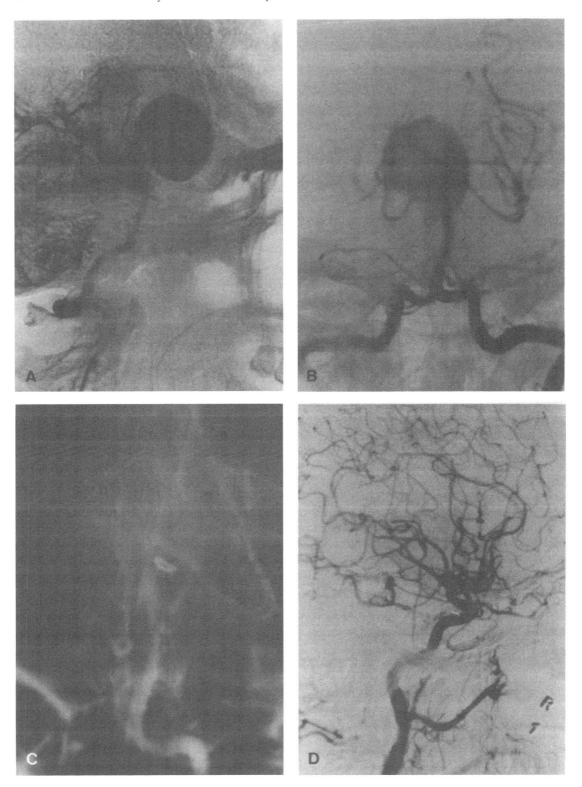

Figure 6.15 A–D. C.L., F, 40, giant basilar bifurcation aneurysm (**A, B**), blind O.S., O.D. 20/400 from subhyaloid hemorrhages. Patient was operated on in Grade 2 34 days after single bleed in December 1984. She tolerated only a severe tourniquet stenosis of basilar artery at clip marker (**C**). Two weeks later spontaneous complete occlusion of the basilar artery has occurred. The carotid fills the upper basilar circulation through small posterior communicating artery under complete thrombosis of aneurysm (**D**). After 5 months, she was able to read newspaper print. Outcome excellent

Upper basilar occlusion was remarkably effective, in long-term freedom from further bleeding and/or increased mass effect even though the thrombosis was incomplete; none of the completely thrombosed aneurysms recurred.

Surprisingly, 6 of the 12 cases with incomplete thrombosis have remained well for 18, 10, 7, 5, 4 and 3 years respectively, although in one there was marked stasis of the dye (Fig. 6.16). Two rebled and died within a month. Two patients suffered infarctions, one surviving for six years in poor condition. In two patients, the clip did not completely occlude the basilar artery, but produced a severe stenosis. Reclipping under one aneurysm which had recanalized after three months resulted in pontine infarction and persistent incomplete thrombosis. In the other, the P1 origin on the side of a fetal PComA was also clipped. The patient has remained well for five years, but with little further thrombosis.

Recurrence after virtually complete thrombosis was only known to have occurred in three cases; one had become hydrocephalic, but shunting and wiring of the residual cavity did not improve her condition. The other slowly developed a hemiparesis over six months in the absence of recanalization. In the third, a "slipped" tourniquet was found to be responsible for deterioration. Repeat angiography showed the basilar artery recanalized and the tourniquet open. At reoperation, the occluding Weck clip was found to have cut through the plastic tube. After removal and clipping of the basilar artery, complete thrombosis occurred with resolution of the brain stem compression.

There was no known recurrence when the thrombosis was complete. The gradual reduction in size of a giant thrombosed aneurysm can be remarkable (Fig. 6.17).

90 Giant Basilar Artery Bifurcation Aneurysms

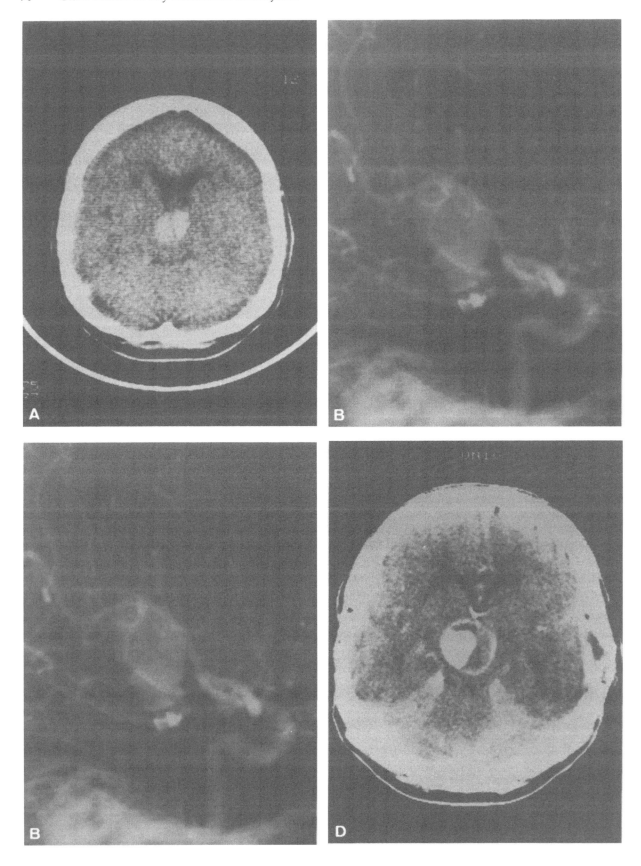

Figure 6.16

Giant Basilar Artery Bifurcation Aneurysms 91

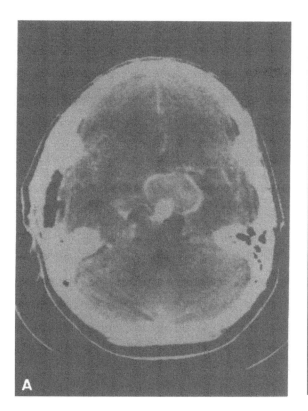 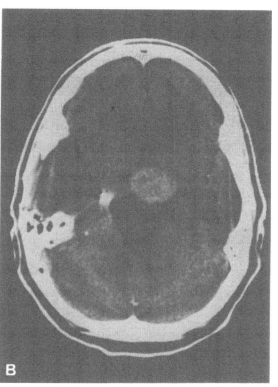

Figure 6.17 A, B. C.V., F, 45, ruptured giant basilar bifurcation aneurysm (**A**). Five days after single bleed in June 1986 in Grade 3 basilar artery clipped. Complete thrombosis of aneurysm was followed by reduction in size of aneurysm from 3.5 cm to 2.75 cm in 6 months (**B**). Preoperative bilateral oculomotor palsy cleared and she made an excellent recovery

←

Figure 6.16 A–D. M.W., F, 59, giant basilar bifurcation aneurysm (**A**), headache. After basilar clip occlusion in October 1983, the aneurysm continued to fill through the single foetal type posterior communicating artery (**B, C**). CT two years later (**D**). With the failure of basilar occlusion the aneurysm has doubled in size. Poor outcome, later lost to follow-up

Table 6.1. Ratio between aneurysmal neck clipping and basilar artery occlusion in giant basilar bifurcation aneurysms

	Pre '79	Post '79
Clipped	20	38
Basilar occlusion	11+3 attempted	40+6 attempted

Table 6.2. Clipping method and outcome in 58 patients with giant basilar bifurcation aneurysms and neck clipping

Operative method	Excellent	Good	Poor	Dead	Total
Single clip	18	10	9	5	42
Multiple clips	2	3	0	1	6
Tandem clips	4	2	2	1	9
Piggy back clips			1		1
Total	24 41%	15 26%	12 21%	7 12%	58 100.0

Table 6.3. Causes of morbidity and mortality in 58 patients with giant basilar bifurcation aneurysms with neck clipping

Cause	Patients	Poor	Dead
Poor grade (grade $\geq$ 3 or severe deficit in unruptured aneurysms)	11	5	4
Intraoperative aneurysm rupture	5	3	0
Perforator injury	7	7	0
Inadvertent arterial occlusion	11	7	2
Postoperative hematoma	4	2	2
Postoperative significant spasm	2	1	0
Rebleeding from treated aneurysm	2	1	0
Sepsis	1	0	1
Meningitis	1	1	0
Cardiorespiratory	4	0	1
Electrolyte disturbances	1	1	0
Pulmonary embolus	1	0	1
Total	32 patients[a]	12 poor	7 deaths

[a] Altogether 13 of 32 patients became good or excellent in spite of the complications.

Giant Basilar Artery Bifurcation Aneurysms

Table 6.4. Results for basilar artery occlusion in 60 patients with giant basilar bifurcation aneurysms

	Total	E	G	P	Dead
Completed basilar artery occlusion					
Clip					
Good risk	16	9	1	4	2
Poor risk	11	8	1	2	0
Total	27	17	2	6	2
Tourniquet					
Good risk	18	10	5	3	0
Poor risk	6	2	1	3	0
Total	24	12	6	6	0
Clip + Tourniquet	51	29	8	12	2
Attempted basilar artery occlusion					
Tourniquet not closed[a]					
Good risk	4	0	0	0	4
Poor risk	5	0	0	3	2
Total	9	0	0	3	6

[a] 5 intolerant.

Table 6.5. Effectiveness of basilar artery occlusion (degree of thrombosis in aneurysm[a]) in 60 patients with giant basilar bifurcation aneurysms

Method	No.	Complete	Residual neck	Residual fundus
Clip occlusion	27	7 23%	10	10 37%
Tourniquet	24	13 54%	3	8 33%
Tourniquet not closed	9	3 33%		6 66%
Total	60	23	13	24

[a] Complete: no visible neck remaining.
Residual neck: only a thin remnant of neck still filling.
Residual fundus: when neck and waist of aneurysm still filling from posterior communicating collateral.

Table 6.6. Preoperative Grade and outcome in 137 patients with giant basilar bifurcation aneurysms

Grade	Excellent	Good	Poor	Dead	Total
0[a]	29	15	24	7	75
0g	*23*	*10*	*10*	*5*	*48*
0p	*6*	*5*	*14*	*2*	*27*
1	16	6	2	3	27
2	6	5	1	1	13
3	6	5	4	1	16
4		1	5		6
Total	57 41.6%	31 22.6%	32 23.4%	17 12.4%	137 100.0%

[a] *0* Unruptured aneurysm or remote hemorrhage (> 1 year). *0g* Good risk without major neurological deficit. *Op* Poor risk patient with major neurological deficit (severe confusion or dementia or stupor or coma, dysarthria or bulbar paralysis, severe dysphasia or severe mono-, hemi-, or tetraparesis).

Table 6.7. Age related to outcome in 137 patients with giant basilar bifurcation aneurysms

Age group (years)	Excellent	Good	Poor	Dead	Total
10–19	2		1		3
20–29	7				7
30–39	4	4	3	1	12
40–49	20	7	7	4	38
50–59	17	15	9	6	47
60–69	7	5	12	4	28
70 or more				2	2
Total	57	31	32	17	137

94 Giant Basilar Artery Bifurcation Aneurysms

Table 6.8. Operative method and outcome in 137 patients with giant basilar bifurcation aneurysms

Operative method	Excel-lent	Good	Poor	Dead	Total
Neck clipping	24	15	12	7	58
Basilar artery occlusion	29	8	12	2	51
Clip	*17*	*2*	*6*	*2*	*27*
Tourniquet	*12*	*6*	*6*	*0*	*24*
Basilar artery occlusion attempted			3	6	9
Vertebral artery occlusion		1			1
Intraluminal thrombosis	1	1	1	1	4
Exploration only	3	6	4	1	14
Total	57	31	32	17	137

Table 6.9. Operative method and result of aneurysm treatment in 137 patients with giant basilar bifurcation aneurysms

Operative method	Total obliter-ation	Resid-ual neck	Resid-ual fundus	No oblit-eration	Not known	Total
Neck clipping	46	5	7			58
Basilar occlusion	20	13	18			51
Basilar occlusion attempted	3		1	4	1	9
Vertebral ligation				1		1
Intraluminai thrombosis			2		2	4
Explora-tion only	1		2	11		14
Total	70	18	30	16	3	137

Table 6.10. Timing of surgery and outcome in 62 patients with giant basilar bifurcation aneurysms

Timing of surgery	Excel-lent	Good	Poor	Dead	Total
0–1 day				1	1
2–3 day	1				1
4–6 day	3				3
7–10 day	3	2	2	2	9
11–30 day	13	8	6	7	34
31–365 day	8	6			14
Total	28	16	8	10	62

Chapter 7

Non-Giant (Small and Large) Basilar Superior Cerebellar Artery Aneurysms

210 Patients

Anatomical Features

This aneurysm arises at the crotch of the origin of the superior cerebellar artery (SCA), but the neck soon takes in all of the narrow lateral portion of the basilar artery between the SCA and the P1. Although the SCAs may be duplicated, aneurysms arising at the lower branching of a duplication have not been seen. On one occasion, this aneurysm seemed to arise from the obtuse inferior angle of the SCA origin with the artery adherent to and coursing *above* the sac. This aneurysm occurs more often on the left side (two-thirds), is common in females (three-fourths), and is often associated with multiple aneurysms (40%). Bilateral aneurysms have been seen three times.

Two-thirds of the SCA aneurysms project laterally; in the remaining third, backward projection was slightly more common. They lie in a shallow bed on the peduncle where they may be quite adherent, particularly the larger sacs. Because of the origin and lateral projection of this aneurysm, the numerous perforators arising from the posterior aspect of the upper basilar artery are seldom on or adherent to the sac, except when it is large or has a posterior orientation.

There is always an intimate relation to the third nerve, which may course above or below the waist of the sac or more commonly be stretched and splayed thin over the dome. This may occur to a remarkable degree on larger sacs without clinical evidence of paresis but third nerve paresis was seen preoperatively in one-fifth of the non-giant cases. Presumably, in contrast to the tethering of this nerve at its exit, where carotid aneurysms compress it, the mobility of the mid section of the nerve spares it longer during enlargement of this aneurysm. It is often stained or even infiltrated with blood from the clot sealing the rent in the dome of a ruptured sac.

In common with posterior-inferior cerebellar artery (PICA) in vertebral-PICA aneurysms, the SCA tends to emerge from the inferior origin of the neck of the aneurysm rather than from the basilar artery, particularly as the sac enlarges, so that a clip must be applied with exquisite accuracy to preserve the orifice of this vessel. This is essential: of the 10 patients with non-giant basilar-SCA aneurysms in whom a SCA was occluded or trapped at or near its origin, inadvertently or deliberately, only four escaped a devastating infarction of the mid brain and cerebellum; two died and four remained severely disabled. Nine non-giant aneurysms arose peripherally along the course of the SCA, from the side of the midbrain to the superior surface of the cerebellum. Peripheral aneurysms, twice multiple, have occurred on enlarged SCAs feeding cerebellar arteriovenous malformations (AVMs) (three patients with six aneurysms). No saccular aneurysm was seen peripherally on the SCA in front of the midbrain, but one dissecting and one fusiform aneurysm have occurred at this site, both in giant size.

Clinical Features

Because of the intimate association with the third nerve, the clinical localizing feature of rupture or enlargement of the SCA aneurysm is an ipsilateral third nerve paresis, as occurs with carotid communicating aneurysms. CNIII paresis is unusual with small aneurysms, having been seen in only 20 of 153 cases, but common with large aneurysms (35%), and usual with giant aneurysms (61%), with or without rupture. Thus, in the presence of a CNIII palsy with mydriasis but with negative carotid angiography, opacification of the upper basilar arterial tree is essential. In one case, due to adherence of a small backward angling dome to the crus, rupture occurred into the lateral midbrain producing a partial Weber's syndrome.

Sixth nerve palsy was present in nine patients, in three bilaterally. Fourth nerve paresis is rare and was never seen in small aneurysms, but has been the only clinical sign with three giant and one large fusiform aneurysm arising from the peripheral SCA. One was on the anterolateral corner of the midbrain; the others were wedged between the edge of the tentorium and the posterolateral corner of the quadrigeminal plate. Eight of the smaller aneurysms peripherally on the SCA and one giant one have produced only subarachnoid hemorrhage (SAH).

Treatment

The subtemporal approach on the side of the projection of the aneurysm is preferred; it is more common on the left side (65%). The suture reflecting down the edge of the tentorium will provide enough exposure for all but exceptionally low or large aneurysms (Illustration 7.V A); then the inner third of the tentorium must be divided as was necessary in 14 out of 210 non-giant aneurysms (Illustration 3.III E). Low lying necks were rather seldom in these aneurysms, only 12% of the necks were 3 mm or more below the posterior clinoid process level.

The anterior aspect of the neck of this aneurysm usually is seen well enough through the transsylvian exposure (which was used in 13% and nearly always with associated aneurysms), even when it projects to the opposite side, providing it is not too low behind the clivus. However, perforators lurking behind large necks may require a subtemporal exposure.

Although it is tempting to approach this aneurysm from the opposite side (was done subtemporally in 10 of the non-giant cases) to avoid a dissection on and around the dome of the aneurysm, it is awkward to work across in front of the basilar

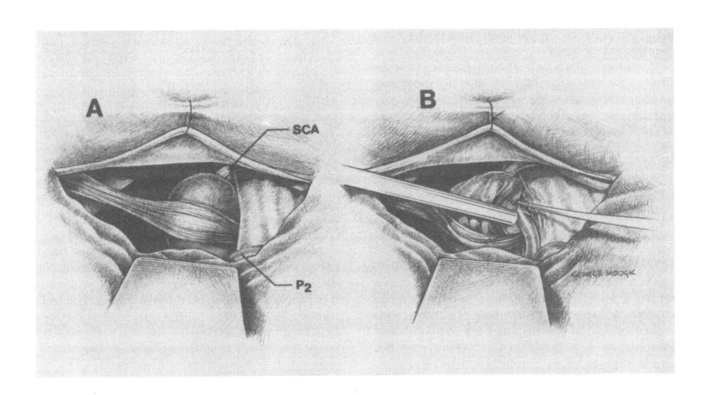

7.V. Operative illustration for basilar SCA aneurysms. **A** An ipsilateral subtemporal approach ordinarily is satisfactory for most basilar SCA aneurysms. There is always an intimate relation to third nerve which may be under or over the neck of the fundus or splayed over the dome as shown here. **B** The dome and waist of large aneurysms may have to be dissected from a pial bed in the peduncle to free them from adherence to P2 and a perforator, even with sharp dissection, in order to see the posterior aspect of the neck, using temporary basilar clipping

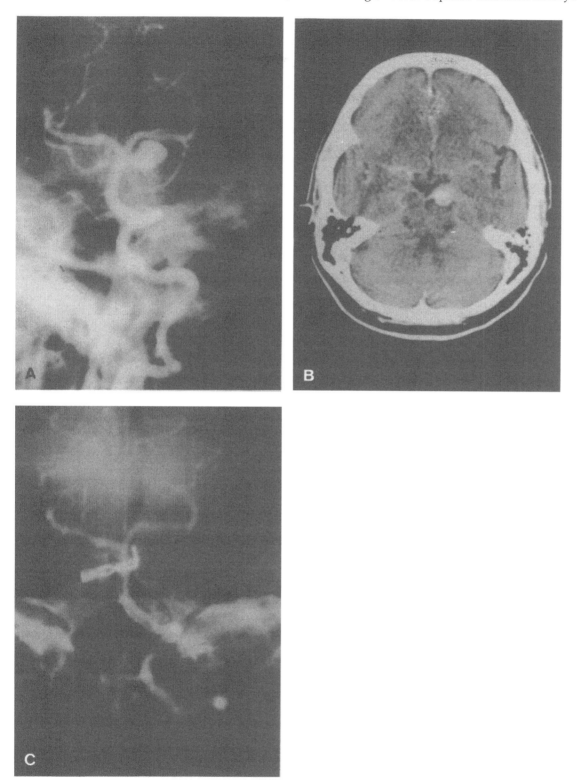

Figure 7.1 A–C. E.S., F, 62, unruptured large calcified left basilar SCA aneurysm with early oculomotor nerve palsy one month (**A, B**). Clipped from opposite side in November 1985 (**C**). Outcome excellent

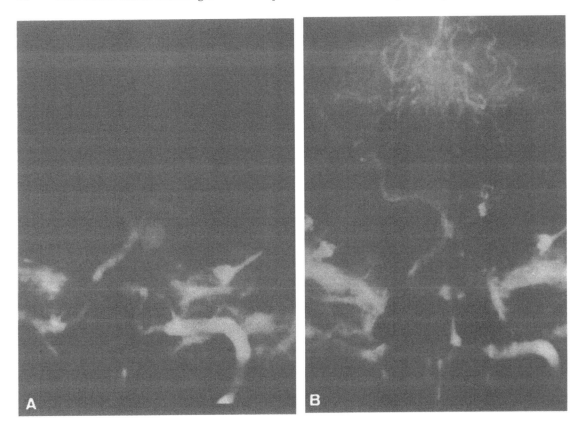

Figure 7.2 A, B. F.M., F, 46, intact small left basilar SCA aneurysm, ruptured middle cerebral artery aneurysm clipped elsewhere 4 months earlier (**A**). Use of curved clip in November 1979 to accommodate origins of P1 and SCA, deep hypotension used (30 minutes 40 mmHg) (**B**). Outcome excellent

artery in the narrow confines behind the clivus and the origin and adherence of the aneurysm to SCA is not seen as clearly. It is more difficult to free the first part of P1, which is frequently adherent to the neck and waist, especially of larger sacs. If a third nerve palsy exists, a blinding bilateral ptosis might occur from manipulation of the intact nerve.

With the development of the fenestrated clip, the *contralateral* approach subtemporally has been rewarding when very large or giant aneurysms have had reasonable necks obscured by a larger thrombosed or calcified mass, but without an oculomotor palsy (nine patients) (Fig. 7.1). It may be a simpler and safer alternative to opening the aneurysm ipsilaterally and evacuating thrombus to see and prepare the neck for clipping. The bulge of larger necks and any perforators, including the origins of SCAs and P1s, can usually be seen in front and behind the basilar artery for the application of a right angled Drake-Sugita clip with the basilar artery in the aperture and the blades properly in the long axis of the parent artery branchings. The base and tips of the blades must close on the neck flush with, but not encroaching on, an adherent SCA or P1. An ordinary angled clip applied with the blades above and below the neck requires separation of P1 and SCA from the neck, and may leave "dog ears" for future regrowth, as well as kink the origin of SCA.

The disadvantages of the contralateral approach have seemed to outweigh those of an approach on the dome of most aneurysms. The latter include an increased risk of intraoperative rupture, and the risk of retraction of the dominant temporal lobe in those cases projecting to the left, although the retraction is less than that required to see basilar bifurcation aneurysms. Inadvertent aneurysm rupture in non-giant SCA aneurysms was not more common than in other locations. The approach over the dome ordinarily is not hazardous as long as it is respected and protected, particularly the fibrin-platelet clot sealing the rent. Only occasionally must the latter be dissected under high magnifica-

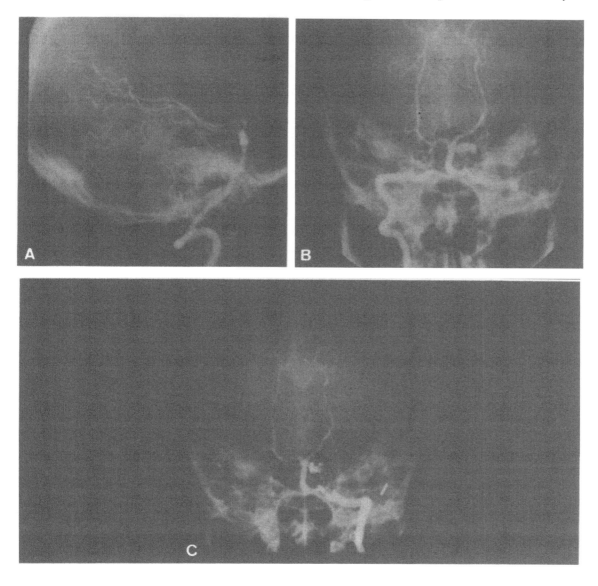

Figure 7.3 A–C. J.H., F, 49, small ruptured typical left basilar SCA aneurysm (**A**, **B**). Curved Scoville clip neck occlusion in July 1977 44 days after single bleed in Grade 1 (**C**). Outcome excellent

tion from an adherence to the crus, tentorium or, rarely, CNIII. Once free, a small patty over the dome offers protection from inadvertent injury. A rupture at the dome can be controlled with the sucker tip for completion of the dissection of the collapsed sac.

Working behind, the aneurysm is gently teased out of its bed in the peduncle using a sucker tip over a small patty to displace the sac forward so as to show the plane of cleavage for blunt or sharp dissection down to the neck. When the aneurysm is freed, then the back of the neck and any nearby perforators can be seen clearly. It takes great care to avoid injury to the third nerve. A third nerve splayed and adherent to the dome can usually be left untouched, but when located over or under the waist, it will have to be freed gently for clip blade placement underneath, especially posteriorly near the root exit where it is nearest the midline. Occasionally, CNIII has had to be placed in the aperture of an angled Drake clip. Rarely, a ligature may have to be used to close the neck under a tense adherent third nerve, or the neck may have to be shrunk with bipolar coagulation. CNIII has been divided deliberately only once, during control of a ruptured large neck; complete long-standing palsy had already existed.

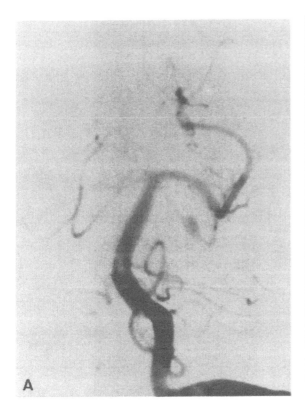 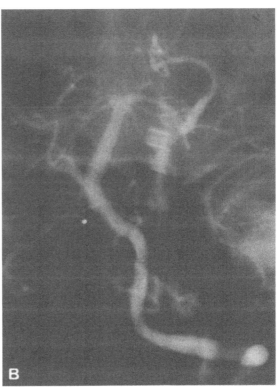

Figure 7.4 A, B. G.B., F, 60, small dissecting (?) fusiform peripheral SCA aneurysm (**A**). Operation in February 1984 three weeks after single bleed in Grade 2. Sundt clip graft encases aneurysm in order to preserve continuity of the artery (**B**). Clearance of postoperative confusion with shunting, good outcome

If necessary, depressing the sac against the peduncle will reveal the neck emerging from the basilar artery and SCA below it. SCA, although partially arising from the neck, is usually free from attachment to small sacs, but may be adherent to the neck and waist of larger aneurysms. An origin of SCA from the very base of the neck must be recognized so that clip placement secures the neck without kinking this branch. P1 may be readily visible too, depending on its course, but if the sac is large, it is often hidden above and behind. Smaller sacs may also be free of P1, but those with an upward angulation, and often larger aneurysms, are quite adherent to the P1 origin. Gentle depression of the sac away from P1 with the sucker tip or over a small patty will show the faint "white line" of the areolar cleavage plane for sharp dissection with the tip of a small knife or tiny scissor blades, taking particular care to recognize the acute angle of the neck origin when it is reached (Illustration 7.V B).

The best clip application is with the blades in front of and behind the neck, in the same axis as the origins of the parent branchings. A curved clip blade often fits nicely into this curve, sparing the origins of P1 and SCA, particularly when the latter arises from the base of the aneurysm (Fig. 7.2). Preliminary bipolar coagulation of the neck, with the forceps placed just outside the origin of SCA, is often helpful in shrinking and thickening the neck for clip application to spare the orifice of this artery. The hazards of a cross axis clip have been mentioned above, but occasionally may have to be accepted (Fig. 7.3).

When P1 is dangerously adherent to the neck and waist of a thin walled aneurysm, or its origin hidden, it is possible to place an angled or curved clip from below. The blades are worked in front of and behind the neck, always inside CNIII, so that with closure they fall just across the upper aspect of the neck, brushing the root of P1 as it comes into view as they close. This "blind" clip application may take several trials for final perfect application.

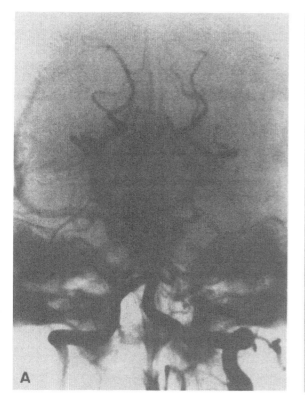 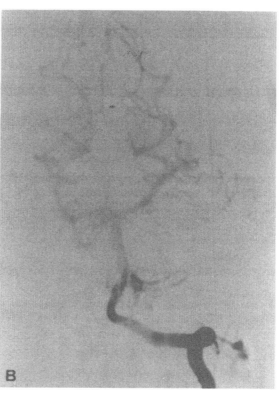

Figure 7.5 A, B. B.R., F, 22, ruptured small dissecting aneurysm of left peripheral superior cerebellar artery (**A**). Operation in August 1983 four days after second bleed, aneurysm clip trapped for biopsy. Good leptomeningeal collateral filling postoperatively (**B**). Preoperative left trochlear and abducens palsies subsided as did postoperative left oculomotor palsy, and she made an excellent recovery

Often when the clip tips encroach on P1, a moment may be taken to separate an adherent P1 from the slack sac before replacement of the clip.

Temporary clips or trapping have seldom been used for this aneurysm (less than 15%) since its exposure and dissection are usually straightforward. However, their success with basilar bifurcation aneurysms may warrant their use more often for large or otherwise difficult SCA aneurysms.

Rarely (11%), this aneurysm projects forward toward, or is adherent to the dorsum sellae. Its obliteration is quite straightforward, for the SCA origin is clear and no perforators are involved. The backward projection demands attention to perforators, as at the basilar bifurcation.

It is customary to aspirate this aneurysm to prove clipping and to ensure decompression of CNIII, which is essential if paresis exists. CNIII seems to have the same potential for recovery as with carotid aneurysms, if the paresis is not long-standing or from operative manipulation only.

Although the sac of a *large* aneurysm obscures the neck region much more, the approach over the dome is still preferred with the same dissection to free the neck. More forceful retraction of the sac forward against the clivus will be necessary to free it both from its bed in the peduncle, and from P1 to expose the neck. P1 tends to be more adherent above and usually must be dissected free with a knife. Coagulation of a thin neck will not only shrink it, but thicken it up for freeing a very adherent vessel. The "blind" clip application described above is most often used for these aneurysms. The third nerve is always displaced and flattened by these large sacs and is more prone to operative injury.

Two small ruptured aneurysms arising on the first part of SCA, one in front of and the other beside the midbrain, have been seen. Both were fusiform; one was a dissection. In order to preserve SCA, the former was encircled with a large Sundt clip graft (Fig. 7.4), but the dissecting aneurysm had to be

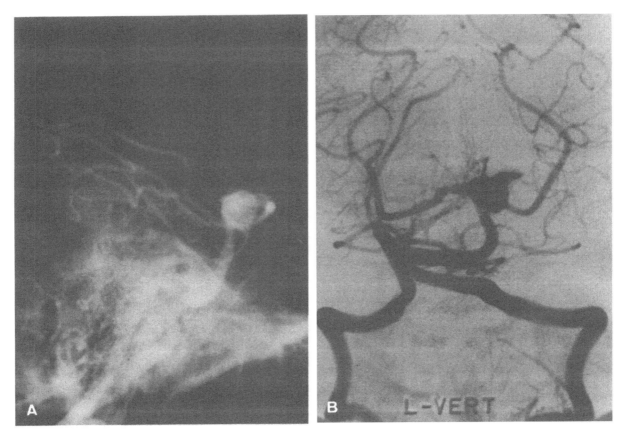
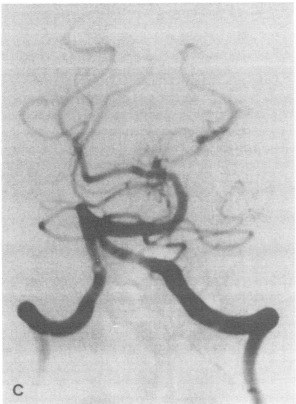

Figure 7.6 A–C. A.H., F, 54, ruptured small fusiform proximal left superior cerebellar artery aneurysm, possibly a dissection (**A, B**). Operation in January 1983 13 days after single bleed; distal SCA occluded except for stump arising from distal sac. No deficit after clip occlusion of SCA and evacuation of the aneurysm (**C**). Outcome excellent

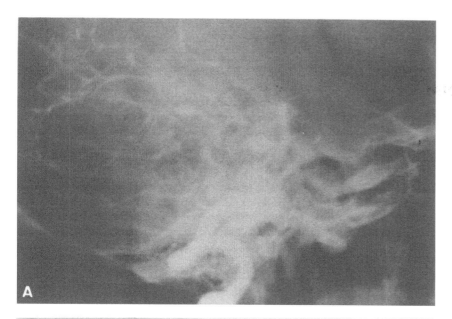
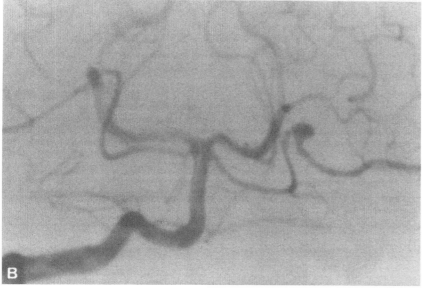
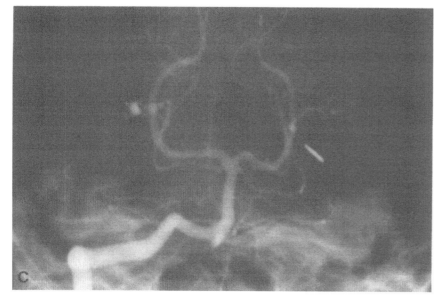

Figure 7.7 A–C. H.S., F, 53, bilateral small distal superior cerebellar artery aneurysms, left ruptured, 11 months after single bleed (**A, B**). Clipping each aneurysm one month apart in Grade 1 in August and September 1976 patient remains well in spite of occlusion of the left SCA at clip site on neck of sac. Outcome excellent

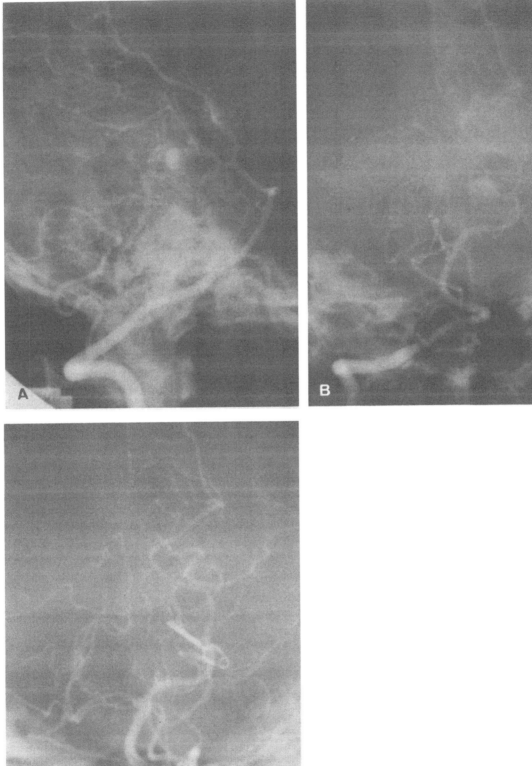

Figure 7.8 A–C. F W., M, 33, intact large peripheral left superior cerebellar artery aneurysm (**A, B**), three weeks of headache and diplopia with trochlear nerve paresis. Feeding SCA artery branch clipped without sequelae in June 1986 (**C**). Outcome excellent

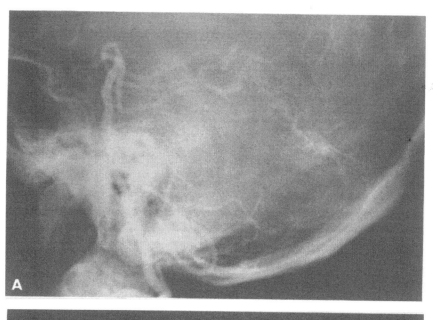
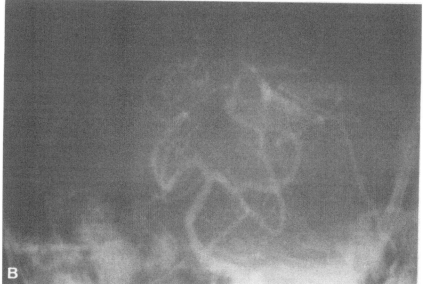
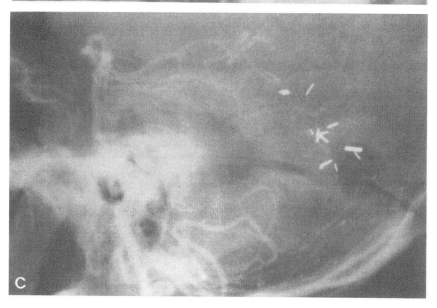

Figure 7.9 A–C. F J., M, 69, three small fusiform peripheral right superior cerebellar artery aneurysm on feeding branch of small cerebellar AVM (**A, B**). Patient was well after excision of ruptured and intact aneurysms and AVM (August 1974, 44 days after second bleed in Grade 2) (**C**) for 10 days when left cerebral infarction occurred with dysphasia and right hemiparesis. He improved and finally had a good outcome. A small ophthalmic artery aneurysm left remained untreated

106 Non-Giant (Small and Large) Basilar Superior Cerebellar Artery Aneurysms

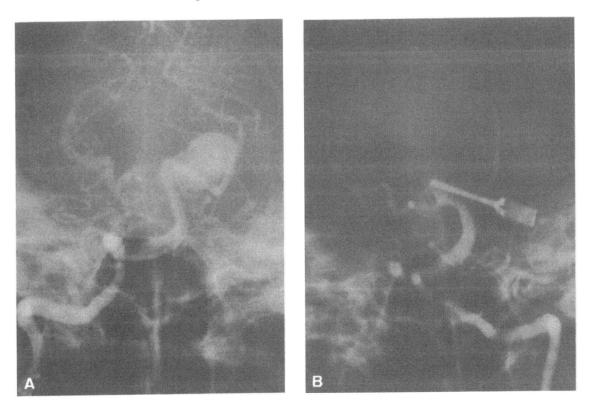

Figure 7.10 A, B. A P., M, 49, ruptured large left basilar superior cerebellar artery aneurysm with SCA emerging from lower neck (**A**). She was operated on five weeks after single bleed in May 1977 in Grade 1. Inadvertent SC artery occlusion by clip on thick yellow neck producing complete Weber's syndrome (**B**). Poor outcome

trapped, fortunately without sequelae (Fig. 7.5). In another larger dissection, only the thrombosed stump of SCA was seen beyond the aneurysm and no deficit resulted from proximal occlusion of SCA (Fig. 7.6). Two more distal SCA aneurysms were placed beside or behind the midbrain (Figs. 7.7, 7.8)

Two small aneurysms arising even more distally on SCA on the superior surface of the cerebellum were approached by a suboccipital-supracerebellar exposure, (one in the sitting position – only used nine times in the whole vertebrobasilar artery aneurysm series). In one of these patients, two intact aneurysms were on the SCA feeder to a small unruptured cerebellar AVM (Fig. 7.9).

The only death in the small SCA aneurysms was due to the tragedy of a postoperative extradural clot. The morbidity was higher in the large aneurysms; in addition to poor grade and vasospasm, inadvertent occlusion of P1 occurred in two and SCA in one (Fig. 7.10). There were only seven perforator injuries, two of them associated with major operative ruptures in one of which a mycotic aneurysm was torn from the basilar artery, necessitating basilar trapping. In two patients with large intact aneurysms, one remained poor from rupture of an associated carotid aneurysm and the other, whose aneurysm was shown to be clipped, died from a basal hemorrhage of unknown cause.

Non-Giant (Small and Large) Basilar Superior Cerebellar Artery Aneurysms

Table 7.1. Preoperative Grade and outcome in 153 patients with small superior cerebellar aneurysms

Grade	Excellent	Good	Poor	Dead	Total
0	26	1			27
1	76	1	1	1	79
2	20	9	3		32
3	6	6	3		15
Total	128	17	7	1	153
	83.7%	11.1%	4.6%	0.7%	100.0%

Table 7.2. Aneurysm site and outcome in 153 patients with small superior cerebellar artery aneurysms

Site	Excellent	Good	Poor	Dead	Total
BA – SCA	125	13	7	1	146
SCA – distal	3	4			7
Total	128	17	7	1	153

Table 7.3. Age related to outcome in 153 patients with small superior cerebellar artery aneurysms

Age group (years)	Excellent	Good	Poor	Dead	Total
10–19		1			1
20–29	11				11
30–39	15	1	1		17
40–49	45	3	2		50
50–59	38	6	1	1	46
60–69	18	4	1		23
70 or more	1	2	2		5
Total	128	17	7	1	153

Table 7.4. Operative method and outcome in 153 patients with small superior cerebellar artery aneurysms

Operative method	Excellent	Good	Poor	Dead	Total
Neck clipping[a]	119	13	6	1	139
Silk ligature	2	1			3
Wrapping	5		1		6
Trapping	1				1
Endovascular		1			1
Excision	1	2			3
Total	128	17	7	1	153

[a] Includes 1 case with a large Sundt clip graft.

Table 7.5. Operative method and completeness of aneurysm treatment in 153 patients with small superior cerebellar artery aneurysms

Operative method	Total obliteration	Residual neck	No obliteration	Total
Neck clipping	131	8		139
Silk ligature	3			3
Wrapping			6	6
Trapping	1			1
Endovascular	1			1
Excision	3			3
Total	139	8	6	153

108 Non-Giant (Small and Large) Basilar Superior Cerebellar Artery Aneurysms

Table 7.6. Timing of surgery and outcome in 126 patients with small superior cerebellar artery aneurysms

Timing of surgery	Excel-lent	Good	Poor	Dead	Total
0–1 day	1				1
2–3 day	3	1	1		5
4–6 day	6	1			7
7–10 day	17	1	1		19
11–30 day	47	10	4	1	62
31–365 day	28	3	1		32
Total	102	16	7	1	126

Table 7.7. Basilar aneurysm projection and outcome in 153 patients with small superior cerebellar artery aneurysms

Basilar projection	Excel-lent	Good	Poor	Dead	Total
Anterior	17	1			18
Lateral	92	8	6	1	107
Posterior	16	4	1		21
SCA distal	3	4			7
Total	128	17	7	1	153

Table 7.8. Relation of superior cerebellar artery aneurysm to the posterior clinoid level and outcome in 153 patients with small aneurysms

Basilar-clinoid	Excel-lent	Good	Poor	Dead	Total
Above	32	3	3		38
At clinoid	35	7	1		43
Below	19	2			21
SCA distal	3	4			7
Not known[a]	39	1	3	1	44
Total	128	17	7	1	153

[a] No bony structures in lateral angiogram tracing in track sheets.

Table 7.9. Preoperative Grade and outcome in 57 patients with large superior cerebellar artery aneurysms

Grade	Excellent	Good	Poor	Dead	Total
0	14	1	1	1	17
1	20	2	3	2	27
2	4	2	1	2	9
3		2	1		3
4			1		1
Total	38	7	7	5	57

Table 7.10. Aneurysm site and outcome in 57 patients with large superior cerebellar artery aneurysms

Site	Excellent	Good	Poor	Dead	Total
BA – SCA	36	7	7	5	55
SCA – distal	2				2
Total	38	7	7	5	57

Table 7.11. Age (years) related to outcome in 57 patients with large superior cerebellar artery aneurysms

Age group (years)	Excel-lent	Good	Poor	Dead	Total
20–29	3				3
30–39	8		1		9
40–49	8	2	2	3	15
50–59	7	2	2	1	12
60–69	11	3	1	1	16
70 or more	1		1		2
Total	38	7	7	5	57

Non-Giant (Small and Large) Basilar Superior Cerebellar Artery Aneurysms 109

Table 7.12. Operative method and outcome in 57 patients with large superior cerebellar artery aneurysms

Operative method	Excellent	Good	Poor	Dead	Total
Clip	32	6	7	3	48
Silk ligature	1	1			2
Hunterian ligation[a]	2			1	3
Trapping	1			1	2
Excision	1				1
Exploration only	1				1
Total	38	7	7	5	57

[a] Basilar artery occlusion 2 and PCA occlusion 1.

Table 7.13. Operative method and completeness of aneurysm treatment in 57 patients with large superior cerebellar artery aneurysms

Operative method	Total obliteration	Residual neck	Residual fundus	No obliteration	Total
Neck clipping	41	5	2		48
Silk ligature	2				2
Hunterian ligation	3				3
Trapping	2				2
Excision	1				1
Exploration only				1	1
Total	49	5	2	1	57

Table 7.14. Timing of surgery and outcome in 40 patients with large superior cerebellar artery aneurysms

Timing of surgery	Excellent	Good	Poor	Dead	Total
2–3 day		1	1	1	3
4–6 day	4	1			5
7–10 day	2	1		2	5
11–30 day	12	3	4		19
31–365 day	6		1	1	8
Total	24	6	6	4	40

Table 7.15. Basilar aneurysm projection and outcome in 57 patients with large superior cerebellar artery aneurysms

Basilar projection	Excellent	Good	Poor	Dead	Total
Anterior	4	1			5
Lateral	23	5	6	4	38
Posterior	9	1	1	1	12
SCA distal	2				2
Total	38	7	7	5	57

Table 7.16. Relation of superior cerebellar artery aneurysm to the posterior clinoid level and outcome in 57 patients with large aneurysms

Basilar-clinoid	Excellent	Good	Poor	Dead	Total
Above	9	5	3	4	21
At clinoid	12	1	3		16
Below	5				5
SCA distal	2				2
Not known[a]	10	1	1	1	13
Total	38	7	7	5	57

[a] No bony structures in lateral angiogram tracing in track sheets.

Chapter 8

Giant Basilar-Superior Cerebellar Artery Aneurysms

56 Patients

Fifty-two giant aneurysms arose from the basilar artery at the origin of the superior cerebellar artery (SCA). Four arose from the SCA itself, two proximally in front of the midbrain and two distally compressing the midbrain posterolaterally. Eighteen were illustrated and described previously (Fig. 8.1).

Anatomical Features

The growth of this aneurysm laterally and posteriorly involves the oculomotor nerve and the cerebral peduncle which it may invade deeply enough to involve the tegmentum of the midbrain, thus explaining the characteristic clinical presentation with varying degrees of Weber's syndrome.

The P1 segment usually curves over the top of the aneurysm, although it may lie in front or behind. The origin of the vessel may become incorporated into the base of the aneurysm as it expands to include the lateral aspect of the basilar bifurcation. The SCA usually arises separately from the necks of these large aneurysms rather than from the parent basilar arteries (Fig. 7.10). Clip placement must not compromise this orifice and it may be necessary to leave open a small wedge of neck just above in order to leave open the origin of the artery. There were nine inadvertent vessel occlusions in this group with two poor results and four deaths: one-third of the mortality in the whole group. The arteries occluded were always unilateral: P1 in 3 patients, SCA in 1 patient, P1 and SCA in 4 patients, and more distally in branches of posterior cerebral artery (PCA) in 1 patient (probably thromboembolic from aneurysm).

Perforators are a lesser problem with this aneurysm although those arising from P1 must be looked for where they may be stretched over the upper aspect of the neck and waist of the sac posteriorly. Perforators from the basilar artery may be adherent behind the neck.

Clinical Features

Twenty-five patients presented with bleeding (7 additional patients had a remote bleed) and in 17, the presence of the aneurysms were previously unsuspected in spite of their large size. In several, the hemorrhage provoked the onset of a Weber's syndrome. Two-thirds had oculomotor palsies: 34 unilaterally and 3 bilaterally. Six patients had trochlear palsy, no other cranial nerves were affected. Two aneurysms were discovered incidentally but the remainder presented as mass lesions, typically with varying degrees of Weber's syndrome, beginning with a hemiparesis or a third nerve paresis (15 patients with partial and 8 patients with complete syndrome). Confusion and dysarthria were seen in six patients.

The one huge proximal SCA aneurysm (Fig. 8.4) presented with Weber's syndrome but the other, almost certainly a dissecting aneurysm, had produced third and fourth nerve palsies with ataxia of the trunk and left limbs. Both more distal giant SCA aneurysms had only fourth nerve palsies.

Explored Only

Three early cases were thought to be unclippable even though two were explored from each side, one of these had gauze reinforcement. In one, the posterior communicating arteries (PComAs) were tiny and basilar artery occlusion was thought to be unfeasible. Another, discovered incidentally and asymptomatic, was found to be densely calcified and the risk of basilar occlusion did not seem warranted. A male aged 47 years had exploration only in 1970. He was for several years self-sufficient but after further decline and clipping of the aneurysm from the contralateral side in 1979, he remained unchanged in poor condition.

In one patient with a partial Weber's syndrome and declining memory with hydrocephalus, the

Giant Basilar-Superior Cerebellar Artery Aneurysms 111

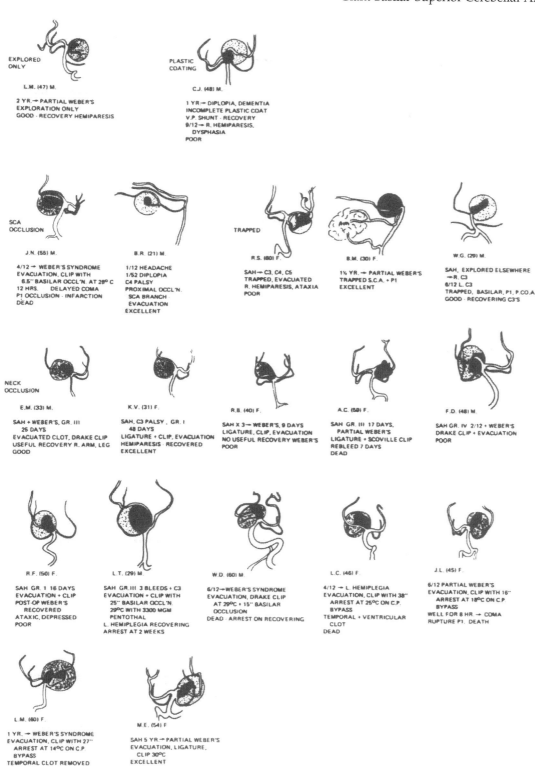

Figure 8.1. The origin, size and shape of giant basilar superior cerebellar artery (SCA) aneurysms and the extent of their mural thrombosis described and illustrated by tracings in the early experience. (Reprinted from Clin Neurosurg 26, 1979, p. 76 by courtesy of Williams and Wilkins)

basilar bifurcation and the aneurysm were partially coated with plastic. Remarkably after shunting he was able to return to work for several years.

Neck Clipping

In contrast to those at the basilar bifurcation, in only three of the giant SCA aneurysms did the neck remain small enough for easy clipping. Most had large bulbous bases often partially filled with clot with the mass embedded in the midbrain and filling the interpeduncular cistern making visualization of the neck difficult. Even so, in another 13 patients, the neck was clipped before evacuation of the sac although it was often a struggle to see the base of the aneurysm. In three the neck was torn and only one of these had a good outcome.

In 16, the aneurysm had to be opened and collapsed by partial clot removal while controlling the bleeding with suction in order to see and clip the neck with reasonable accuracy (Fig. 8.2). Even then it was often difficult to place a clip to avoid compromise of the origins of P1 or the SCA or even both.

Early in this series, six were operated upon under hypothermia, three at moderate and three at deep levels using cardiopulmonary bypass. Only one in each group had a good outcome. Moderate hypothermic levels (29–30°C) were used for longer temporary basilar clipping and more extensive and careful preliminary sac evacuation. The first man with severe atherosclerosis died suddenly during rewarming for unexplained reasons except that the SCA was found occluded by the clip. The other fatality was tragic in a 29 year old man with a complete hemiplegia and intractable headache. He survived tearing of the neck off the basilar artery when the last bit of mural thrombus was being removed, by repair of the basilar opening with a clip graft which included both superior cerebellar and P1 origins. Relieved of his headache, he succumbed suddenly 12 days later from respiratory arrest after unrecognized plugging of a ventricular drain for his acute hydrocephalus.

Two of the three patients done during cardiac arrest on cardiopulmonary bypass at 14–16°C developed massive temporal lobe hematomas originating under the retractor sites during closing.

Remarkably one of these patients with one of the largest aneurysms had a good outcome. The third death resulted from bleeding from a pinhole opening in P1 after the patient had been well for 8 hours. This was thought to be related to incomplete neutralization of the heparin.

In the other 10 later cases where the aneurysm was first partially evacuated of clot under normothermia, 8 had good outcomes. The postoperative coma in a man who was bedridden and on dialysis for renal cystic disease was unexplained by postoperative angiography. The other poor result occurred when the P1 was inadvertently clipped after a tear occurred in the neck in a poor grade patient who did not improve and died suddenly of unknown cause one month later.

In most cases, an attempt was made to evacuate the aneurysm either to facilitate clipping or reduce mass effect. Before ultrasonic suction, tearing into giant necks during removal of mural thrombus was not infrequent requiring exquisitely accurate clip placement. This was the cause of bad outcome in two other cases. Further, teasing out firm adherent clot with a dissector and pituitary rongeurs undoubtedly hurt brain stems from tugging movements on the embedded capsule. Even so, the results varied directly with the preoperative condition of the patients (Table 8.1).

Basilar Artery Occlusion

In nine patients, all in reasonably good preoperative condition but with huge impossible necks, basilar artery occlusion proximally seemed the only reasonable solution. This was accomplished in seven by clipping the basilar artery. All had a good outcome except one who was in quadriplegic coma postoperatively in spite of one large and one smaller PComAs and whose aneurysm still filled. Thrombosis was complete in two and incomplete in the other three, but who have had extended good outcomes. One of the latter had the aneurysm clipped two years later (Fig. 8.3).

In three with marginal PCom collateral, the tourniquet was used, but in none could the artery be occluded. Two patients were much worse after only the exploration and application of the tourniquet, both survived less than a year. The sac became 50% thrombosed in the first and he had inexplicable left hemiplegia and bulbar palsy. In the second, the basilar artery and the aneurysm were both occluded above the open tourniquet whose placement may have produced a dissection of the artery. The

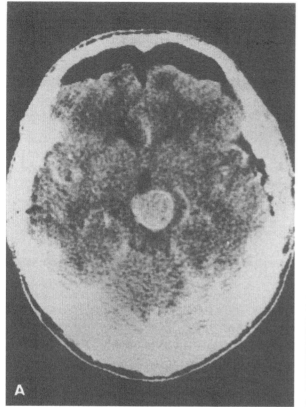
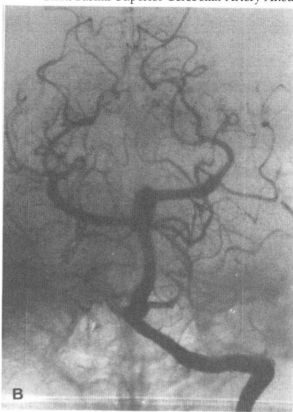
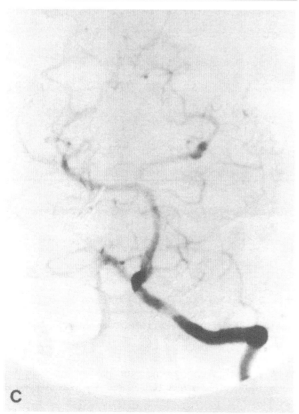

Figure 8.2 A–C. A.P., M, 53, giant left basilar SCA aneurysm (**A, B**), ruptured four years earlier, explored elsewhere (right sided clip), partial Weber's syndrome. Left subtemporal tic craniectomy with single neck clip occlusion in June 1983 after evacuation (**C**). Good outcome

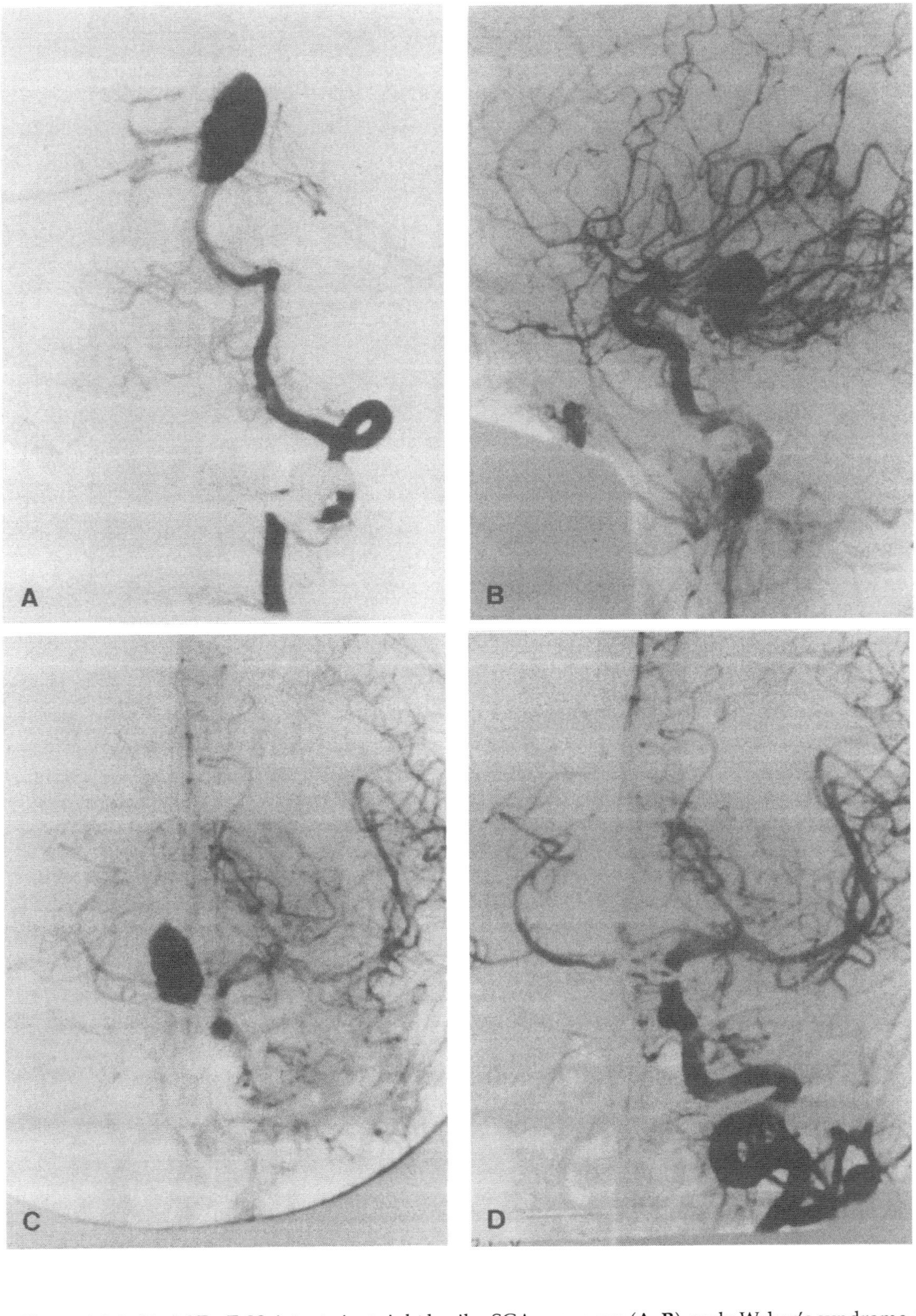

Figure 8.3 A–D. M.D., F, 38, intact giant right basilar SCA aneurysm (**A, B**), early Weber's syndrome. Basilar artery clipped in July 1980. Aneurysm continued filling from large left posterior communicating artery (**C**). Aneurysm was clipped in February 1982 from left side with Drake-Sugita clip (**D**). Excellent outcome

Giant Basilar-Superior Cerebellar Artery Aneurysms 115

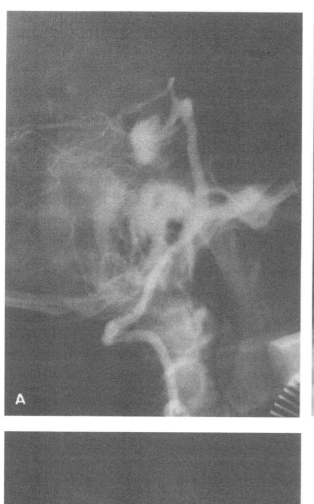
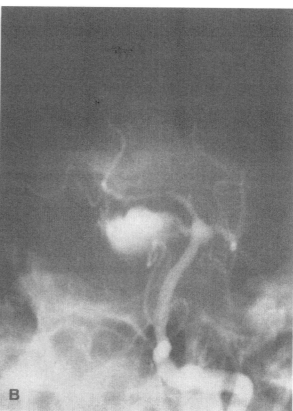
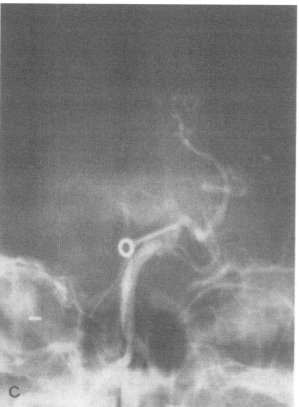

Figure 8.4 A–C. J.N., M, 53, intact giant fusiform right SCA aneurysm (**A, B**), Weber's syndrome over four months. After temporary basilar artery clip in February 1974, sac evacuated but tear in SCA origin which was clipped with endaneurysmorraphy. Decline after initially good, in spite of removal of extradural clot. Clip also occludes P1 (**C**). Died 6 days after operation

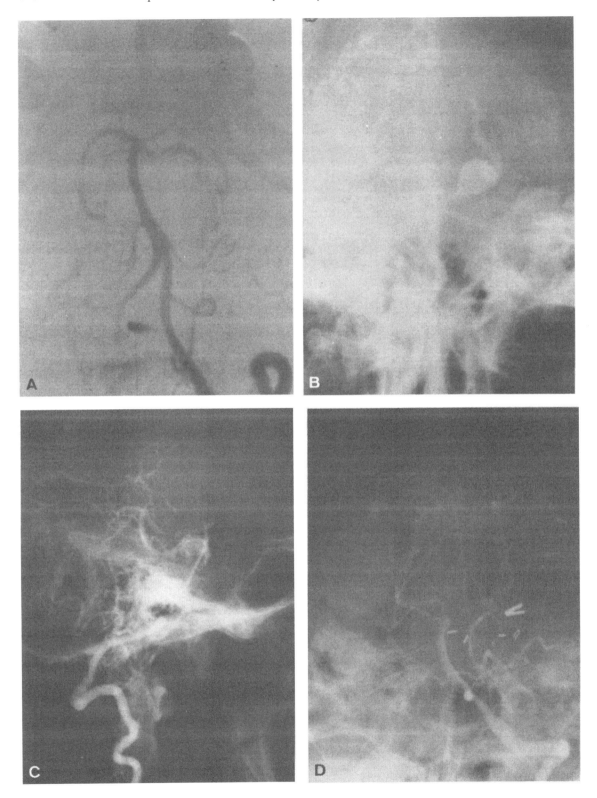

Figure 8.5 A–D. R.S., F, 60, enlarging SCA dissecting aneurysm, five weeks headache and diplopia with trochlear nerve palsy, and oculomotor palsy for one day. Dissecting aneurysm of superior cerebellar artery (**A**). **B** and **C** show enlargement of dissection in four weeks. A 3 cm aneurysm trapped and evacuated in January 1974 (**D**), postoperatively she had Weber's syndrome with ipsilateral cerebellar incoordination. Poor outcome

third patient did not tolerate occlusion of the tourniquet and refused P2 bypass, she was well only for one year before death.

SCA occlusion was used for the peripheral aneurysms combined with trapping in two. The origin of the largest aneurysm in a patient with a complete Weber's syndrome was first thought to be from the basilar artery (Fig. 8.4). Only at operation was the fusiform origin from the beginning of the SCA recognized. While removing most of the thrombus, a small tear in the neck occurred but the Scoville clip placement on the neck stopped the bleeding. He was well for several hours before becoming stuporous when angiography revealed occlusion of P1 as well although review of the tape showed the tips to be clear of it at closure. Removal of a shallow extradural did not prevent a fatal decline. Autopsy was refused. The other proximal aneurysm almost certainly was a dissection and was trapped with disastrous consequences following a SCA territory infarction (Fig. 8.5).

Both distal SCA aneurysms had good outcomes. One was treated by clip proximal occlusion and the other trapped and evacuated. Complete recovery of fourth nerve function did not occur.

In two patients the aneurysm was trapped, one by occluding the basilar artery above and below the aneurysm and the other by occluding both the origin of P1 and the SCA . Remarkably, both had good outcomes. In the first, previously explored, the surgeon had somehow caused occlusion of the basilar bifurcation above a smaller aneurysm which enlarged rapidly over a few weeks and re-bled causing bilateral third nerve palsies. The other patient had a large temporal-occipital arterio-venous malformation (AVM) whose exuberant collateral undoubtedly was a factor in the good outcome.

Table 8.1. Preoperative Grade and outcome in 56 patients with giant superior cerebellar artery aneurysms

Grade	Excellent	Good	Poor	Dead	Total
0ᵃ	11	8	5	7	31
0g	*10*	*3*	*2*	*3*	*18*
0p	*1*	*5*	*3*	*4*	*13*
1	4	6	1	1	12
2	4	1	1	1	7
3	1	1		2	4
4			2		2
Total	20	16	9	11	56
	35.7%	28.6%	16.1%	19.6%	100.0%

ᵃ *0* Unruptured aneurysm or remote hemorrhage (> 1 year). *0g* Good risk without major neurological deficit. *0p* Poor risk patient with major neurological deficit (severe confusion or dementia or stupor or coma, dysarthria or bulbar paralysis, severe dysphasia or severe mono-, hemi-, or tetraparesis).

Table 8.2. Age related to outcome in 56 patients with giant superior cerebellar artery aneurysms

Age group (years)	Excellent	Good	Poor	Dead	Total
0–9	2				2
20–29	3	1		1	5
30–39	4	1			5
40–49	2	3	1	3	9
50–59	5	5	4	3	17
60–69	4	5	4	3	16
70 or more		1		1	2
Total	20	16	9	11	56

118   Giant Basilar-Superior Cerebellar Artery Aneurysms

Table 8.3. Operative method and outcome in 56 patients with giant superior cerebellar artery aneurysms

Operative method	Excellent	Good	Poor	Dead	Total
Clip	6	14	5	7	32
Silk ligature + Scoville clip	1			1	2
Wrapping		1			1
Hunterian ligation	6	1	1	2	10
Clip	*5*	*1*	*1*		*7*
Tourniquet	*1*[a]			*2*	*3*
Explorative	3		2		5
Trapping[b]	4		1	1	6
Total	20	16	9	11	56

[a] Died 13 months later.
[b] Includes two proximal occlusions of SCA with opening of aneurysm.

Table 8.4. Operative method and completeness of aneurysm treatment in 56 patients with giant superior cerebellar aneurysms

Operative method	Total obliteration	Residual neck	Residual fundus	No obliteration	Total
Neck clipping	29	1	2		32
Silk ligature	1		1		2
Wrapping				1	1
Hunterian ligation	4	1	4	1	10
Trapping	6				6
Explored only				5	5
Total	40	2	7	7	56

Table 8.5. Outcome as related to timing of surgery in 25 patients with giant superior cerebellar artery aneurysms

Timing of surgery	Excellent	Good	Poor	Dead	Total
0–1 day			1		1
2–3 day	1				1
4–6 day	1			1	2
7–10 day	1			1	2
11–30 day	4	4	2	1	11
31–365 day	2	4	1	1	8
Total	9	8	4	4	25

Chapter 9
Midbasilar Trunk Aneurysms
44 Patients

There is a distinct group of aneurysms which arise from the basilar artery trunk *between* the origins of the superior and anterior inferior cerebellar arteries. These and basilar-AICA aneurysms are the rarest on the basilar circulation in this series, 44 and 41 respectively.

The first basilar aneurysm operated upon by the senior author was at this site. A male farmer, aged 50, spoke incoherently on the telephone on December 21, 1958. In the local hospital with headache and diplopia, he suddenly collapsed on December 29. After negative carotid angiograms, submastoid vertebral angiography revealed a small bilocular aneurysm on the upper part of the basilar trunk (Fig. 9.1). But basilar artery aneurysms were said to be inoperable except with great hazard. However the more his angiograms were examined the more operable this one appeared to be if a satisfactory approach could be worked out. In the post-mortem room the subtemporal route seemed most direct and the tentorium could be divided if necessary. It had been anticipated that the frontotemporal exposure would provide the best view of the upper basilar, as seen after removal of a suprasellar tumour, but under normal brain it seemed too narrow beside the carotid even when the Sylvian fissure was split.

Then the family refused consent for what they considered to be an experimental operation.

Meanwhile he improved but a third coma-producing hemorrhage occurred on January 7, 1959, and the family, recognizing the gravity of his illness, requested the operative procedure. This was done, on January 8th, under moderate hypothermia through a subtemporal exposure. During temporary carotid and vertebral artery occlusion, the neck of the aneurysm was occluded with an Olivecrona clip. He made excellent recovery, a slight third nerve palsy subsided in one week. This early case has been classified through the years as a small superior cerebellar artery (SCA) aneurysm (also in the database), but examination of the lateral angiogram of this case, only recently found, shows it to be clearly a high midbasilar (Fig. 9.1)!

Curiously two other patients with basilar trunk aneurysms (1 midbasilar and 1 AICA aneurysm) were among the first 14 patients with vertebrobasilar artery aneurysms in the London, Ontario experience. A small midbasilar aneurysm was ligated successfully with a McKenzie clip on July 12th, 1963 (Case 8, J.S.) under deep hypothermia. An associated pontine arteriovenous malformation (AVM), fed by SCA was packed with hammered muscle on its surface but bled fatally five hours after operation. Ten days later, a large AICA aneurysm was ligated with silk (Case 10, G.Mc.). This patient made an excellent recovery in spite of poor preoperative grade and early surgery within 24 hours after recurrent bleed.

Twenty-three midbasilar aneurysms were small and 21 were large. Those rare aneurysms arising immediately proximal to SCA and in close relationship to this vessel (2) are reported with SCA aneurysms, and not included in this series.

Anatomical Features

In 44 patients, no significant branch artery crotch of origin has been identified. In three of them, the aneurysm arose from the proximal carina of a short mid basilar fenestration (Figs. 9.2 and 9.3). Usually the aneurysm projects laterally or anteriorly, seldom posteriorly (6). The necks of five aneurysms were located clearly above and six at the posterior clinoid process level, the rest being clearly below this level. Two small and one large aneurysms arose proximally from an artery feeding a small AVM. The sixth nerve was free of the small aneurysms but compressed medially by the larger sacs.

Seven aneurysms were fusiform, and four were found to be dissecting, the rest being saccular ex-

120 Midbasilar Trunk Aneurysms

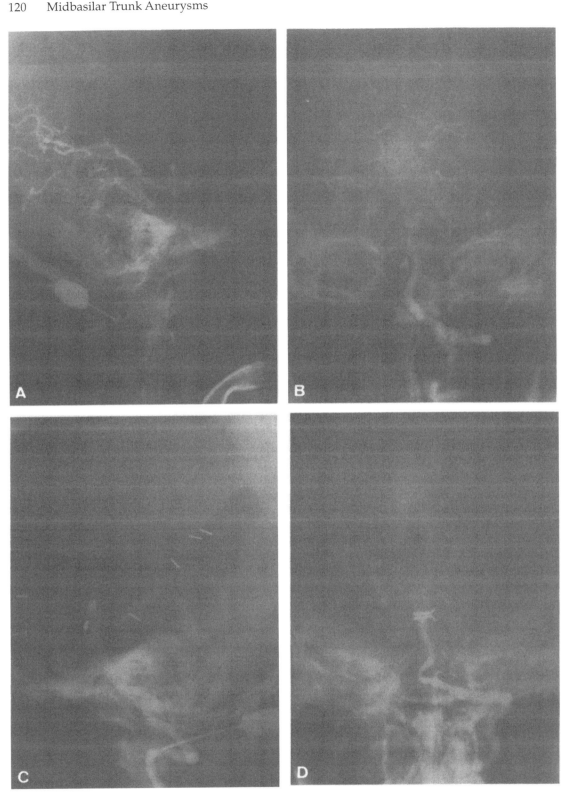

Figure 9.1 A–D. A.N., M, 53, the first basilar artery aneurysm operated on by the senior author: midbasilar artery aneurysm (**A, B**). The operative procedure was done one day after a third coma-producing bleed in Grade 3 on January 8, 1959 under moderate hypothermia through a subtemporal exposure. During temporary carotid and vertebral artery occlusion, the neck of the aneurysm was occluded with an Olivecrona clip (**C, D**). He made excellent recovery, a slight third nerve palsy subsided in one week

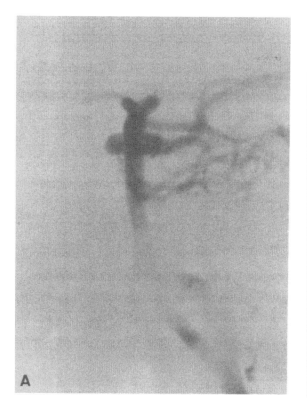 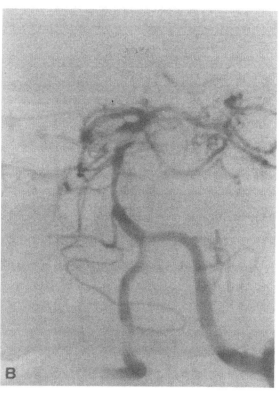

Figure 9.2 A, B. A.C., M, 40, ruptured butterfly anterior and posterior midbasilar artery aneurysms (**A**). Both sacs were clipped four days after single bleed in Grade 1 in September 1991. Fenestration is seen above clip blades (**B**). Outcome excellent

cept one large aneurysm which was undoubtedly false and traumatic (Fig. 9.4). Headache began about one year after transsphenoidal surgery for prolactinoma which was complicated by brisk arterial bleeding from behind which stopped with packing. After a successful pregnancy she began to complain of headache. After producing a tear in the fragile neck of this large aneurysm during dissection, the basilar artery had to be clipped below, but with an excellent outcome with complete thrombosis of the aneurysm.

Clinical Features

Remarkably only six patients had sixth nerve paresis, two of them bilaterally. Six patients had oculomotor palsy, one bilaterally. No other cranial nerves were affected preoperatively. Headache was a common feature in the six intact and large aneurysms, probably from impingement on the clival dura. Further all except one of these six patients had transient ischemic attacks but none presented with cranial nerve paresis. A boy aged 12 had headaches after carotid ligation for a giant carotid cavernous aneurysm. In repeat angiograms four years later, a large midbasilar aneurysm was detected and treated with basilar artery occlusion. Two small aneurysms had ruptured more than one year ago and were graded as unruptured aneurysms.

Approach

Division of the inner third or more of the tentorium is nearly always required for their exposure. This is usually done through a generous posterior temporal bone flap on the side of their projection, so as to obtain good line of sight behind the dorsum sellae and clivus in front of the pons (see Basilar AICA Aneurysms). However, in one-third, a bone flap was unnecessary: the inner tentorial division could be done through a tic craniectomy, or there was no need for tentorial division as the basilar artery

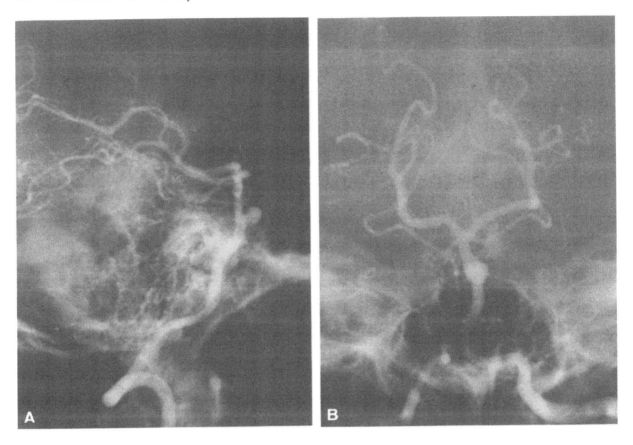
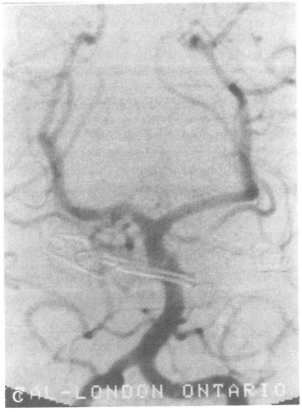

Figure 9.3 A–C. E.B., M, 50, intact midbasilar artery aneurysm (**A, B**), ruptured left carotid aneurysm operated on 17 days earlier. Fenestration seen above clip blades, also clip on ruptured carotid aneurysm (**C**). Outcome excellent

Midbasilar Trunk Aneurysms   123

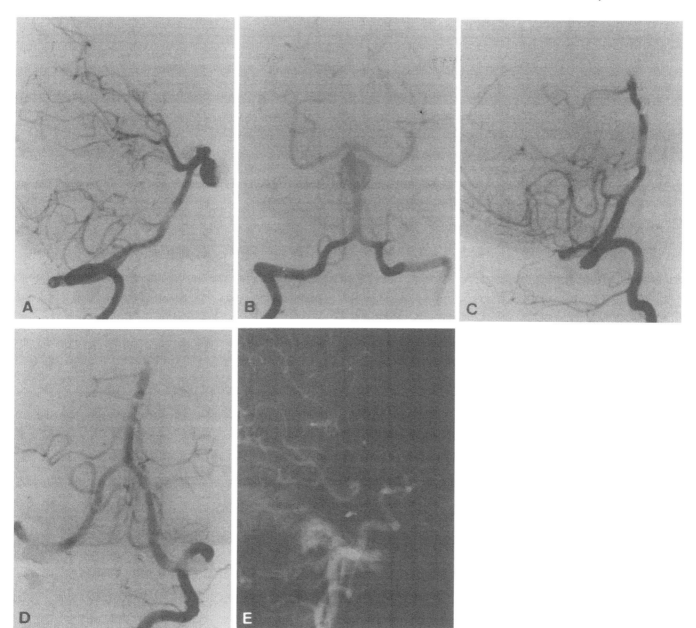

Figure 9.4 A–E. S.M., F, 30, midbasilar false aneurysm (**A, B**), transsphenoidal prolactinoma resection in February 1985 was complicated by arterial bleeding. Postoperative cerebrospinal fluid leak for three weeks. Subsequently, successful pregnancy (!), but after delivery onset of headache, and in summer 1987 episodic blurring of vision. CT scan for recurrent tumor, angiography revealed a 2 cm false aneurysm. Clipping proved to be impossible in August 1987, after a tear in the sac a basilar clip was left in place, this produced an inadvertent severe basilar stenosis (**C, D**). Postoperatively left hemiplegia with a pontine low density in CT scan. Later she made a complete recovery, and the aneurysm thrombosed (**E**). Outcome excellent

124 Midbasilar Trunk Aneurysms

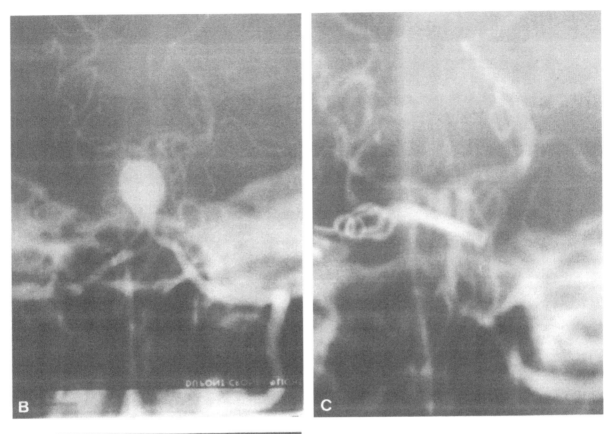
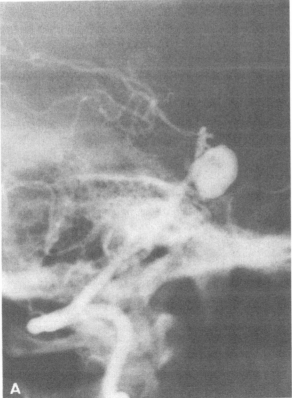

Figure 9.5 A–C. D.V., F, 36, ruptured large midbasilar artery aneurysm (**A, B**), amnestic with bilateral abducens nerve palsy. Aneurysm clipped with two clips one month after single bleed in Grade 3 in May 1986 (**C**). Aneurysm was shown to arise at fenestration at operation. Postoperative dysarthria remained, good outcome

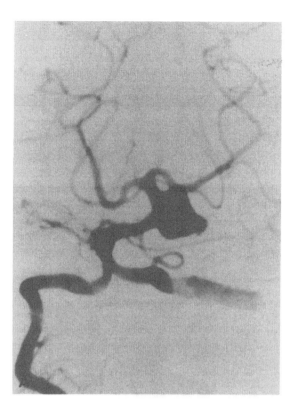 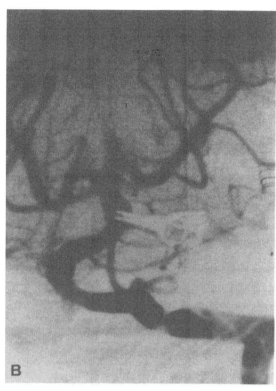

Figure 9.6 A, B. R.G., F, 64, ruptured large left midbasilar artery aneurysm (**A**), left oculomotor nerve palsy, mild right hemiparesis. Blind after angiogram, recovered. Virtual complete clipping 10 days after single bleed in Grade 1 in September 1981 (**B**). Outcome excellent after 13 years

origin was high. It is not usually necessary to divide the petrosal vein which will be near the lateral end of the tentorial cut. These aneurysms can be exposed by working *medial* to the fifth nerve and usually on one or both sides of the slender fourth nerve. But the fifth nerve tends to hide some as well as the lower basilar artery for a temporary clip. The long Drake temporary clip applied from lateral the trigeminal nerve is helpful in keeping the clip handle out of the way and easier to place and remove. In those arising from a fenestration and those with a forward projection (11) the domes, with the sealing clot, was often adherent to the clivus. Clip application should be perfect the first time so that if the dome is pulled away from its attachment, bleeding during a reapplication is avoided. Intraoperative aneurysm rupture occurred more frequently than in other locations (10 patients).

Larger sacs, like those at AICA, often were adherent to the pontine pia, the integrity of which could not always be preserved during the dissection to free the neck (Figs. 9.5, 9.6, and 9.7).

Four large mid trunk aneurysms, one ruptured, three intact and three of which were fusiform in character, were treated by basilar artery clip occlusion and three had good outcomes. All had complete thrombosis in the sac. One had clipping of the vertebrobasilar junction after a left dominant vertebral clip slipped off the artery. The poor result with quadriparesis and dysarthria resulted from thrombosis of the basilar artery under the neck of a saccular aneurysm where two large perforators arose (Fig. 9.8). Basilar occlusion was used when it was not possible to clip the neck without kinking the perforators with the hope that they might be irrigated retrogradely.

126 Midbasilar Trunk Aneurysms

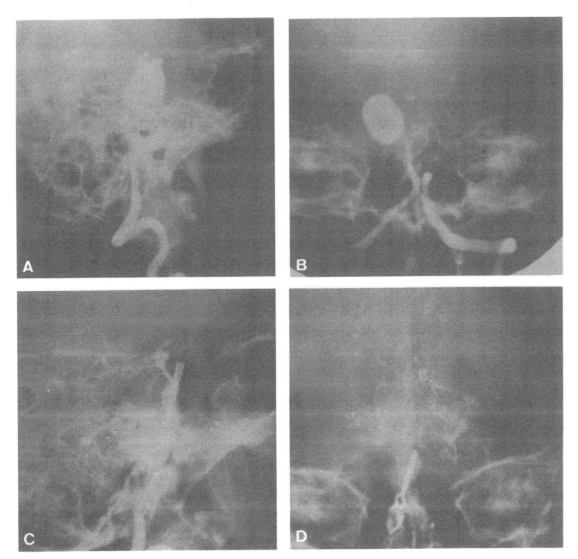

Figure 9.7 A–D. F.F., F, 57, ruptured large right midbasilar artery aneurysm (**A, B**). Right subtemporal approach with clipping 17 days after third bleed in Grade 1 in June 1975 (**C, D**). Postoperatively poor, acute extradural clot removed. Residual severe left hemiparesis from clot or dissection of sac from midbrain and pons. Poor outcome

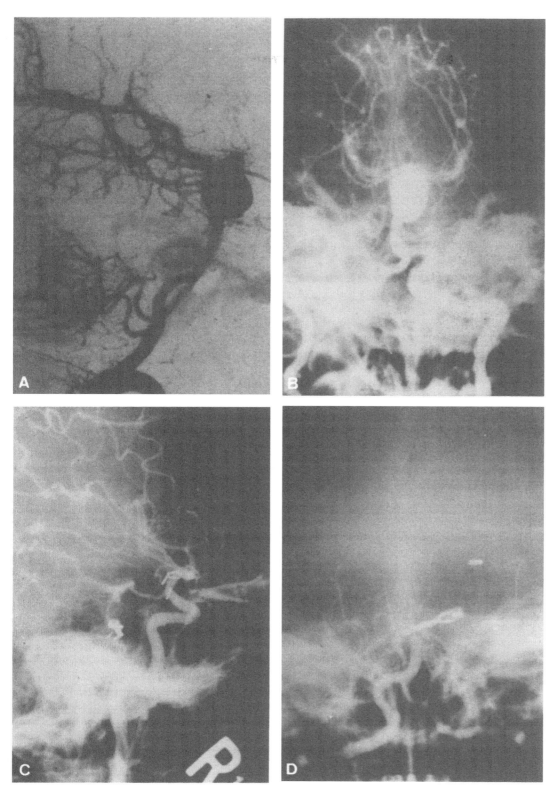

Figure 9.8 A–D. C.M., F, 36, ruptured large midbasilar artery aneurysm (**A, B**). Basilar artery clip one month after single bleed in Grade 1 in May 1983. Postoperatively stupor and quadriplegia. Right carotid angiogram shows retrograde filling of upper basilar artery down to upper neck of aneurysm. Then a thin streak of filling of posterior basilar artery opposite neck. CT showed pontine infarct, probably the result of thrombus in neck partially occluding basilar artery and perforators (**C, D**). Poor outcome

Results

Results can be seen in Tables 9.1 to 9.6. Although these aneurysms were somewhat easier to expose than those lower at AICA and no arterial branch of origin could be identified for special protection, the operative morbidity was higher.

There were 6 deaths and 3 poor results in the 44 non-giant aneurysms. A hemiplegia occurred from a clip on a wide neck of a small aneurysm which severely crimped and ultimately occluded the basilar artery (Fig. 9.9). Two deaths were in patients with midbasilar dissecting aneurysms. One was wrapped but died three days later from temporal lobe venous infarction from the only major tear of the vein of Labbé in the whole series of vertebrobasilar aneurysms. Another woman died after an uneventful neurological course at 36 days from lupus nephritis. The fourth death occurred in a woman already demented and paraparetic from rupture of a small aneurysm arising from a mid basilar branch feeding a small AVM. The artery was clipped proximally but the trigeminal and brain stem AVM was only partially excised. Another death in the small aneurysm group occurred from a brain stem hemorrhage from a small intact AVM after the aneurysm had been clipped under deep hypothermia with cardiac bypass and circulatory arrest.

One death in the large aneurysms occurred from brain swelling after hemiplegic infarction from vasospasm which had nearly occluded the carotid artery, in spite of an operation at 21 days (Fig. 9.10). The other was in a Grade 5 state from recurrent bleeding, although the enlarging dissecting aneurysm was nearly completely obliterated by endovascular coil placement. One poor result occurred after basilar artery clip occlusion (vide supra) but the other's hemiplegia probably resulted from a difficult dissection of the 2.4 cm sac from the pons. Four patients were operated on in the first week after bleeding, three of them died (Table 9.7)! The patient with excellent outcome was in Grade 1 preoperatively, the deaths occurred in Grades 2, 3 and 5.

Ten intraoperative aneurysm ruptures resulted in two deaths and one poor result. Temporary clipping was used in 3 of these 10 patients with 2 excellent results and 1 death.

Two of the deaths occurred in dissecting aneurysms, but the deaths were not related to basilar ischemia, rather to poor grade and an injury to the vein of Labbé (Table 4). Two of the fusiform aneurysms could partially be clipped. The number of nonsaccular aneurysms is extraordinarily high in this location. The types of aneurysm and treatment are scrutinized in Table 9.8.

Midbasilar Trunk Aneurysms 129

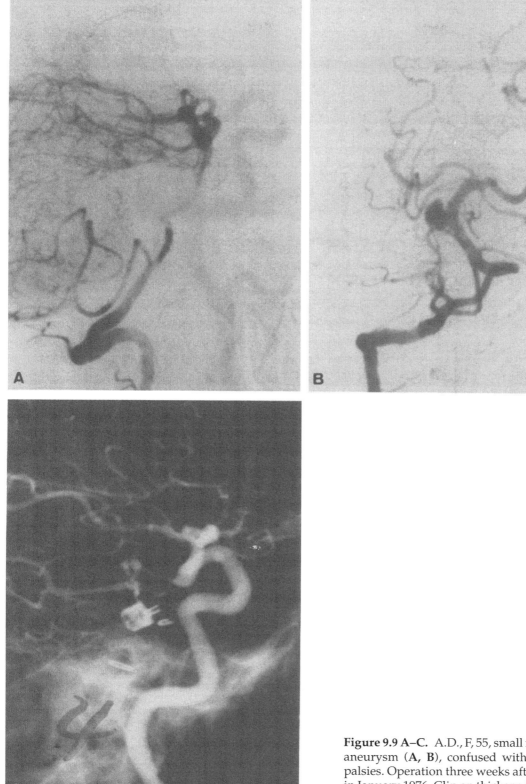

Figure 9.9 A–C. A.D., F, 55, small ruptured midbasilar artery aneurysm (**A, B**), confused with bilateral abducens nerve palsies. Operation three weeks after second bleed in Grade 3 in January 1976. Clip on thickened lower neck has slipped to occlude basilar artery causing left hemiplegia (**C**). Poor outcome

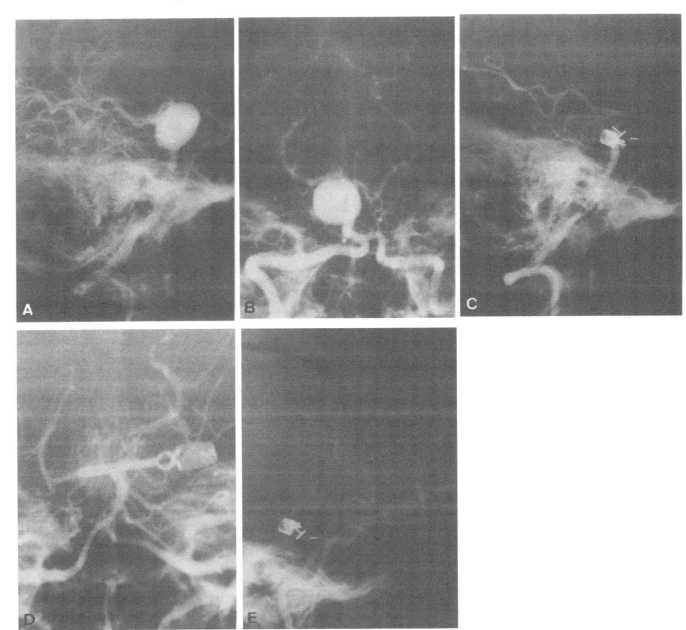

Figure 9.10 A–E. C.S., F, 38, large ruptured midbasilar artery aneurysm explored elsewhere (**A, B**). Operation three weeks after bleed in Grade 1 in May 1977, initially good outcome with only a slight hemiparesis in spite of severe basilar artery clip stenosis (**C, D**). Day 6 decline to death with severe right carotid vasospasm producing massive hemisphere swelling seen in exploration (**E**)

Table 9.1. Preoperative Grade and outcome in 44 small and large basilar trunk aneurysms

Grade	Excellent	Good	Poor	Dead	Total
0	6	2			8
1	21	3	1	3	28
2	1	1	1	1	4
3		1	1	1	3
5				1	1
Total	28	7	3	6	44

Table 9.2. Aneurysm size and outcome in 44 small and large basilar trunk aneurysms

Size	Excellent	Good	Poor	Dead	Total
Small	16	2	1	4	23
Large	12	5	2	2	21
Total	28	7	3	6	44

Table 9.3. Age related to outcome in 44 small and large basilar trunk aneurysms

Age group (years)	Excellent	Good	Poor	Dead	Total
10–19	1	1			2
20–29	2				2
30–39	6	2	2	1	11
40–49	7	2		3	12
50–59	8	2	1		11
60–69	4			2	6
Total	28	7	3	6	44

Table 9.4. Aneurysm type related to outcome in 44 small and large basilar trunk aneurysms

Type	Excellent	Good	Poor	Dead	Total
Saccular	21	5	2	4	32
Fusiform	5	1	1		7
Dissecting	1	1		2	4
Traumatic	1				1
Total	28	7	3	6	44

Table 9.5. Operative method and outcome in 44 patients with small and large midbasilar trunk aneurysms

Operative method	Excellent	Good	Poor	Dead	Total
Clip	23	4	2	3	32
Wrapping	3			1	4
Hunterian ligation	2	2	1		5
Trapping				1	1
Endovascular				1	1
Exploration only		1			1
Total	28	7	3	6	44

132 Midbasilar Trunk Aneurysms

Table 9.6. Operative method and result of aneurysm treatment in 44 patients with small and large basilar trunk aneurysms

Operative method	Total obliter-ation	Resid-ual neck	Resid-ual fundus	No oblit-eration	Total
Clip	26	5	1		32
Wrapping				4	4
Hunterian ligation	4		1		5
Trapping	1				1
Endo-vascular			1		1
Exploration only				1	1
Total	31	5	3	5	44

Table 9.7. Timing of surgery and outcome in 36 patients with small or large midbasilar trunk aneurysms

Timing of surgery	Excel-lent	Good	Poor	Dead	Total
0–1 day				1	1
2–3 day				1	1
4–6 day	1			1	2
7–10 day	3				3
11–30 day	9	3	2	1	15
31–365 day	9	2	1	2	14
Total	22	5	3	6	36

Table 9.8. Operative method used in different aneurysm types in 44 patients with small and large midbasilar trunk aneurysms

Operative method	Saccular	Fusiform	Dissecting	Traumatic
Neck clipping	30	2		
Wrapping		2	2	
Hunterian ligation	1	3		1
Explorative			1	
Trapping	1			
Endo-vascular			1	
Total	32	7	4	1

Chapter 10

Basilar Anterior Inferior Cerebellar Artery Aneurysms
41 Patients

Basilar anterior-inferior cerebellar artery (AICA) aneurysms are rare lesions: detection and treatment of one single aneurysm has been reported only in recent years. In 1989, Kamii described 1 personal case and collected 33 cases in the literature. One year later with another personal, Russegger was able to find 26 cases in the literature. The first case done in our series in 1963 was described in detail (Case 10, G.Mc., cf. Chapter 9, p. 119).

Anatomical Features

These aneurysms arise in the crotch of the origin of AICA over the lower reaches of the middle third of the clivus, about 1 cm above the vertebrobasilar junction. In two patients the aneurysm, however arose on the proximal side of this junction. They tend to project laterally, but one-fourth have been anteriorly against the clivus or even posteriorly to indent the pons (three cases). There is always a close or intimate relationship to the sixth nerve. Six patients had an associated arteriovenous malformation (AVM): in two, the aneurysm arose from the basilar artery, once proximally and three times distally from AICA. In five instances, the aneurysm was responsible for bleeding. Three additional proximal and one distal AICA aneurysms were seen.

Twenty aneurysms were located on the right, 18 on the left and 3 posterior projecting in the middle position. Ten aneurysms were large, and 31 were small. Two aneurysms were fusiform: an unruptured fusiform aneurysm in a 40 year old male was wrapped with acrylic, but a large bilocular basilar aneurysm at the origin of both AICAs in a 59 year old female could be treated with a combination of a long straight Sugita clip and a Drake-Sugita clip. Mean age in those 34 patients with aneurysms located on the basilar artery was 10 years lower than in those patients with aneurysms proximally or distally on AICA.

Clinical Features

Two-thirds of the patients (27) were females, with a mean age in both sexes of 44 years (range 10–71). A 32 year old patient operated on abroad (China) was in late pregnancy with a bleed from her very distal aneurysm (without AVM). A healthy daughter was delivered on the same day as the aneurysm was trapped. Both made excellent recoveries.

Five basilar AICA aneurysms were unruptured: two were buried in the pons with some mass effect (hemiparesis and diplopia), two presented with headache, diplopia and vertigo and one with a right-sided visual loss. An unruptured proximal AICA aneurysm was associated with a large ruptured AVM. Half of the patients with ruptured aneurysms (17/35) had multiple bleeds.

Localizing features were absent in the majority. Ten patients had cranial nerve symptoms preoperatively. As might be expected, sixth nerve palsy was the most frequent occurring in five patients, bilaterally in two. Other cranial nerves were involved in three patients on the side of the aneurysm. One patient with a ruptured peripheral aneurysm associated with a large AVM had fifth to tenth cranial nerves completely paralyzed. One patient with bilateral "butterfly" aneurysms had unilateral complete sixth, seventh and eighth cranial nerve palsies. One female, aged 34, explored elsewhere both suboccipitally and subtemporal-transtentorially, had on the side of the aneurysm facial nerve paresis, unilateral deafness and CNIX and CNX completely paralyzed; her aneurysm was clipped uneventfully and finally she made an excellent recovery. Hemiplegia followed the hemorrhage in five, but was temporary in four patients. Two patients were dysarthric. No intra-axial hemorrhage was seen.

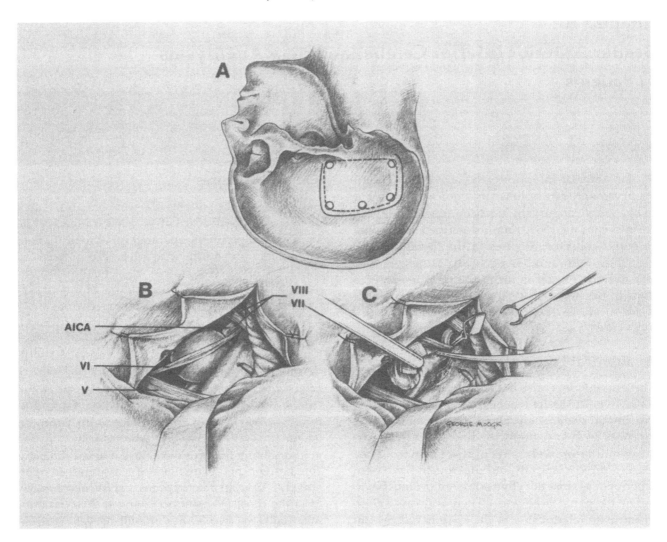

10.VI. Illustration for the subtemporal-transtentorial approach to the basilar AICA and vertebrobasilar junction aneurysms. **A** The temporal bone flap should be extended posteriorly in order to gain line of sight down the posterior slope of the petrous bone through the divided tentorium. After division of the tentorium about 1 cm. from the petrous ridge from the incisura to its lateral extremity and division of the petrosal vein, the exposure is over and down the pons between CNV above and CNVII and CNVIII below. **B** With small aneurysms the sixth nerve usually lies free of the sac and can be laid up against the clivus or under the tip of the retractor on the pons. The pontine pia seems more fragile and it may be difficult to dissect free a larger partially buried sac while preserving its integrity; but the origin of AICA must be seen and cleared from the neck before clipping which is best along the axis of the basilar artery, either from below or above. **C** Because of the depth, application and removal of a small temporary clip may be difficult especially if the handle of a clip on the aneurysm overlies. The use of a long temporary Drake clip with the handle just outside the field simplifies this problem. The closing strength of a Drake clip may be reduced greatly for temporary clipping by repeatedly springing the blades until the tips just close

Approaches

The *approach* is in one of three ways: *subtemporal-transtentorial* (Illustration 10.VI, p. 134), *lateral suboccipital* (Illustration 14.VIII, p. 202) or, in unusual circumstances, the *transmastoid-transpetrosal* (Illustration 12.VII, p. 172) might be used. Ordinarily, most aneurysms arising on the basilar artery trunk down to AICA are approached transtentorially, while those at posterior-inferior cerebellar artery (PICA) and up to the vertebral-basilar junction are exposed by the lateral suboccipital-subcerebellar approach. But both AICA and vertebral-basilar junction aneurysms can be exposed by either route if necessary. The choice of approach depends on the height of the aneurysm on the clivus, its size and projection, and certain other disadvantages of each approach. These are:

(1) from above – the possibility of injury to the cranial nerves, fourth to eighth, and, if necessary, an approach under the dominant temporal lobe near the vein of Labbé.
(2) from below – injury to cranial nerves 10 and 11.

While the use of temporary basilar artery clipping has relieved much of the danger of an approach over or beside the dome of the sac, the exposure should be that which will best expose the neck and the origin of AICA. The transoral-transclival approach has been abandoned for aneurysms, as it is too narrow and confining and poses the risk of meningitis, and it is now unnecessary. The region behind the lower third of the clivus is no longer a "no-man's land" since with experience it can be exposed from the more lateral approach from below or even from above through the tentorium.

The subtemporal-transtentorial approach requires a temporal bone flap which extends well posterior because the edge of a smaller flap will interfere with the line of sight down the posterior slope of the petrous bone (Illustration 10.VI A). The mid temporal lobe is elevated to display the edge of the tentorium *beside* the midbrain. It is most important to preserve the integrity of the vein of Labbé during this maneuver; in one case (midbasilar dissection), when it was torn, a fatal temporal venous infarction occurred postoperatively. With the microscope, it is possible to work on one or the other side of an inferior temporal vein or even between the two veins inserting separately into the dural floor while carefully monitoring the retractor pressure and vein stretching.

The tentorial edge is picked up 1 cm or so behind the exit of the fourth nerve for insertion of a suture which is also passed under a bit of dura in the floor of the middle fossa for later tying. The tentorium may be divided from medial to lateral, vice versa or beginning centrally. Preferred is to make the first opening centrally with a sharp hook and a knife in an avascular portion about 1–2 cm behind the petrous ridge. Bleeding from tentorial venous sinuses with further division medially is easily seen and controlled with coagulation or clipping. Nearing the tentorial edge, the position of CNIV underneath must be identified so that the edge is divided safely about 1 cm behind the exit of the nerve into the triangular ligament. The divided tentorial artery usually requires a clip on the anterior edge. The tentorium can then be tied forward with the suture to the dura of the floor of the middle fossa, with care not to put undue tension on CNIV. Division of the lateral tentorium behind the petrous ridge to a point near the sigmoid-lateral sinus confluence may be done with a knife cutting over a blunt hook as it lifts the tent from the cerebellum. It may be necessary to avoid a large venous lake along this line. The remainder of the anterior tentorial leaflet can be reflected forward on its attachment to the ridge and tied firmly with one or two more sutures to the more lateral dura of the middle fossa. The edge of the posterior leaflet is thoroughly coagulated for hemostasis and shrinking out of the way. The fourth and fifth nerves will be exposed medially under the arachnoid and midway the petrosal vein, which may be one or several bridging from the petrosal sinus to the anterior cerebellum. The vein(s) is divided after careful coagulation, then the arachnoid is opened and more cerebral spinal fluid evacuated.

With a slack brain, very little retraction of the temporal lobe is required, as the tip of the same retractor is worked down over the edge of the anterior cerebellum and over the divided petrosal vein stump just lateral to CNV. As the tip is advanced gently to retract the pons from the petrous bone and clivus, the bundle of the seventh and eighth nerves will come into view laterally, and are not to be put on stretch. The final exposure for the lower basilar artery will be in this opening between CNV medially and CNVII and CNVIII laterally.

At first this space may seem too confined, but with suction and further advance of gentle retraction, it will open up considerably to reveal the sixth nerve and its insertion into the clivus. For AICA aneurysms, it may be wise to get an idea of the position of the aneurysm by finding the basilar artery well above by proceeding past the sixth nerve; this nerve ordinarily is slack enough that it can be laid up against the clivus or held under the retractor tip gently on the pons. Handled gently, the sixth nerve, like the third nerve, has a remarkable propensity for complete recovery of function. The arachnoid sheet in front of this space can be a nuisance, repeatedly plugging the sucker tip; splitting it with the scissors avoids this problem. If there is much clot in the cistern, it is best to suck it away in a direction away from the presumed position of the dome of the aneurysm. Forward projecting aneurysms are commonly adherent to the clivus and those projecting laterally or posteriorly are shallowly embedded in the pons.

AICA will be recognized laterally by its loop in proximity to the bundle of CNVII and CNVIII at the porus (Illustration 10.VI B). The base of the aneurysm is disclosed by following AICA medially, but as soon as the basilar artery is seen, it should be freed below AICA for temporary clipping. The long Drake temporary clip (a long Drake clip which has been sprung often enough so that the tips just close together lightly) is useful here since it may be difficult to apply a shorter clip and especially to remove it (Illustration 10.VI C). The handle and long blades can be tucked away laterally in front of the cerebellum. Then the neck and waist of the aneurysm can be dissected free for clipping, taking great care to preserve the origin of AICA. If the dome is adherent to the clival dura, the first clip application should be in perfect position for occasionally the closure of the aneurysm neck will tug the dome away from the adherent clot sealing the rent. If not in the best position, another clip can be placed out on the collapsed dome to prevent

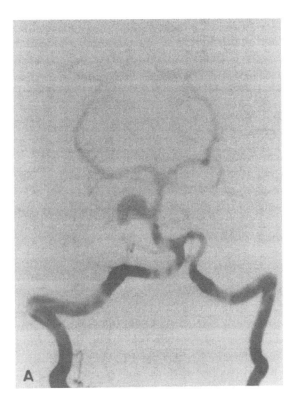
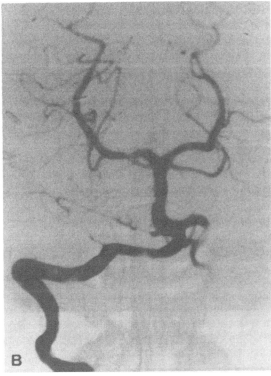

Figure 10.1 A, B. E.R., F, 43, large ruptured right basilar-AICA aneurysm with small neck (**A**). Clipping 10 days after bleed in Grade 1 in June 1981 (**B**). Outcome excellent

bleeding while the original clip is replaced accurately.

For posteriorly projecting sacs, it is quite possible to work behind and underneath the basilar artery to free the perforators and the neck.

Laterally projecting aneurysms usually have to be freed from their pial bed in the pons especially if they are large. With temporary clipping, the dome can be displaced forward against the clivus with the sucker tip on a patty, as it is freed from the pia down to its base with fine or sharp dissection. For a large dome unduly adherent to the pia, it has been possible to free only the neck from the pons and apply an angled clip from above, or even from below by directing the applier beneath CNVII and CNVIII (Fig. 10.1).

Rupture of the sac is frustrating because of the narrow exposure and multiple cranial nerves which can be injured with suction or frantic dissection; but the dissection must be completed before clipping after reapplication of the temporary clip. Preservation of AICA is essential. Inadvertent rupture occurred five times resulting in one death and one poor result.

Bilateral aneurysms arising from the basilar artery at AICA have been seen once (as well at the superior cerebellar artery) ("butterfly" aneurysms) (Fig. 10.2). In each case, it has been possible to clip both aneurysms, but doing the opposite sac first, with a clip whose blades or handles do not interfere with the placement of the second clip. It has meant working behind the basilar artery on two occasions to clip a posteriorly projecting sac on the opposite side. The origin of the opposite AICA must clearly be identified before such clip placement.

Most large, bulbous aneurysms have been approached transtentorially, although coming down on the dome of an upward projecting sac may be precarious because it obscures the neck and must be freed from the pontine pia. Because of this, in two early cases, the neck was approached through a tentorial opening on the side opposite to dissect on the neck across the midline in front of and behind the basilar artery. While it was feasible to dissect around the basilar artery, the visualization of the neck was not as clear and in one case, the basilar artery too was inadvertently occluded by the clip, although without effect (Fig. 10.3). Temporary basilar or nearby bilateral vertebral artery clipping makes manipulation of larger adherent domes

much easier and safer (was used five times). It is a matter of working down the sides of the sac and displacing the waist of the aneurysm with either the sucker tip on a small patty, a spatula or even a narrow retractor blade which will free both hands for suction and dissection. The origin of AICA may be difficult to see under the neck of a large sac, and considerable displacement may be required to be certain the clip has not compromised this vital vessel.

Clip application on basilar trunk aneurysms can be awkward especially with larger sacs, because of the angle of clip application and the nose of the clip applier is large enough to obscure vision. Angled blades and the smallest low profile applier tips are helpful.

In this series, the subtemporal-transtentorial approach was used in all but nine patients; seven were suboccipital, another was suboccipital after transtentorial exploration. The last was begun as a transmastoid-transpetrosal in a patient who had been explored before suboccipitally. However, when the sigmoid sinus was found thrombosed, it, instead of the petrosal sinus, was divided for the exposure. One patient had a frontotemporal approach for associated aneurysms, but the AICA aneurysm was treated subtemporally.

Clip occlusion was used for most AICA aneurysms arising from the basilar artery. Two were wrapped in gauze and soaked in plastic. One was a blister off a fusiform enlargement of the basilar artery and the other aneurysm was intact and partially buried in the pons so that the neck could not be easily freed; this wrapping was incomplete. Both have had long term good survival without known recurrence. In one patient, a large aneurysm was only explored: clipping proved to be impossible as over 1 cm of the basilar artery was incorporated into sac. As the posterior communicating arteries were tiny, temporary basilar occlusion produced apnea, and both vertebral arteries were of equal size, no proximal vessel occlusion was possible. However, she made an excellent recovery, and has remained so for 20 years!

Two of the three peripheral AICA aneurysms, without an AVM, were clipped but one with a broad neck was treated by proximal AICA clipping without consequence (Fig. 10.4)! In one of the clipped aneurysms, AICA was occluded, but filled distally from a PICA-AICA anastomosis. Unfortunately,

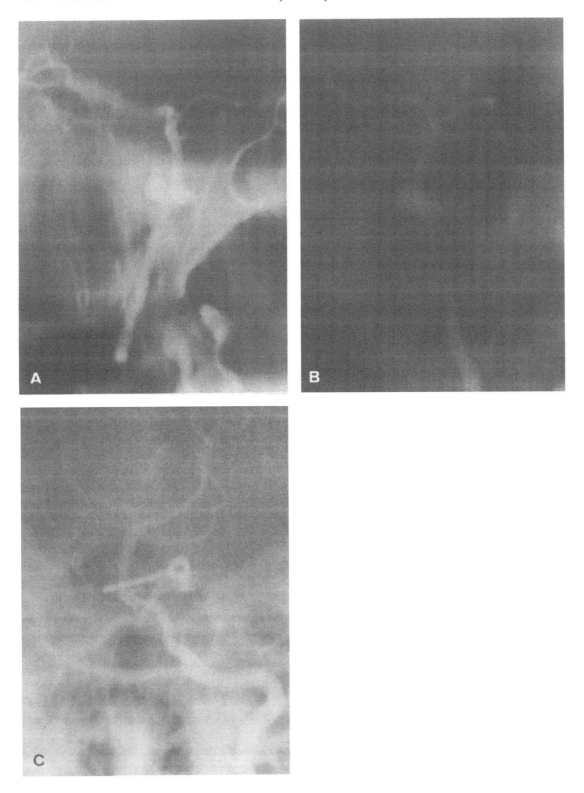

Figure 10.2 A–C. G.H., M, 19, bilateral "butterfly" aneurysms at basilar-AICA seen with autotomography, left one had ruptured one month earlier twice, Grade 1 (**A, B**). Left-sided subtemporal transtentorial approach with clipping of separate sacs in May 1973 (**C**). Postoperatively left Horner's syndrome, abducens and facial nerve paresis and right hemiparesis. All subsided except a slight abducens paresis, outcome excellent

Basilar Anterior Inferior Cerebellar Artery Aneurysms 139

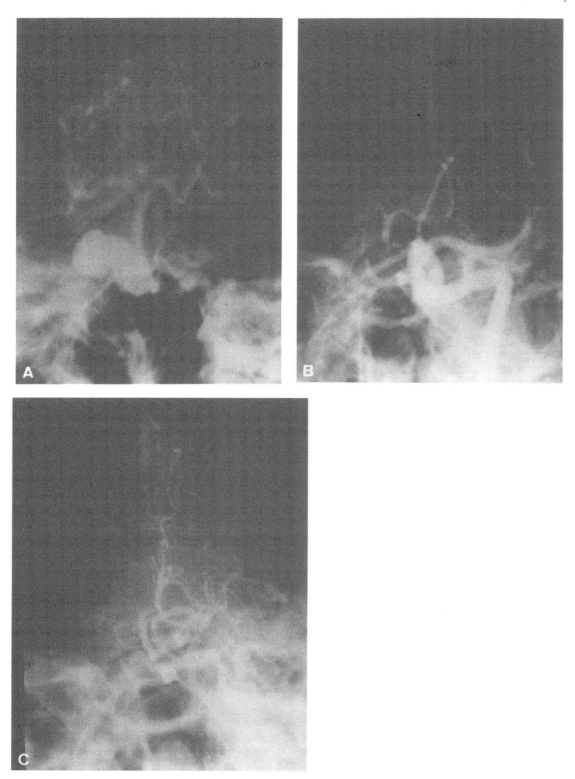

Figure 10.3 A–C. R.K., M, 21, large ruptured right basilar-AICA aneurysm (**A**), bleeding nearly four months before. After transtentorial clipping from *opposite* side in December 1971. In postoperative angiogram clip had slipped off aneurysm, redone same night. Later angiograms show the basilar artery is also occluded, but without sequelae (**B, C**). Transient abducens nerve palsy, excellent outcome

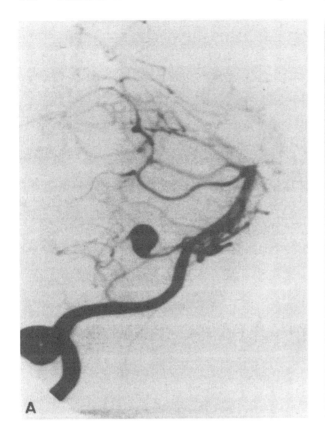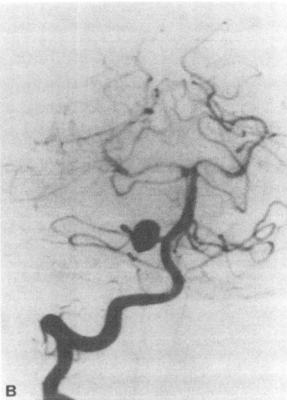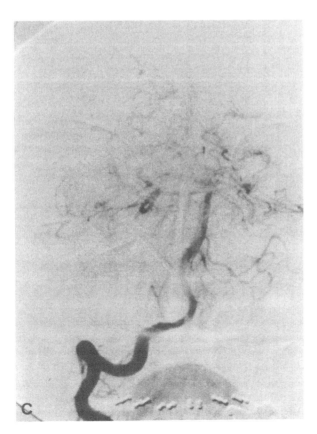

Figure 10.4 A–C. G.J., F, 71, intact peripheral fusiform right AICA aneurysm (**A, B**), headache and diplopia. AICA clipped proximally in October 1987. PICA small with faint collateral filling of AICA (**C**). Preoperative abducens nerve palsy subsided, excellent outcome

she became a poor result from a postoperative cerebellar hematoma. Two further peripheral aneurysms, one proximal and one more distal, were trapped with excellent results in both.

Of six aneurysms with an AVM, four were clipped and two were excised with the AVM. Although the AVM was felt to be completely excised, one of these patients had a poor outcome after removal of a large postoperative cerebellar hematoma.

Results

The two poor results in good grade patients were from a hemiplegia with severe carotid vasospasm and a postoperative clot after clipping a peripheral aneurysm. One Grade 3 patient remained mute but otherwise intact for unknown reasons.

One of the patients with a large aneurysm died from massive unrecognized bilateral retroperitoneal bleeding from the needle punctures in the femoral arteries for repeat angiography. Another had a pre-existing hemiplegia but the other remained poor (and died later) after evacuation of a huge temporal lobe clot, undoubtedly from retractor injury.

Table 10.1. Preoperative Grade and outcome in 41 patients with small and large AICA aneurysms

Grade	Excellent	Good	Poor	Dead	Total
0	4	2			6
1	21	2	2	1	26
2	4	1		1	6
3	1	1	1		3
Total	30	6	3	2	41
	73.2%	14.6%	7.3%	4.9%	100.0%

Table 10.2. Aneurysm size and outcome in 41 patients with small and large AICA aneurysms

Size	Excellent	Good	Poor	Dead	Total
Small	23	5	3		31
Large	7	1		2	10
Total	30	6	3	2	41

Table 10.3. Aneurysm site and outcome in 41 patients with small and large AICA aneurysms

Site	Excellent	Good	Poor	Dead	Total
Basilar AICA	25	5	2	1	33
AICA proximal	2		1	1	4
AICA distal	3	1			4
Total	30	6	3	2	41

142 Basilar Anterior Inferior Cerebellar Artery Aneurysms

Table 10.4. Age related to outcome in 41 patients with small and large AICA aneurysms

Age group (years)	Excellent	Good	Poor	Dead	Total
10–19	2				2
20–29	2	3	1		6
30–39	7				7
40–49	7	1	1		9
50–59	10	2			12
60–69	1		1	2	4
70 or more	1				1
Total	29	6	3	2	41

Table 10.5. Operative method and outcome in 41 patients with small and large AICA aneurysms

Operative method	Excellent	Good	Poor	Dead	Total
Clip	23	5	3	2	33
Silk ligature	1				1
Wrapping	2				2
Trapping	2				2
Excision	1	1			2
Exploration only	1				1
Total	30	6	3	2	41

Table 10.6. Operative method and result of aneurysm treatment in 41 patients with small and large AICA aneurysms

Operative method	Total obliteration	Residual neck	Residual fundus	No obliteration	Total
Neck clipping	29	3	1		33
Silk ligature	1				1
Wrapping				2	2
Trapping	2				2
Excision	2				2
Exploration only				1	1
Total	34	3	1	3	41

Table 10.7. Timing of surgery and outcome in 35 patients with small and large AICA aneurysms

Timing of surgery	Excellent	Good	Poor	Dead	Total
0–1 day	1		1		2
4–6 day	1				1
7–10 day	3				3
11–30 day	13	2	2	2	19
31–365 day	8	2			10
Total	26	4	3	2	35

Chapter 11

Giant Basilar Trunk Aneurysms

59 Patients

Since the original 13 cases were described and illustrated (Fig. 11.1) another 46 patients with giant truncal aneurysms have been operated upon for a total of 59 cases.

Anatomical Features

Most of the saccular aneurysms probably originated from smaller aneurysms at the anterior-inferior cerebellar artery (AICA) although in many the central portion of the basilar artery was widely expanded into the base of the aneurysm. In some, AICAs could be seen arising from the sac. Another group arose from the artery above the AICAs but below the superior cerebellar arteries (SCAs), probably from the site of a smaller midbasilar aneurysm (Chapters 9 and 10). Many (half of all, and 11 of 16 cases in patients below age 20) were fusiform but non-atherosclerotic in a younger age group, probably from an unknown arteriopathy in the basilar artery. Since perforators to the midbrain and pons emerge from the basilar artery throughout its length, there is a constant danger of brain stem infarction from occlusion of these vessels either during clipping or from extension of thrombosis from within the sac after proximal basilar artery occlusion.

Only four typical S-shaped fusiform aneurysms, atherosclerotic in origin and associated with hypertension, were subjected to operation. These patients usually have irregular elongated and ectatic carotid arteries intracranially including their bifurcation and the proximal middle and anterior cerebral arteries. The origin of brainstem deficits was often sudden suggesting thromboembolic perforator occlusion rather than mass effect.

Clinical Features

Four patients had oculomotor palsy preoperatively (two of them with Weber's syndrome), 11 had sixth nerve palsies, and two had fourth nerve palsies. Seven patients had facial paresis and three unilateral hearing loss. Four patients had CNIX-CNX paresis, two of them bilaterally. Two-thirds of the giant aneurysms (37) were unruptured, all with mass effect. No definite syndrome emerged from mass effect as Weber's did for giant basilar SCA aneurysms. Pontine invasion predominated except that with larger aneurysms the midbrain and medulla became involved, even both. Headache, becoming severe, was a common complaint, perhaps because of early infringement on the clival dura. Diplopia and facial paresthesia occurred more often than flagrant fifth (4) or sixth nerve paresis, although the latter was the most common cranial nerve palsy (11), bilateral in three patients. Disconjugate gaze with INO also occurred rarely. One-third of the patients without hemorrhage had varying degrees of ataxia, often incapacitating, and hemiparesis, occasionally sudden in onset. Diplopia, dysarthria and dysphagia were common complaints and quadriparesis with bulbar palsy was usual with the largest aneurysms; a number were bedridden, two were on respirators. Decline in mentation was often associated with hydrocephalus and emotional lability; syncopal episodes and drop attacks occurred in a few.

Seventeen patients presented with unheralded subarachnoid hemorrhage (SAH) alone but which occasionally precipitated focal findings such as a hemiparesis and sixth nerve palsy.

The syndromes were not very different with the four atherosclerotic fusiform aneurysms which were subjected to operations, except that in two the hemiplegia was of sudden onset.

Treatment

In three, no treatment was possible after exploration (Table 11.3). One in Grade 4 after hemorrhage had an irreversible cardiac arrest after opening the

144 Giant Basilar Trunk Aneurysms

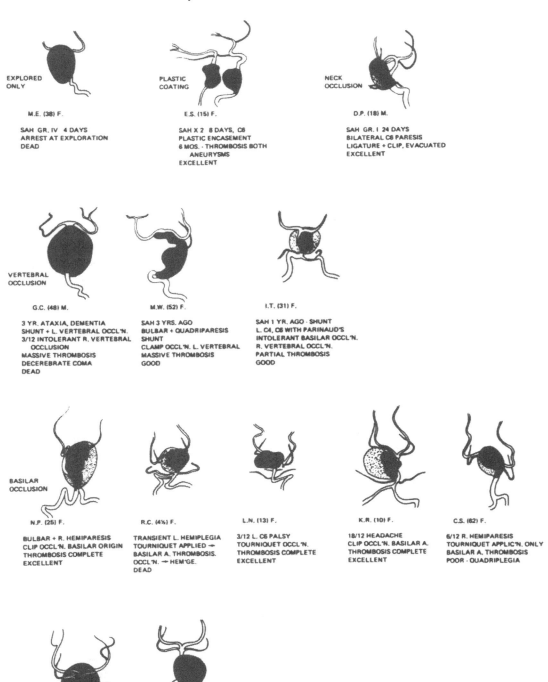
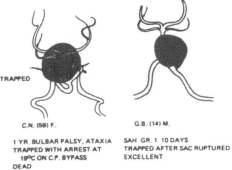

Figure 11.1. The origin, size and shape of giant basilar trunk aneurysms and the extent of their mural thrombosis described and illustrated by tracings in the early experience. (Reprinted from Clin Neurosurg 26, 1979, pp. 82 by courtesy of Williams and Wilkins)

tentorium. The second patient had been explored previously but suffered a postoperative wound infection. Intense meningeal scarring prevented an attempt at extracranial-intracranial (EC-IC) bypass to P2 preliminary to a proposed basilar artery occlusion below the aneurysm. He died from rupture of the intact sac 10 months later. The third aneurysm was found to give origin to both AICAs and several perforators, a situation deemed too dangerous at the time for basilar artery occlusion. She was well for 8 days before declining to her death at 12 days from angiographic evidence of progressive thrombosis in the aneurysm presumably related to the manipulation of the sac.

One patient, 66, with early dementia, headache, ataxia and drop attacks from a wide atherosclerotic aneurysm of the upper two-thirds of the basilar artery, had remarkable recovery of her mind and memory after ventriculoperitoneal shunting of her hydrocephalus. One-fourth of the patients in this group of giant aneurysms had shunt operations.

Neck Clipping

Only seven of these aneurysms could be clipped (Fig. 11.2). The subtemporal approach with suture reflection of the tentorial edge sufficed to show the neck of two higher aneurysms but the tent had to be divided in four cases in order to visualize the lower origin of the aneurysms. For the other, the lateral suboccipital exposure was used. Worrisome was the dissection of these large sacs from their beds in the pons in order to free the neck and the perforators for placement of a clip. Although the sac can generally be displaced forward against the clivus, it may not be possible to maintain the integrity of the pontine pia completely. Particular care is necessary to avoid injury to one or other of the fifth to eighth cranial nerves which may be draped over the mass and impede access to the base. Three patients had good outcomes. One patient with Weber's syndrome remained unchanged but two had immediate postoperative hemiplegias, presumably from perforator injury, although one was severely hemiparetic and -anesthetic before. One patient was deeply unconscious after operation when a postoperative extradural clot was removed but she remained severely disabled.

In two patients, a small portion of the bulbous neck was still filling in postoperative angiograms.

One remains well but the other returned 11 years later after rebleeding from a large recurrent sac found proximal to the original ligature and clip (vide infra under vertebral occlusion for the excellent outcome).

Parent Artery Occlusion

Forty-six patients had some form of parent artery occlusion of the basilar or one or both vertebral arteries. In 29, occlusion of the basilar artery was attempted either by clip or tourniquet depending on the angiographic potential of the posterior communicating arteries (PComAs).

Fifteen of the 19 patients with basilar artery clipping fared well (Table 11.3). Two others suffered brain stem infarcts with hemiplegia and bulbar paresis from perforator occlusion by the thrombosing aneurysm. One death resulted from rupture of the previously intact sac in the recovery room after wakening unchanged and it was shown that the clip blades did not completely cross the basilar artery.

All the other aneurysms were completely obliterated by thrombosis and it is remarkable that in many of the successful outcomes pontine perforators were seen to be arising from that portion of the basilar artery involved in the aneurysm wall. It must mean that deep unseen brain stem collateral to these vital vessels was sufficient to prevent pontine infarction.

The tourniquet was placed on the basilar artery below the aneurysm in 10 cases where the PComA calibre seemed marginal. Closure of the artery was completed only in four, three of whom had good outcomes (Figs. 11.4, 11.5). In one of these, a basilar clip had been placed but inadvertently or by slipping it did not completely cross the artery. A tourniquet occlusion was done nine days later uneventfully. The fatality was a girl, $4\,^1/_2$, who was alert in her preoperative condition, 24 hours later when angiography revealed that the basilar artery was occluded at the site of the open tourniquet and the aneurysm was thrombosed (Case R.C., Fig. 11.1). A decision was made to close the tourniquet to prevent recanalization. Fifteen minutes later she became abruptly unconscious with arterial blood emerging from and beside the tube. Postmortem was refused but the artery must have been torn by the snare, presumably by rupture of a dissection

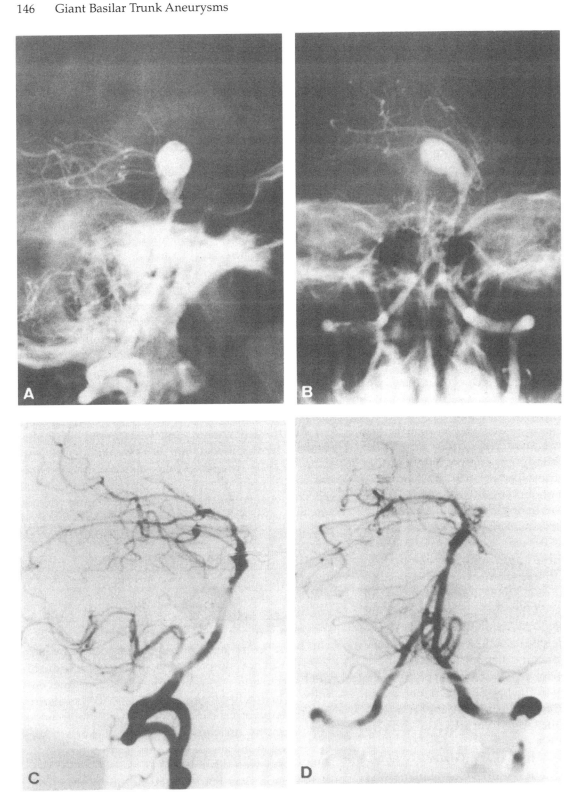

Figure 11.2 A–D. D.H., M, 19, ruptured giant basilar trunk aneurysm (**A, B**). After opposite *left* transtentorial approach in August 1980 in Grade 1 one month after bleed, single neck clipping revealed basilar ectasia at clip site (**C, D**). Outcome excellent

caused by practice occlusions in the operating room as was verified in another case on the vertebral artery (Fig. 6.14).

Three patients were intolerant of complete basilar occlusion, rapidly becoming comatose after four minutes in one and five hours in the others. The latter two died from rupture of their previously intact aneurysms, one patient eight hours after opening the snare and then producing a severe basilar stenosis, the other after bleeding repeatedly six days after opening. The third intolerant patient with barely visible PComAs had been explored and the aneurysm was found to be unclippable. As the sac and P1 and SCA collapsed with a temporary basilar clip, a bypass was deemed necessary and the tourniquet was placed and an interposition vein graft from external carotid to P2 was performed. He became stuporous four minutes after tourniquet closure but the graft was occluded. He tolerated a 95% stenosis only for two hours but did tolerate an 80% stenosis and was discharged. He returned after three months having developed a left third nerve palsy and the aneurysm was much larger. An occipital artery – P2 bypass also became occluded. Yet he tolerated now a severe basilar stenosis and the bulk of the aneurysm thrombosed except for the base where the basilar artery expanded into the sac. Only a trickle of dye passed the stenosis and no filling of basilar branches above was seen. That he remained well appeared to be due to excellent PICA and AICA collateral which filled both SCAs and the left PComA which had enlarged slightly and now filled the left posterior cerebral artery (PCA).

Another two patients were shown to have a severe stenosis at the tourniquet sites although both snares had been left open in the operating room. Probably an angulation of the tubing was responsible. One aneurysm thrombosed virtually completely and the patient has remained well. The other, already hemiparetic, came around mute and akinetic with hemiplegia and has remained poor.

The last non-occlusion of the basilar was deliberate since the tourniquet could only be placed below large AICAs as the artery above was obscured by the mass. However, the patient tolerated a severe stenosis and the aneurysm thrombosed completely except for a minor channel through it which filled the upper basilar circulation (Fig. 11.6). He has returned to work as an aircraft dispatcher for over six years.

Three were treated with single vertebral artery occlusion (Table 11.3) in two of whom only one vertebral filled the basilar artery angiographically. One woman, 31, developed gasping respiration after a temporary basilar clip, so only the large right vertebral artery was clipped. A postoperative quadriparesis recovered in one week and she has remained well for 17 years, although there was little thrombosis in the sac which still filled from a left vertebral artery (Fig. 11.7).

The second patient, 18, had a giant lower basilar artery aneurysm neck occlusion by ligature and clip in 1973 at age 18 leaving a small residual neck (Case D.P., Fig. 11.1). He had remained well for 11 years when 30 minutes of coma followed a seizure. The residual neck had enlarged to form another giant aneurysm with the original clip at its apex. Another attempt at clipping was thwarted by hard atheroma at the base with the right AICA emerging from it. He tolerated tourniquet occlusion of the left vertebral artery. The right vertebral artery which previously seemed to end in posterior-inferior cerebellar artery (PICA) now formed a tiny channel beyond filling the lower basilar artery and AICA and PICA. The aneurysm underwent virtually complete thrombosis and he remains well over seven years later.

The third patient, 52, bedridden with quadri- and bulbar paresis was presumed to have a huge tortuous atherosclerotic aneurysm involving most of her basilar artery. No PComAs were identified and the right vertebral artery seemed to end in PICA. Selverstone clamp occlusion of the left vertebral in the neck was followed by remarkable recovery. In postoperative studies, the right vertebral artery faintly filled a portion of the sac but no definite filling of any of the upper basilar branches could be seen (Fig. 11.8)! She recovered to "90% perfect" and has remained so for 20 years. This was the only successful outcome in the four attempts using proximal occlusion for fusiform atherosclerotic aneurysms. Her long survival may suggest that it was non-atherosclerotic. We have been in despair about the treatment of this aneurysm. Unilateral vertebral occlusion should have little therapeutic effect were the other to be present. Bilateral vertebral occlusion in the presence of one or both larger PComAs would certainly alter the dynamics within the aneurysm but unless thrombosis of the channel within it could be prevented, massive brain stem thrombosis will almost certainly occur.

Figure 11.3 A–D

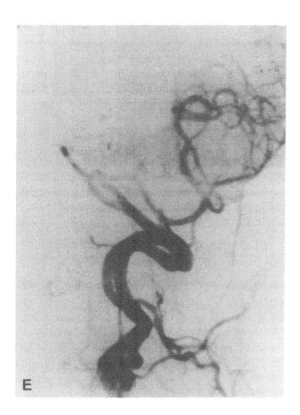 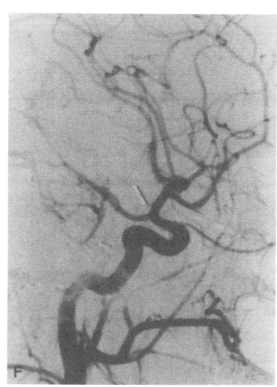

Figure 11.3 E, F

Figure 11.3 A–F. D.H., M, 13, ruptured (?) giant basilar trunk aneurysm, headache for three years, sudden severe headache five and three weeks ago. CTs done by father, a radiologist, reveal giant aneurysm (**A, B**). Lateral and AP angiograms show one large posterior communicating artery (**C, D**). Clip occlusion of basilar artery above AICAs in May 1983 (**E**). Good upper basilar irrigation from carotid artery (**F**). Outcome excellent

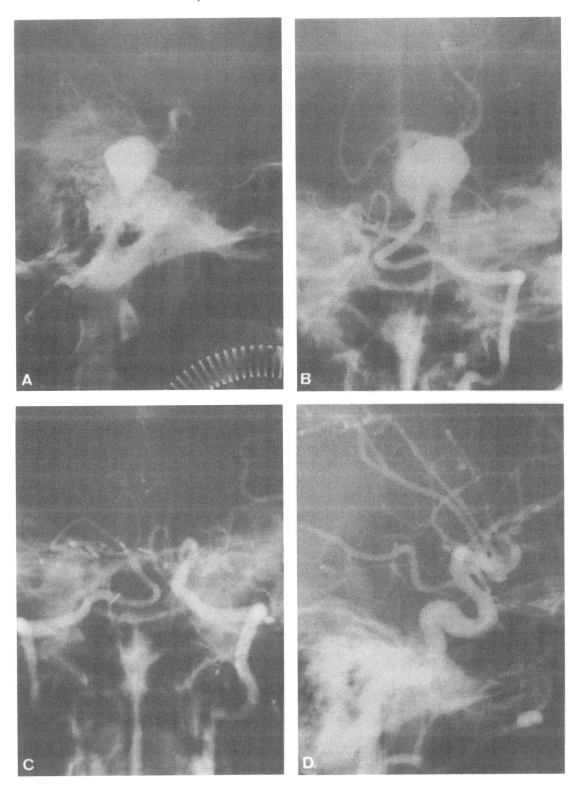

Figure 11.4 A–D. L.N., F, 13, ruptured giant basilar trunk aneurysm, severe headache three months ago and now for five days, found to have left abducens nerve palsy. Lateral and AP angiograms show giant basilar trunk aneurysm (**A, B**). Tourniquet occlusion of basilar artery above AICAs in October 1975 (**C**). Large right posterior communicating artery fills upper basilar circulation (**D**). Outcome excellent

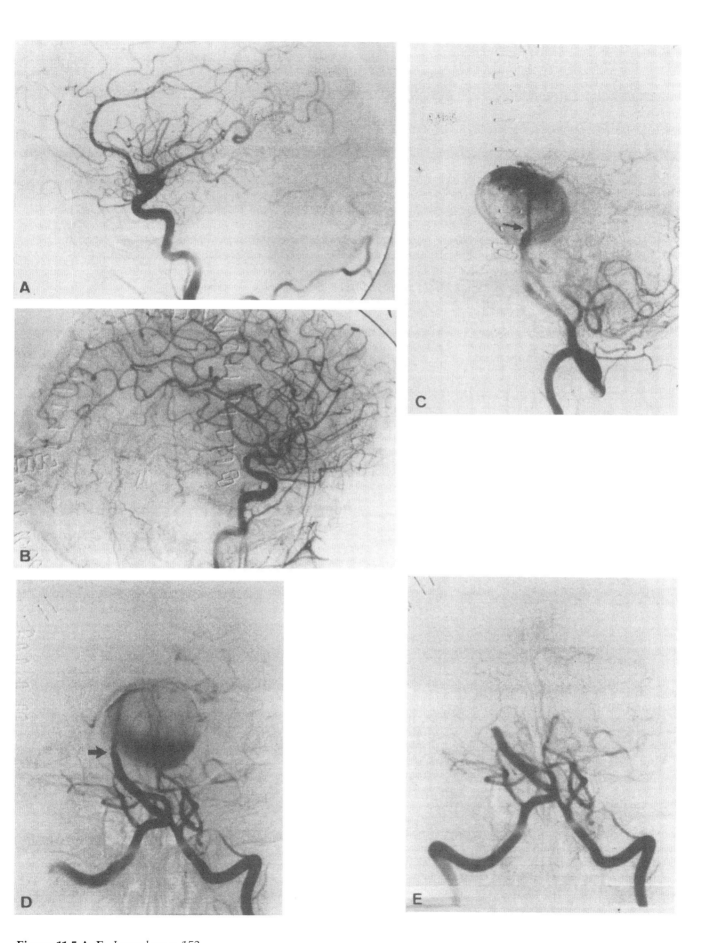

Figure 11.5 A–E. *Legend see p. 152*

152   Giant Basilar Trunk Aneurysms

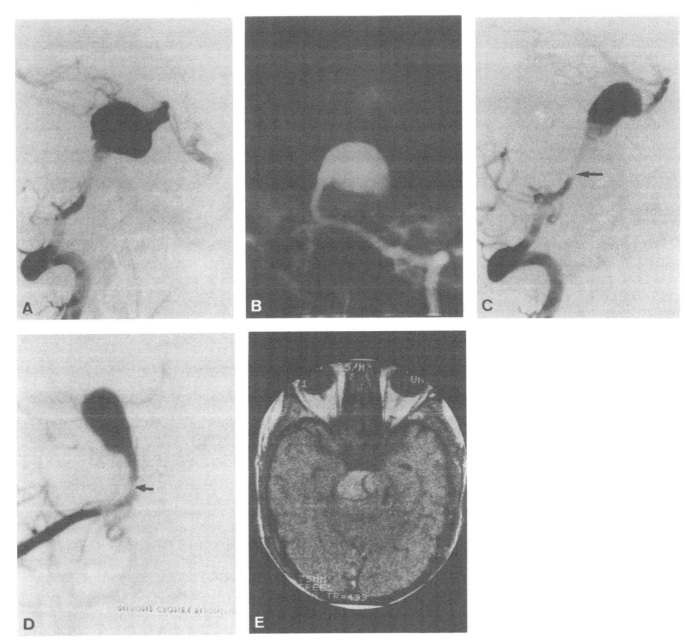

Figure 11.6 A–E. J.M., M, 36, giant upper basilar trunk aneurysm, headache, bulbar paresis, ataxia. Good posterior communicating arteries with Allcock's test (A, B). Severe tourniquet stenosis of basilar artery just below AICAs in August 1985 (C, D, arrow). It was not possible to see the basilar artery above AICAs for basilar clipping. MRI one year later (E). Thrombosis in aneurysm virtually complete except for narrow channel through it centrally for basilar circulation. Virtual complete recovery except for mild left dysmetria, working

←

Figure 11.5 A–E. H.C., M, 46, giant upper basilar trunk aneurysm, headache and diplopia six months. No posterior communicating arteries demonstrated on right or left carotid angios with Allcock's test (A, B). Aneurysm enlarging in spite of 66% stenosis with tourniquet in May 1991 (C, D, arrows). In spite of failure of ECIC-P2 and occipital-P2 bypasses, complete occlusion of basilar artery was tolerated in September 1991 probably because of remarkable PICA–AICA–SCA and posterior cerebral artery leptomeningeal collaterals (E). Needed hypertension for several days. Outcome excellent (see p. 151)

Giant Basilar Trunk Aneurysms 153

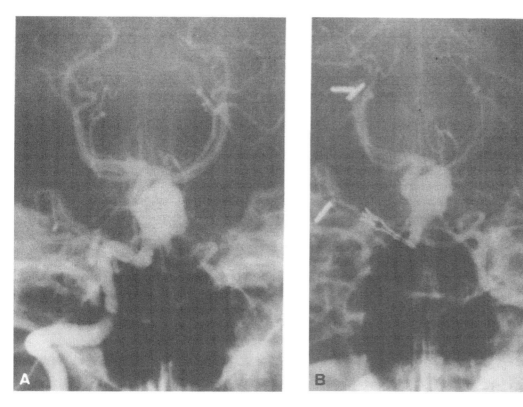

Figure 11.7 A, B. I.T., F, 30, ruptured giant midbasilar trunk aneurysm (**A**), bleeding nine months earlier, originally hemiparetic but improved after shunting. Intolerant of temporary bilateral vertebral occlusion at operation in September 1974, larger right vertebral artery clipped. In spite of continued filling of the aneurysm from smaller left artery (**B**) she has remained well for 20 years. Good outcome

154 Giant Basilar Trunk Aneurysms

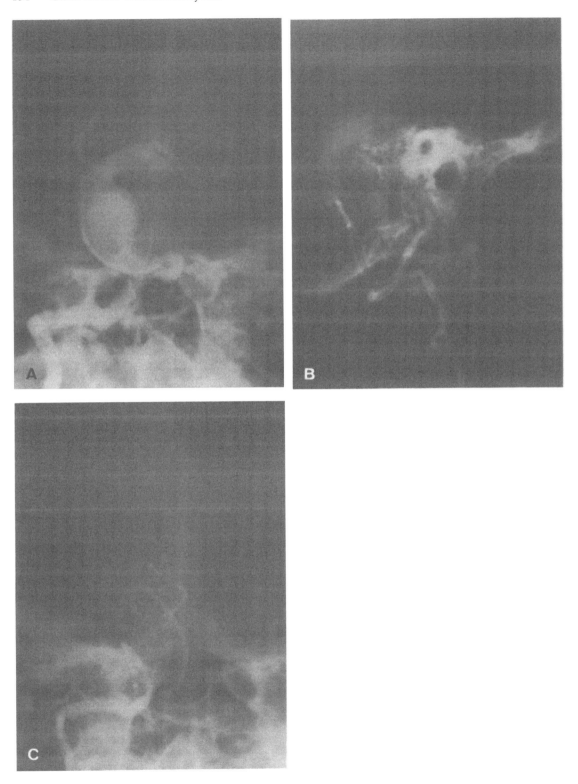

Figure 11.8 A–C. M.W., F, 56, giant atherosclerotic basilar trunk aneurysm, bleeding three years before sudden hemiplegia, but with "90%" recovery. Right vertebral artery filling presumed atherosclerotic basilar aneurysm (**A**). Left vertebral artery ended in PICA. Selverstone clamp occlusion of right vertebral artery in December 1971. Reconstitution of vertebral artery by deep cervical collaterals but no filling of the aneurysm (**B, C**) Remarkably in spite of no reflux from either carotid into vertebral artery she has remained well for 23 years despite no basilar artery circulation seen in any of the postoperative angiograms!

Bilateral vertebral instead of basilar artery occlusion was used in seven patients when the origin of the aneurysm was so low as not to allow easy or safe application of clip or tourniquet to the basilar artery or when there was uncertainty of PComA collateral (Fig. 11.9). In most, one vertebral artery was clip occluded above PICA at exploration and occlusion of the other vertebral was attempted in the awake patient by a tourniquet placed at the operation or by detached balloon in the upper cervical segment or in the lower neck by Selverstone clamp (Table 11.4). The latter was used when no or tiny PComAs. were demonstrated and reconstitution of the vertebral by deep cervical collateral was felt necessary to provide some diminished flow to irrigate the basilar system. In three later cases, balloons detached just extracranially in the artery at the sulcus arteriosus of the atlas were used to occlude the second vertebral. Test occlusion can be used for 30–45 minutes and an open operative procedure is avoided.

The failure of clamp occlusion of the vertebral artery in the neck by reconstitution of its flow from deep cervical collateral was demonstrated in a 23 year old woman who had balloon occlusion of the left vertebral at the axis (Fig. 11.10). After nine months, the reconstituted right vertebral flow caused significant enlargement of the aneurysm with increasing hemiparesis. After clip occlusion of the basilar artery she was bulbar – and quadriparetic. Incomplete thrombosis of the aneurysm occurred because it still filled partially through remarkable collateral from PICA to AICA which even perfused the basilar artery above. However, she made a remarkable recovery over several months and although left with right hemiparesis she remains reasonably self-sufficient for 12 years.

In one case, detached balloons were used on both sides at the atlas when overlap of the vertebrobasilar junction area by the mass made intracranial exploration unlikely to be rewarding (Fig. 11.11).

The aneurysm in a 12 year old girl refilled and enlarged after right vertebral clipping beyond PICA and a severe Selverstone clamp stenosis of the other in the neck. When refilling and enlargement occurred, tourniquet occlusion of the left vertebral in the sulcus arteriosus was tolerated but then the snare slipped. Detached balloon occlusion of the vertebral at the same site was followed by virtual occlusion of the sac except superiorly where a little filling persisted from retrograde flow down the basilar. She remains well for 12 years.

The morbidity was all due to brain stem infarction not always because of diminished flow but rather subsequent thrombosis in the large aneurysm sacs several hours later which obliterates perforating arteries to the brain stem. Before one of the deaths, a respiratory arrest was reversed on opening the tourniquet but quadriplegia occurred 17 hours later. Another lower basilar trunk aneurysm thrombosed completely even though he was intolerant of the second vertebral occlusion. His death was due to a basilar artery occlusion just above the AICAs by a presumed embolus from the sac. Evacuation of the lower two-thirds of a large thrombosed atherosclerotic sac to reduce the mass after bilateral vertebral occlusion by clip and tourniquet had no effect on the declining neurological state (Fig. 11.12). The bilateral Selverstone clamp occlusion was in a 48 year old man with ataxia and bulbar palsy who was first shunted for declining memory and then the left vertebral was clamp occluded in the neck. When he failed to improve, a clamp was placed on the right vertebral. Three hours after the second right vertebral occlusion, he became drowsy with a right hemiplegia but this reversed after opening the clamp. Suddenly one day later, deep decerebrate coma occurred from massive thrombosis within the sac which included a long segment of the basilar artery involved in the aneurysm. Death occurred three weeks later (G.C. in Fig. 11.1).

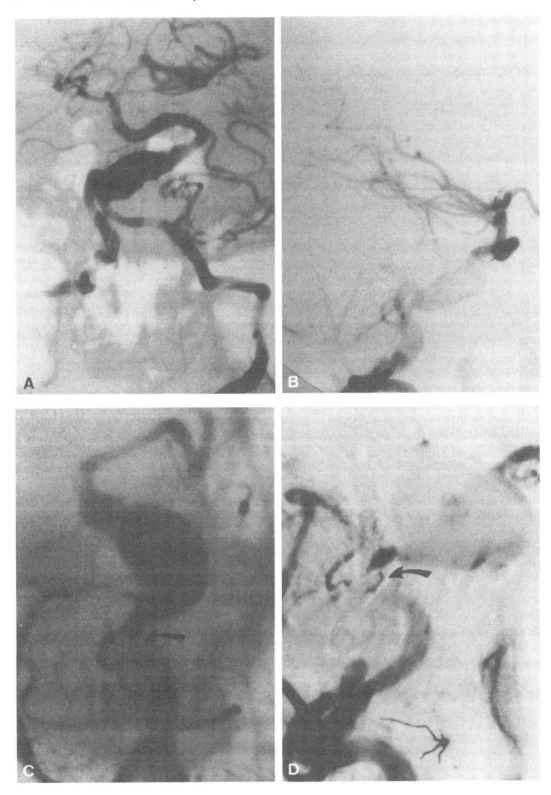

Figure 11.9 A–D

Giant Basilar Trunk Aneurysms 157

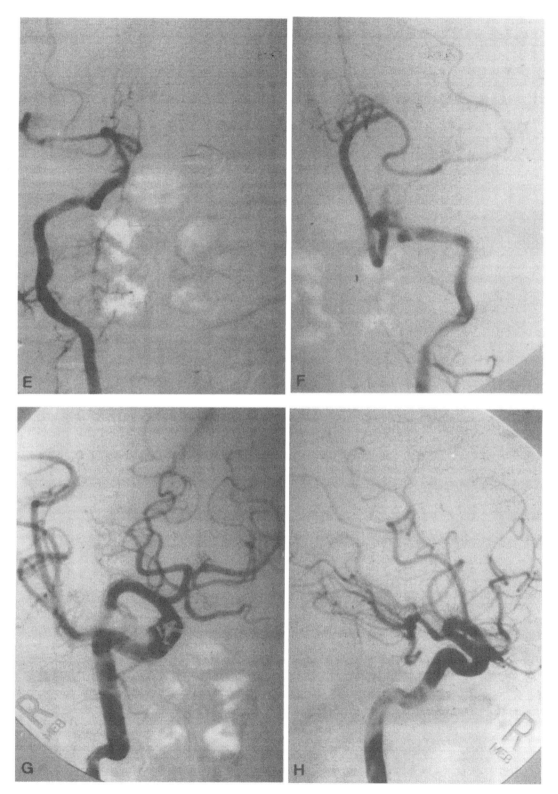

Figure 11.9 E–H

Figure 11.9 A–H. K.S., M, 21, giant fusiform basilar trunk aneurysm (**A, B**), two years headache, vertigo and left paresthesia. In April 1984 suboccipital approach. After clip occlusion of terminal left vertebral and 60% clip stenosis of terminal right vertebral artery (**C**, arrow). After one week stenosis increased to 80% (**D**, arrow). Four months later, spontaneous complete bilateral vertebral occlusion (**E, F**) with good retrograde filling of basilar artery and complete thrombosis of aneurysm (**G, H**). Outcome excellent

158 Giant Basilar Trunk Aneurysms

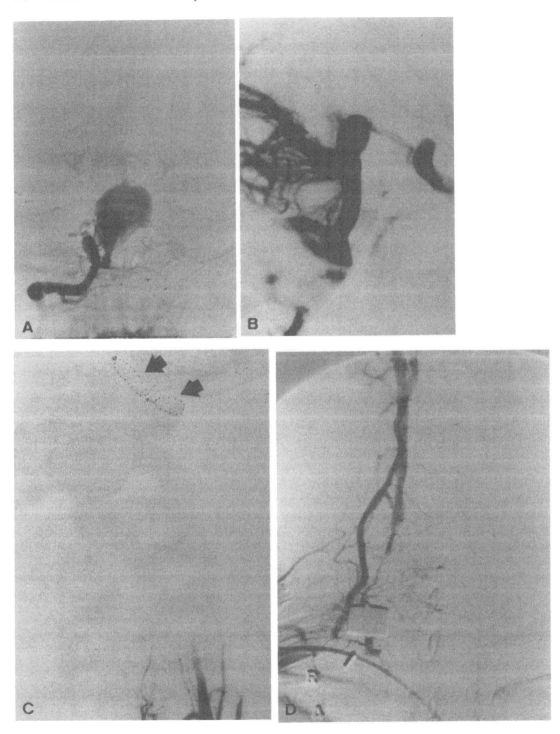

Figure 11.10 A–D

Figure 11.10 A–H. C.C., F, 23, giant lower basilar trunk aneurysm (**A**), mild left hemiparesis. Only tiny posterior communicating arteries seen with Allcock's test (**B**). Double balloon occlusion of left vertebral artery at atlas (**C**, arrows) and Selverstone clamp occlusion of right vertebral artery which became reconstituted by deep cervical collateral (**D**). Eight months later headache, aneurysm filling by reconstituted flow in right vertebral had increased in size (**E, F**). After transpetrosal lower basilar clipping in March 1983 she was poor with bulbar palsy and quadriparesis. Angiograms revealed that the aneurysm was still filling partially through remarkable collateral from PICA to AICA (**G**, arrow) and then (**H**) the basilar artery beyond. After six months her recovery was gratifying with subsidence of the bulbar palsy and left hemiparesis but with a palsied right arm

Giant Basilar Trunk Aneurysms

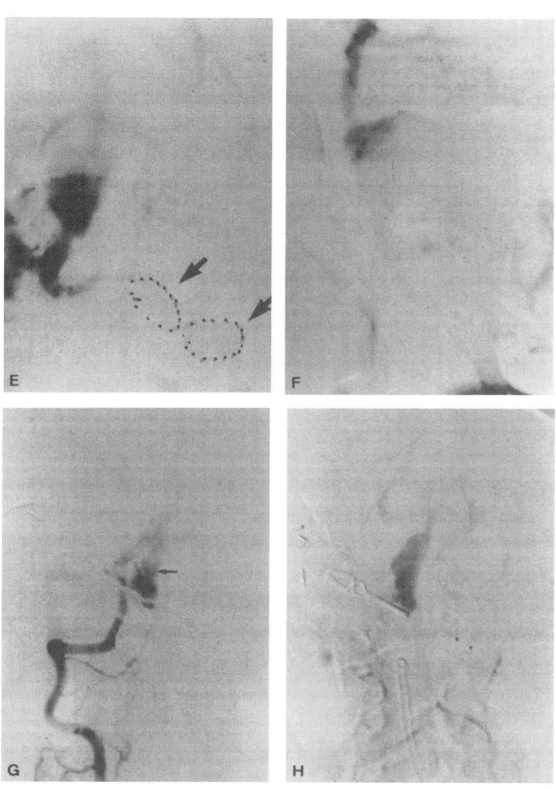

Figure 11.10 E–H

160 Giant Basilar Trunk Aneurysms

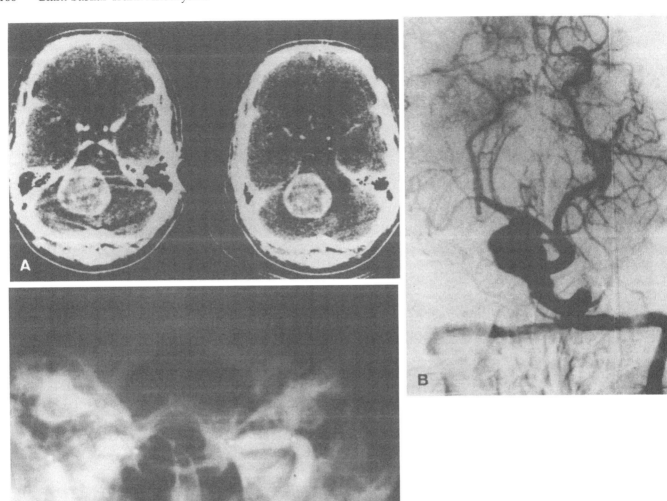

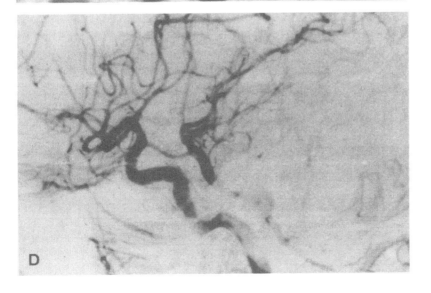

Figure 11.11 A–D. J.H., M, 29, giant basilar trunk aneurysm, five years slowly progressive right cerebellopontine angle syndrome with right-sided complete facial palsy and loss of hearing, ataxia and spastic quadriparesis. CTs and angiogram show huge right-sided aneurysm (**A, B**). In November 1982 double balloon occlusion of each vertebral artery in sulcus arteriosus of atlas one week apart (**C**). Nearly complete thrombosis of aneurysm with filling of PICAs retrograde by narrow channel through base of sac (**D**). Good outcome

Giant Basilar Trunk Aneurysms 161

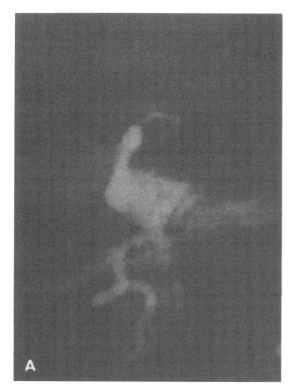
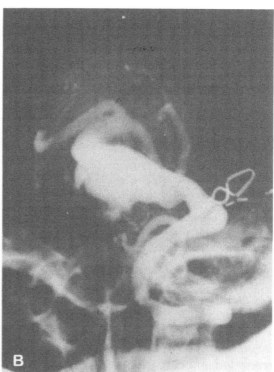
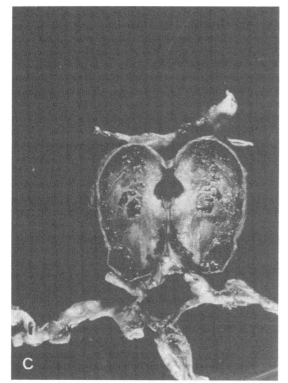

Figure 11.12 A–C. B.L., M, 57, giant basilar trunk aneurysm, in one year decline to ataxia, bulbar palsy and sudden left hemiplegia. Large partially thrombosed atherosclerotic basilar aneurysm (A). After clip occlusion of larger right vertebral artery and tourniquet application to left vertebral artery in February 1980 (B). He was "locked in" in spite of good posterior communicating arteries and had only partial recovery. The right vertebral was clip occluded in March 1980 when the tourniquet tore the artery and the aneurysm was partially evacuated. At death three months later there was massive brain stem infarction from complete thrombosis of the aneurysm and branch and perforator occlusion(C)

Trapping

Trapping was used in seven patients, in six to reduce the mass compression of the brain stem. Of the two originally described, one had a good outcome from emergent trapping when the sac ruptured but the other died of massive brain stem infarction when both AICAs and several perforators were shown to arise from the sac (Fig. 11.1).

Of the five more recent cases two had good outcomes. A 17 year old boy, with a four month history of headache was admitted on a respirator after rapid decline to bulbar palsy and quadriparesis 16 days after a probable hemorrhage (Fig. 11.13). He was basically "locked in" with little response to command. After tourniquet occlusion of the lower basilar artery he improved rapidly with more movement in his limbs and he could protrude his tongue (Fig. 11.13 C). Five days later when the aneurysm was thrombosed, it was trapped with a basilar clip above the sac and the aneurysm was evacuated and collapsed after control of some pesky bleeding from the interior with brief packing (Fig. 11.13 D). Thereafter, improvement was dramatic and became virtually complete within a few weeks with only some restriction of right gaze and he leads a normal life.

Incomplete trapping, using severe arterial stenosis rather than complete occlusion was used in the other. This woman, 45, had had two procedures to clip a basilar trunk aneurysm but a small residual neck remained (Fig. 11.14 A, B). She returned seven years later with headache and signs of brain stem compression and now had a giant aneurysm from regrowth of the residual neck (Fig. 11.14 B, C). After the basilar clip stenosis there was miniflow through the stenosis with thrombosis of all but the base of the aneurysm (Fig. 11.14 D). In addition to the incomplete basilar clipping, a tourniquet had been placed on the left P1 and after creating a severe stenosis of this artery to prevent backflow, virtual complete thrombosis of the aneurysm occurred. The right P1 and SCA filled through the basilar stenosis while the left P1 and SCA filled via the left PComA (Fig. 11.13 E, F).

Three trappings proved fatal although two were in extremis with bulbar and hemi- or quadriparesis. One female, 54, done under deep hypothermia and bypass remained unchanged until demise four months later (C.N. in Fig. 11.1). The other man, 54, had a huge atherosclerotic fusiform aneurysm and worsened after left vertebral occlusion. Six days later, the aneurysm was trapped by right vertebral and upper basilar occlusion but he remained unresponsive until death three days later. The third patient had only headache with a severe ataxia but remained "locked-in" after bilateral intracranial vertebral clipping in spite of good PComAs. Upper basilar clipping and evacuation of the aneurysm did not prevent death two days later.

In these sacs of giant size, neck clipping is always difficult and in most cases impossible. The proximal or Hunterian ligation of the parent artery in these circumstances is an effective and usually safe alternate method of treatment in those patients coming electively to surgery. Trapping, while occasionally dramatically successful, had a high morbidity. The disappointing results in a few patients with complex lesions have made us cautious about attempting proximal vessel ligation in the immediate week following acute SAH. The high mortality for early operation in these cases suggests that the risk of delay may be acceptable. In the same way surgery on aged patients carries higher risks, and conservative management should be cautiously weighed.

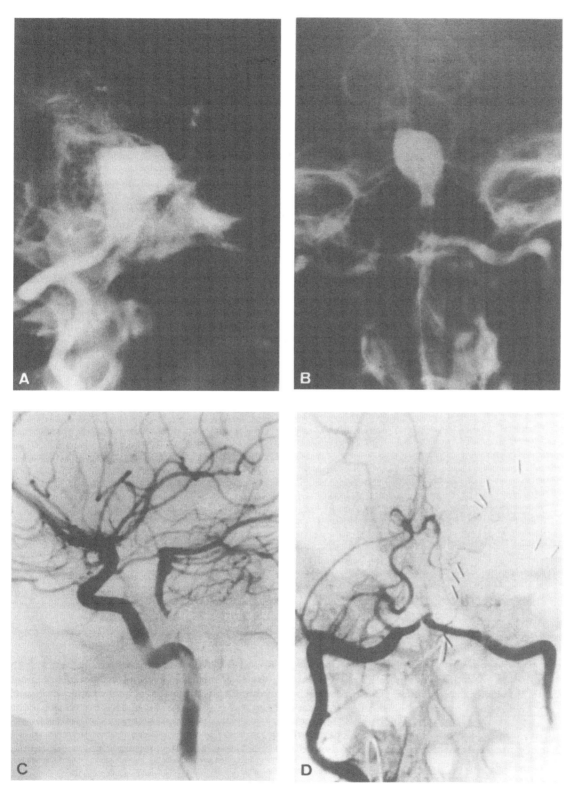

Figure 11.13 A–D. S.D., M, 17, ruptured giant basilar trunk aneurysm (**A, B**), in Grade 4 with bulbar palsy and quadriplegia. Tourniquet occlusion of lower basilar artery in February 1980 16 days after bleed followed by rapid partial recovery (**C**). Trapping and evacuation of aneurysm after basilar clip above one week later, virtual complete recovery (**D**). Excellent outcome

164 Giant Basilar Trunk Aneurysms

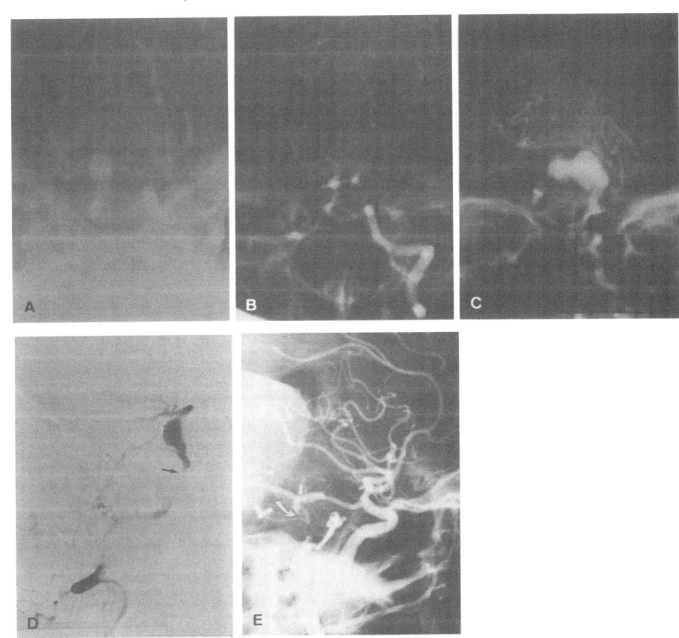

Figure 11.14 A–E. K.R., F, 45, ruptured small basilar trunk aneurysm clipped in 1978 16 days after bleed in Grade 1, with small residual neck (**A, B**), two procedures one month apart. Seven years later residual neck had expanded into giant partially thrombosed aneurysm with the clip on its apex (**C**). She had pseudobulbar signs and right hemiparesis. There was only one large posterior communicating artery which filled the aneurysm retrogradely so it was decided to stenose the basilar artery below by a clip and then P1 above by tourniquet. The aneurysm underwent massive thrombosis and there was miniflow through the basilar stenosis filling the right P1,P2 and SCA (**D**, arrow). The left P1 and SCA filled through the P1 stenosis (**E**, arrow). She became headache free but without early recovery of the brain stem compression. Good outcome

Table 11.1. Preoperative Grade and outcome in 59 patients with giant basilar trunk aneurysms

Grade	Excellent	Good	Poor	Dead	Total
0[a]	15	7	6	9	37
0g	*13*	*3*	*2*	*3*	*21*
0p	*2*	*4*	*4*	*6*	*16*
1	11	3	1	1	16
2		1			1
3	1	1	1		3
4				1	1
5				1	1
Total	27	12	8	12	59
	45.8%	20.3%	13.6%	20.3%	100.0%

[a] *0* Unruptured aneurysm or remote hemorrhage (> 1 year). *0g* Good risk without major neurological deficit. *0p* Poor risk patient with major neurological deficit (severe confusion or dementia or stupor or coma, dysarthria or bulbar paralysis, severe dysphasia or severe mono-, hemi-, or tetraparesis).

Table 11.2. Age related to outcome in 59 patients with giant basilar trunk aneurysms

Age group (years)	Excellent	Good	Poor	Dead	Total
0–9	1	1		1	3
10–19	10		1		11
20–29	5	3		1	9
30–39	6	2	1	2	11
40–49	1	3	2	2	8
50–59	3	2	4	2	11
60–69	1	1		4	6
Total	27	12	8	12	59

Table 11.3. Operative method and outcome in 59 patients with giant basilar trunk aneurysms

Operative method	Excellent	Good	Poor	Dead	Total
Neck clipping	3	4			7
Silk ligature	1				1
Wrapping	1				1
Hunterian ligation	19	10	3	7	39
Basilar clip	*12*	*3*	*2*	*2*	*19*
Basilart tourniquet	*4*	*2*		*4*[a]	*10*
Vertebral					
– one		*3*[b]			*3*
– both	*3*	*2*	*1*	*1*	*7*
Trapping	2	1	1	3	7
V-P Shunt	1				1
Explorative		1		2	3
Total	27	12	8	12	59

[a] In one case tourniquet not closed.
[b] Two had only one vertebral artery.

166 Giant Basilar Trunk Aneurysms

Table 11.4. Operative method and result of aneurysm treatment in 59 patients with giant basilar trunk aneurysms

Operative method	Total obliteration	Residual neck	Residual fundus	No obliteration	Not known	Total
Neck clipping	6		1			7
Silk ligature			1			1
Wrapping				1[a]		1
Hunterian ligation	28	1	9		1	39
Basilar a.	*22[b]*	*1*	*5*		*1*	*2*
1 Vertebral	*1*		*2*			
2 Vertebrals	*4*	*1*	*2*			*7*
Trapping	7					7
V-P shunt				1		1
Exploration only				3		3
Total	41	1	11	5	1	59

[a] Thrombosed later spontaneously totally.
[b] In one case tourniquet not closed.

Table 11.5. Timing of surgery and outcome in 22 patients with ruptured giant basilar trunk aneurysms

Timing of surgery	Excellent	Good	Poor	Dead	Total
0–1 day				1	1
4–6 day		2		2	4
7–10 day	3		1		4
11–30 day	5		1		6
31–365 day	4	3			7
Total	12	5	2	3	22

Chapter 12
Vertebral-Basilar Junction Aneurysms
77 Patients

Anatomical Features

Because intracranial saccular aneurysms ordinarily arise at the carina of a bifurcation on which the higher velocity, axial arterial stream impinges, it would seem incongruous for aneurysms to arise in the region of the union of the vertebral arteries that forms the basilar artery. What has been realized is that in most cases they do not arise at that carina projecting downward, but rather arise at the lower carina of a fenestration at the origin of the basilar artery, pointing upward. The occurrence of aneurysms at proximal carinae of fenestrations here at the basilar origin, on the mid-basilar, and on other arteries is compelling additional evidence for the hemodynamic factor in the origin of intracranial aneurysms. Even where a fenestration was not evident in the angiogram, small or even incomplete clefts have been recognized at operation. Fenestration was verified in X-rays or at operation in 32 cases, with increasing frequency in the last half of the time period. In five where one vertebral artery ended in PICA, the aneurysm seemed to arise on the side of the basilar artery where the vertebral union would have been.

We believe it is likely that a complete, or incomplete, fenestration exists at the origin of all vertebral-basilar junction aneurysms.

In 14, "butterfly" aneurysms existed, with one saccule pointing backward and the other forward. In several of the small aneurysms, it seemed that two separate aneurysms arose at the proximal fenestration (Figs. 12.1, 12.2). The larger ones were probably bilocular, but the locularity was not caused by pressure against the distal carina, for the upper portion of the fenestration was usually open.

One patient, in whom a large forward projecting sac had been clipped eight years before, had recurrent hemorrhage from a similar sac projecting backward. This may have arisen from a bit of neck left proximal to the clip on the other side of the proximal carina or perhaps there had been a tiny unseen separate saccule.

The aneurysm had its origin from a persistent hypoglossal artery in one patient (Fig. 12.3).

Clinical Features

Most patients had no localizing features. Transient or persisting sixth nerve palsy was seen in 10 and was bilateral in 7. CNV and CNVII palsies, dysarthria and conjugate gaze palsy were each seen once. Three patients had unilateral hearing loss, two patients unilateral CNIX-CNX paresis and two further patients CNXII affected unilaterally. Mild hemiparesis was seen in 10 patients. Severe hemiparesis in six patients was transient in four. Two patients were dysarthric. All patients operated on on the day or next day of recurrent bleedings were Grade 4 (Table 12.7).

Approach

The vertebral-basilar union usually overlies the junction of the lower and middle thirds of the clivus. Earlier this region was approached subtemporally through the tentorium but most were done through the lateral posterior fossa or the combined transpetrosal approach.

The subtemporal-transtentorial exposure is now seldom used unless another higher basilar aneurysm is to be obliterated too. The pontine retraction must be extended lower and just lateral to the origin of anterior-inferior cerebellar artery (AICA) and there is more manipulation of CNVII and CNVIII. Often the ipsilateral vertebral artery is seen under the filaments of CNX, but if the vertebral-basilar aneurysm is larger and projects forward (one-third of the cases), only glimpses of the opposite vertebral may be obtained until the neck is

168 Vertebral-Basilar Junction Aneurysms

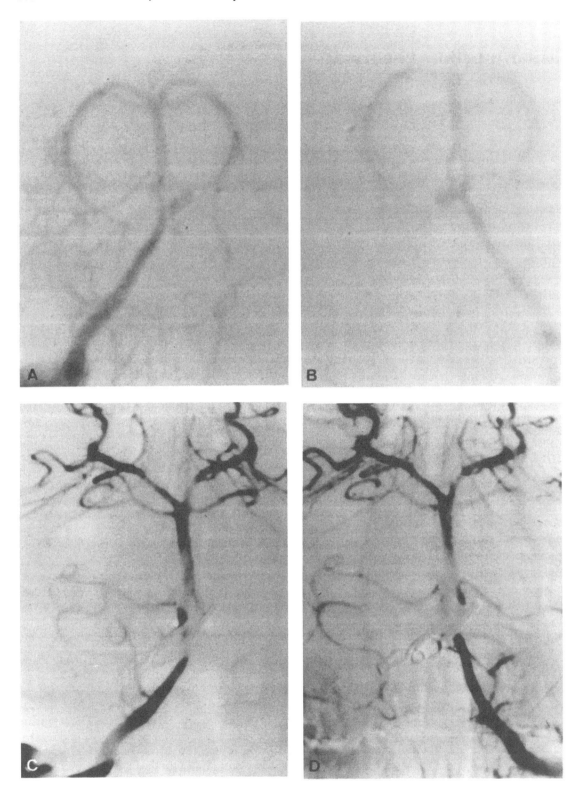

Figure 12.1 A–D. D.N., M, 22, ruptured small vertebrobasilar junction aneurysm, in Grade 1 after bleed. AP and oblique views to show bilateral ("butterfly") aneurysms arising at fenestration above V-B junction, left ruptured (**A, B**). Both aneurysms have been clipped through a right suboccipital approach 22 days after bleed in October 1985 (**C, D**). Outcome excellent

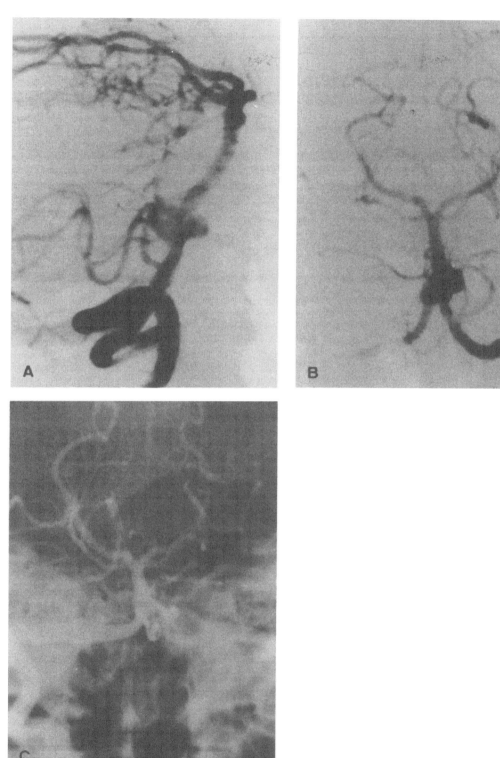

Figure 12.2 A–C. M.B., F, 30, ruptured large "butterfly" vertebrobasilar junction aneurysm at fenestration above V-B junction (**A, B**). Clipping of both aneurysms 13 days after bleed in Grade 1. Fenestration seen best in postoperative AP view (**C**)

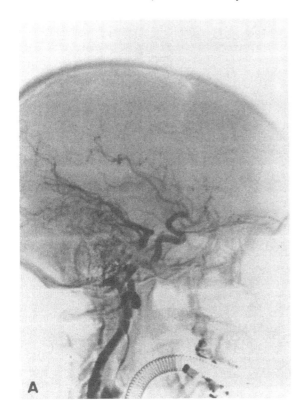 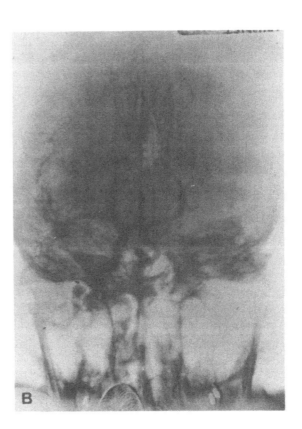

Figure 12.3 A, B. T.H., F, 52, lateral and AP of basilar artery origin from primitive hypoglossal artery with aneurysm arising at or near the origin of the basilar artery (**A, B**). This 13 months earlier ruptured small aneurysm was completely wrapped in cottonoid in November 1967 and she has remained well for over 25 years

clipped. The rewards of temporary clipping are such that it is imperative that both vertebral arteries are easily available, if need be, by exposure on either side of the medulla.

That 10 of the first 14 aneurysms were approached transtentorially was because of early experience suboccipitally, where the jugular tubercle seemed to obstruct the midline exposure of the lower third of the clivus with the overlying medulla and lower cranial nerves. With experience, however, this promontory can be bypassed by a more lateral angle so that virtually all later vertebral-basilar junction aneurysms are done by the lateral suboccipital approach (59 of 77 in this series) (Illustration 14.VIII, p. 202 and Fig. 12.4). The greatest care must be taken not to injure the medullary filaments of CNXI for, arising from the nucleus ambiguus, injury of even one will result in dysphagia and dysarthria. Fortunately, this distressing and dangerous complication is rarely persistent, although a temporary tracheostomy may be required.

The "park bench" position has been used routinely for the lateral posterior fossa approach (Illustration 14.VIII, A, p. 202). It allows the surgeon to sit, while giving a nice angle for the dissection alongside, then under the brain stem. It reduces the risks of air embolism and allows a combined subtemporal-transtentorial or transmastoid-transpetrosal exposure, if necessary.

The lateral suboccipital approach is satisfactory for most vertebral-basilar and vertebral-PICA aneurysms that underlie the medulla. An inverted midline "hockey stick" incision usually allows a generous lateral suboccipital craniectomy that exposes the medial edge of the sigmoid sinus. The horizontal limb of the incision should stop just short of the occipital nerves to preserve sensation in the scalp above. The paramedian "S" incision is satisfactory too, although the occipital nerves cannot always be saved (Illustration 14.VIII, B, p. 202). Removal of the foramen magnum is done for identification of the origins of the vertebral arteries on

Vertebral-Basilar Junction Aneurysms 171

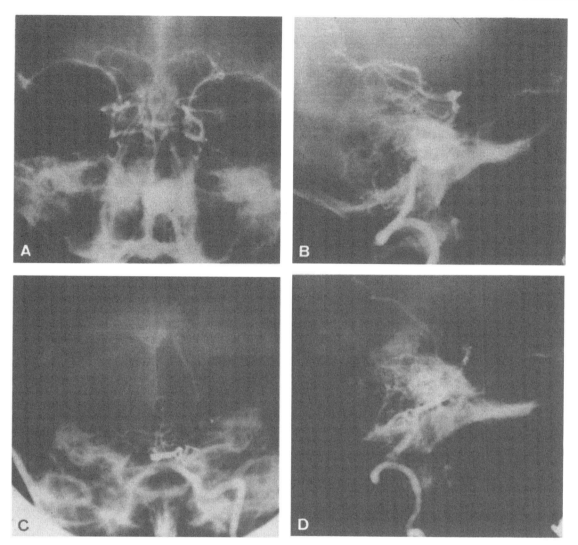

Figure 12.4 A–D. D.G., F, 35, ruptured large vertebrobasilar junction aneurysm (**A, B**). Suboccipital clipping (16 mm Drake clip) of aneurysm 11 days after bleed in Grade 2 in February 1977 (**C, D**). Postoperatively lethargic with weak left arm and hand and right leg. Good outcome

both sides for bilateral temporary clipping. The temporary clip on the opposite vertebral can be left in place until neck clipping is completed, using brief periods of ipsilateral vertebral clipping when desired to slacken off the aneurysm.

The cerebellum is made slack by opening the cistern. Its elevation with the retractor at the base of the tonsil exposes the lateral medulla, the vertebral artery as it emerges from under the first dentate ligament, the caudal loop of PICA and then the lower cranial nerves CNXII, CNXI with its tiny important filaments that arise from the medulla, and the lower filaments of CNX (Illustration 14.VIII, C, p. 202). Rarely, when the vertebral-basilar (V-B) junction or vertebral aneurysm is unusually high, it is necessary to separate CNX and CNIX from the flocculus and choroid tuft at the foramen of Luschka, so that the exposure of the aneurysm is between CNIX and CNVIII.

The vertebral artery is followed upward and medially to where it disappears under the medulla. The remainder of the exposure under the medulla usually can be done just below CNX or between the medullary filaments of CNXI. The importance of recognition and preservation of these filaments from the nucleus ambiguus cannot be overemphasized. Fortunately, they are not tense, and are attenuated enough to allow dissection in between with

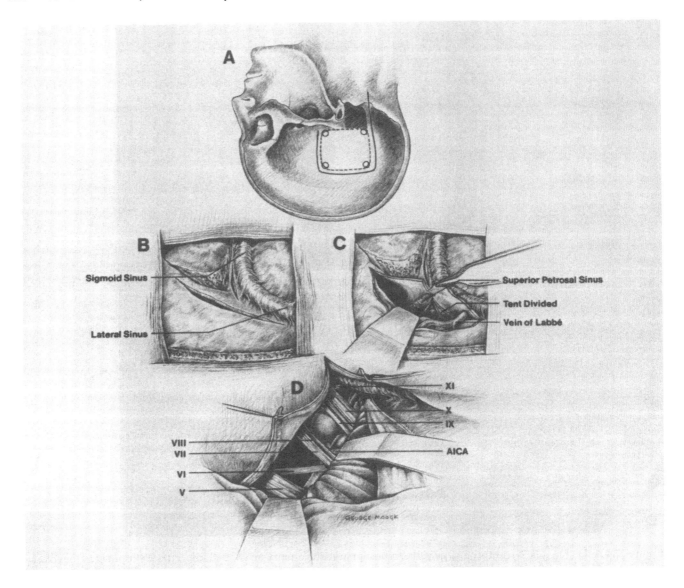

12.VII. The transmastoid transpetrosal approach which avoids the hazards of lateral or sigmoid sinus division, provides similar excellent exposure of the mid and lower basilar artery to the vertebrobasilar junction. **A** A posterior temporal craniotomy is combined with a lateral suboccipital craniectomy which exposes the lateral sinus. **B** The confluens and sigmoid sinus are skeletonized by removal of the posterior two-thirds of the mastoid and the outer petrous ridge which should expose 5–10 mms of the presigmoid dura so that sutures can be placed for water tight closure, even though the mastoid air cells are waxed. **C** Through a temporal dural opening the insertion of the vein of Labbé into the lateral sinus *behind* the confluens must be verified. **D** The presigmoid dura is opened to glimpse the anterolateral cerebellum and this incision and that completely dividing the tentorium are carried as near as possible to the insertion of the superior petrosal sinus into the confluens. The trifoliate leaf of dura containing this sinus is then divided using clips or ligatures. This mobilizes the sigmoid and lateral with their confluence for retraction posteriorly with the anterolateral cerebellum for wide exposure of the angle. As the approach is centred on the bundle of CNVII and CNVII nerves, great care with retraction must be exercised to avoid their injury since the basilar artery must be exposed either above or below them. Shown here is the initial exposure of a vertebrobasilar junction aneurysm arising at a fenestration. In adhering to the principle of clipping in the long axis of the parent artery, the clip on many of these aneurysms had to be placed from below using an angled clip applier worked under the fibres of CNX and directed rostrally. – It is wise to prepare for prevention and control of inadvertent rupture of the aneurysm by visualization of a segment of each vertebral artery below. Usually both can be seen in this field but if not, consideration should be given to exposure of the opposite artery beside the medulla by extending the incision and suboccipital craniectomy to the midline

Vertebral-Basilar Junction Aneurysms   173

gentle manipulation. The side of the approach to the V-B junction varies with the size and direction of the aneurysm. The right is preferred if the sac points primarily forward or backward, but if laterally projecting and not large enough to obscure the neck, then an approach on the dome side is preferred. This is usually quite safe with temporary bilateral vertebral clipping, although dissecting an unusually adherent aneurysm from the medulla can be interesting (16 cases had a backward projection). A large lateral aneurysm may have to be approached from the other side when the dome obscures the neck ipsilaterally, when provision for bilateral suboccipital craniectomy, sitting or prone, should be made. Although awkward, it is possible to free and clip the neck working across the V-B junction (Fig. 12.4). Temporary trapping with another clip on the basilar artery above has been used in trying situations.

Sometimes it is quite simple to expose the vertebral artery junction when the retroclival space is wide. But in others, the medulla seems plastered over the arteries against the clivus. Here the angle of attack narrows sharply and to get better line of sight to the V-B junction region, the "far lateral" subcerebellar exposure is helpful. This uses retraction that begins far out on the anteroinferior aspect of the cerebellum near or at the sigmoid sinus, gradually displacing the cerebellum out of the lower lateral posterior fossa.

Removal of the lateral rim of the foramen magnum and posterior third of the condyle has not been used, although it should increase the exposure. At first, as with transtentorial pontine retraction, the inexperienced surgeon will feel that there is just not enough room to get under the brain stem to the V-B junction. But with patience, suction and gentle retraction of the medulla using a narrow dissector between CNXI filaments, the medulla can be displaced gradually to open the region so that the vertebral artery can be followed to the union and the aneurysm. In difficult exposures, spontaneous breathing is often used as the best guide to retractor pressure and medullary ischemia.

Clipping can be awkward in the narrow exposure, in that the clip applier jaws and the clip handle, which must be worked in between the CNXI filaments safely, then obscure the view of the aneurysm neck. Often it is a matter of using the lowest profile applier and moving the angle of the

microscope upward or downward so as to see more of the clip blades. Or, if the clip applier can be guided below or between the lower filaments of CNXI, then the advance of the clip blades can be seen more clearly, including their positioning over the aneurysm neck. Further, application more along the axis of the basilar artery is less likely to leave tags of neck or "dog-ears" which might lead to recurrence. The upper portion of the fenestration is usually quite evident. For backward projecting sacs, even though the origin of the neck is at a fenestration, one or more perforators may arise here and must be searched for and preserved if present. In several cases where the origin of the neck at the fenestration was quite expanded, taking one limb of the fenestration with the blades made the clipping more complete. With large aneurysms, one vertebral artery may be included in the clip on the neck to simplify the procedure (Fig. 12.5).

Pricking the sac with the stylet of a 22 gauge needle should indicate whether the clipping is complete after which needle aspiration can collapse the sac for more detailed inspection. If the clip needs to be replaced, bleeding from a needle hole in the sac will always stop with suction over a tiny patty, so that re-application can be done in a dry field.

Recently more use has been made of the transmastoid-transpetrosal approach (5 cases) for the large or complex V-B aneurysms and second attempts (Illustration 12.VII). It provides wider exposure while avoiding division of the lateral or sigmoid sinuses. Division of these sinuses, especially on the right carries major risk unless there is sure knowledge that the confluens is widely patent. The transpetrosal approach avoids this hazard and provides nearly the same exposure. The posterior limb of the incision for a small posterior temporal bone flap is carried down over the mid suboccipital region so that a lateral suboccipital craniotomy can be combined with the temporal flap to uncover the lateral sinus. If there is any doubt about the ease with which the contralateral vertebral artery may be seen for temporary clipping under the brain stem, then this incision should be curved over to the midline so that, after removal of foramen magnum and C1 lamina, the opposite vertebral artery may be freed for temporary clipping beside the medulla. Removal of the posterior half to two-thirds of the mastoid and outer lateral petrous apex will uncover the sigmoid sinus, its confluence with the lateral

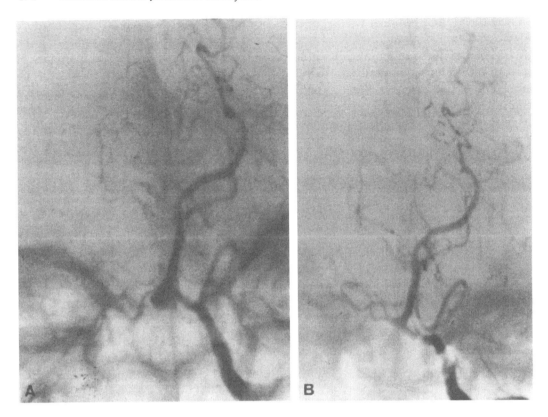

Figure 12.5 A, B. J.V., F, 31, ruptured large partially thrombosed vertebrobasilar junction aneurysm (**A**). Subtemporal transtentorial clipping of aneurysm 26 days after bleed in Grade 1 in June 1977, clipping of neck and small right vertebral artery (**B**). Outcome excellent

sinus and enough of the presigmoid dura so that tight dural closure is possible to prevent cerebral spinal fluid (CSF) leakage into the mastoid cells (Illustration 12.VII B). The dural sheath of the sigmoid sinus is extremely thin and fragile and must be carefully preseparated as the overlying bony canal is removed. Small tears can be repaired with pin sutures.

The tentorium is completely divided a centimeter or so behind the petrous ridge to near the end of the superior petrosal sinus. The dural opening in the presigmoid dura is carried up to the same point so that the petrosal sinus can be divided after clipping or ligature. This frees the confluence so that it and the adjacent lateral and sigmoid sinus can be retracted posteriorly with the anterolateral cerebellum for wide exposure of the angle. A virtual prerequisite to this approach is that the vein of Labbé enters the lateral sinus *behind* the confluence. When it enters the dura over the lateral petrous apex, it may be spared by separation of the dural slip containing it from the floor of the skull over to the lateral sinus. The exposure is centered on the seventh and eighth cranial nerves so that the basilar artery must be exposed above or below this nerve bundle. Even so, the whole of the basilar artery from near its apex to the V-B junction can be seen and usually both terminal vertebral arteries for temporary clip control.

Results

Methods other than neck clipping were: packing 4, single vertebral occlusion 1, bilateral vertebral occlusion 1, basilar occlusion 1 and trapping 1. One was explored only since clipping produced apnea – she rebled one week later and died. Three early cases were packed in gauze including the aneurysm with the hypoglossal artery origin. Remarkably, this patient and one other have remained well for over 20 years. The third remained dysphasic and finally died from the consequences of a postoperative extradural clot. A more recent packing was over a ruptured bleb on a hard yellow fusiform aneurysm.

The vertebral artery was occluded once under a large bilocular sac whose origin at a fenestration could not be seen clearly. The other vertebral was tiny and the aneurysm thrombosed except for a millimeter of its base.

Another man arrived with one vertebral clipped. Postoperative scarring prevented adequate visualization of the aneurysm and the other vertebral was balloon occluded at the atlas without consequence.

For another small bilobular sac, the lower limbs of the fenestration (and thus the basilar artery) were occluded at their origin uneventfully, when it proved not possible to clip both lobules.

Failure to prepare *both* vertebral arteries for temporary clipping resulted in two poor results from rupture of one small and one large aneurysms before complete dissection. The large aneurysm had to be trapped by bilateral vertebral and basilar occlusions when premature and uncontrollable rupture occurred at the neck before the opposite vertebral artery was prepared for a temporary clip. A poor outcome resulted from bulbar paresis and hemiplegia. Premature rupture before exposure accounted for another poor result when temporary trapping had to be used during extreme hypotension from blood loss. Poor grade accounted for the other bad outcomes. One death after uneventful clipping of an intact V-B junction aneurysm resulted from operative rupture of a large (and ruptured) associated basilar bifurcation aneurysm when that clip occluded the opposite P1.

Clips slipped completely off three large aneurysms which had been needled and collapsed. Two survived the rebleeding and reclipping but the other died on day three.

One death occurred from avulsion of an adherent middle cerebral branch when the bone flap was raised with torn adherent dura and in spite of evacuation of a huge Sylvian clot. The aneurysm was not approached (in Table 12.6 classified as exploration only).

Table 12.1. Preoperative Grade and outcome in 77 patients with small and large VB junction aneurysms

Grade	Excellent	Good	Poor	Dead	Total
0	3		1		4
1	38	4	2	1	45
2	11	3	3	3	20
3	1	3			4
4		2	1	1	4
Total	53	12	7	5	77
	68.8%	15.6%	9.1%	6.5%	100.0%

Table 12.2. Aneurysm size and outcome in 77 patients with small and large VB junction aneurysms

Size	Excellent	Good	Poor	Dead	Total
Small	36	5	4	1	46
Large	17	7	3	4	31
Total	53	12	7	5	77

Vertebral-Basilar Junction Aneurysms

Table 12.3. Known fenestration and outcome in 77 patients with small and large VB junction aneurysms

Site	Excellent	Good	Poor	Dead	Total
No fenestration	31	4	5	4	44
Fenestration	21	8	2	1	32
Hypoglossal artery	1				1
Total	53	12	7	5	77

Table 12.4. Age related to outcome in 77 patients with small and large VB junction aneurysms

Age group (years)	Excellent	Good	Poor	Dead	Total
10–19	1				1
20–29	13	1		1	15
30–39	15	4	1		20
40–49	8	1	1	1	11
50–59	14	4	3	3	24
60–69	2	2	1		5
70 or more			1		1
Total	53	12	7	5	77

Table 12.5. Operative method and outcome in 77 patients with small and large VB junction aneurysms

Operative method	Excellent	Good	Poor	Dead	Total
Clip	50	10	4	3	67
Wrapping	1	1	2		4
Hunterian ligation	2	1			3
Trapping			1		1
Exploration only				2	2
Total	53	12	7	5	77

Table 12.6. Operative method and result of aneurysm treatment in 77 patients with small and large VB junction aneurysms

Operative method	Total obliteration	Residual neck	Residual fundus	No obliteration	Total
Clip	53	12	2		67
Wrapping				4	4
Hunterian ligation	3				3
Trapping	1				1
Exploration only				2	2
Total	57	12	2	6	77

Table 12.7. Timing of surgery and outcome in 73 patients with small and large VB junction aneurysms

Timing of surgery	Excellent	Good	Poor	Dead	Total
0–1 day		1	1	1	3
2–3 day	2	3			5
4–6 day	5				5
7–10 day	5	1			6
11–30 day	22	5	3	4	34
31–365 day	16	2	2		20
Total	50	12	6	5	73

Chapter 13

Giant Vertebrobasilar Junction Aneurysms
39 Patients

Thirty-nine giant aneurysms arose at the vertebral-basilar (V-B) junction. Twelve were illustrated and described previously (Fig. 13.1). Most probably had their origins from small aneurysms which usually arise at the proximal crotch of a fenestration at the beginning of the basilar artery. That the fenestration was seldom seen in angiograms was presumably because the expansion of the necks of these masses would obliterate the fenestration, although in three the remnant of the fenestration could be seen in the angiogram and/or at operation. Two patients had only one vertebral artery, the other ending in posterior-inferior cerebellar artery (PICA). In nine cases, the aneurysm was obviously fusiform, probably having origin from an unknown arteriopathy.

Most patients presented with headache and mass effect featuring varying degrees of bulbar (14), hemi- or quadriparesis with ataxia (13). Less than half (19) patients had no cranial nerve deficits. Two patients had oculomotor palsy, the one with severe hemiparesis (Weber's syndrome). Eight patients had trigeminal affection, in three of them bilaterally. Sixth nerve paresis was seen in six patients. Cerebellopontine angle syndromes were frequent (14) with varying involvement of CNV through CNIX and CNX. A few patients had accessory (3) or hypoglossal (4) nerve affected. Two had papilledema with hydrocephalus and one each had hemifacial spasm, sleep apnea and transient attacks of hemiparesis. Six were recognized only after recent subarachnoid hemorrhage (SAH) and in five others with mass effect, there was a recent (2) or remote (3) history of bleeding. Those patients with remote bleeding are graded as unruptured aneurysms (Table 13.1).

Treatment

In two patients, both in very poor condition, the aneurysm was only explored. The first then refused vertebral artery occlusion in the neck and the other who had been quadriplegic was discharged in a comatose state.

The neck of the aneurysm could be clipped only in eight patients using multiple tandem clips in two (Table 13.4). Suboccipital exposure was used in three, subtemporal-transtentorial in three and the combined transmastoid-transpetrosal in two. Four had good outcomes (Fig. 13.2). An early case, a man 36, from overseas, was unchanged from his preoperative hemiplegia although the aneurysm was evacuated but he remained ambulatory for five years. Even though the clip deliberately occluded the larger right vertebral as well, a stump of the neck remained filling from the left which enlarged to another mass which caused his death six years later. In retrospect, an attempt at occlusion of the second vertebral artery should have been advised. The other poor result was a tetraparetic lady, 46, who had uneventful tandem clipping after temporary trapping but who became "locked in" 12 hours after operation. The aneurysm was occluded but the clip had caused severe basilar artery stenosis.

The two who died were also well postoperatively for 12 hours before suddenly becoming "locked in" from brain stem infarction. In one, the V-B junction was occluded by the clipping but presumably tolerated until strangely, retrograde thrombosis of the left vertebral artery back to C2 occurred. In the other, a severe basilar artery stenosis had been produced by the clip.

178 Giant Vertebrobasilar Junction Aneurysms

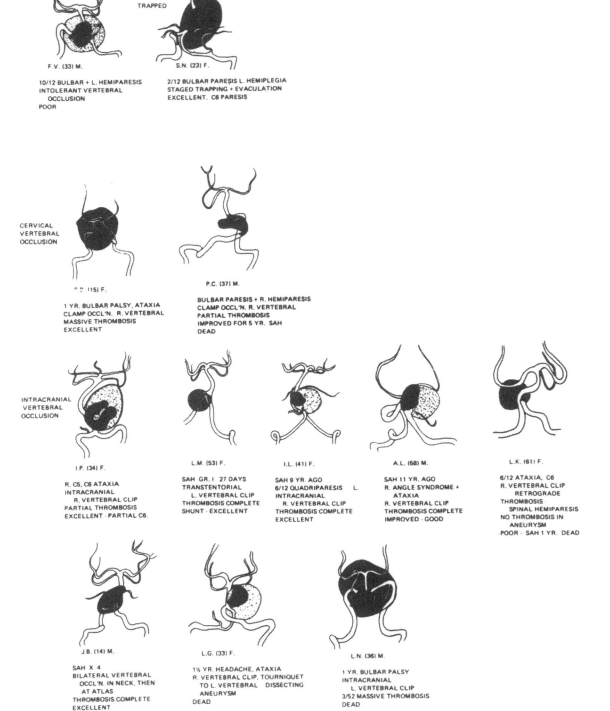

Figure 13.1. The origin, size and shape of giant vertebrobasilar junction aneurysms and the extent of their mural thrombosis described and illustrated by tracings in the early experience. (Reprinted from Clin Neurosurg 26, 1979, pp. 86 by courtesy of Williams and Wilkins).

Giant Vertebrobasilar Junction Aneurysms 179

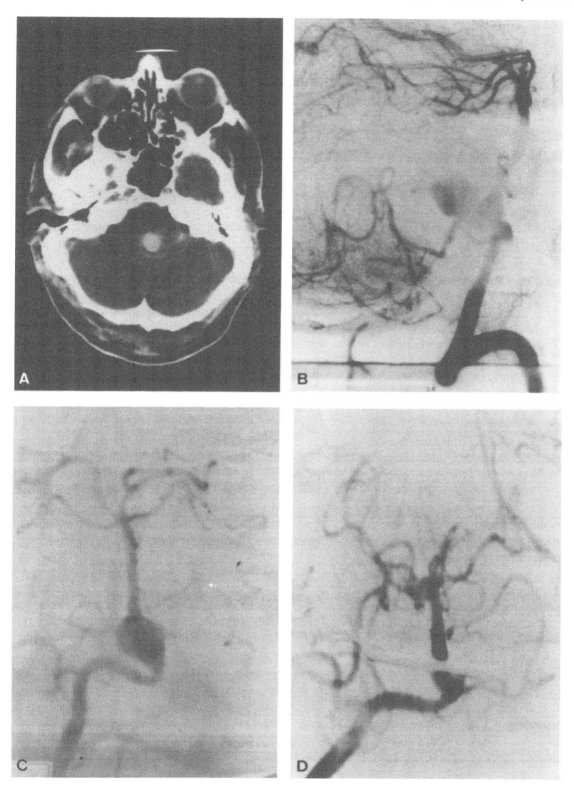

Figure 13.2 A–D. R.E., M, 51, giant partially thrombosed vertebrobasilar junction aneurysm (**A–C**), headache, ataxia, dysphagia, also Charcot-Marie-Tooth disease. After suboccipital temporary clip trapping and evacuation in April 1984, a single long clip occluded the neck of the aneurysm (**D**). Outcome excellent

180 Giant Vertebrobasilar Junction Aneurysms

Vertebral Artery Occlusion

Twenty-seven patients were treated by proximal vertebral artery occlusion in the neck or intracranially or in combination; unilateral in 11 and bilateral in 16.

Unilateral Vertebral Occlusion

Two early cases had Selverstone clamp occlusion of the dominant vertebral artery in the neck. The aneurysm, in a girl, 14, with bulbar paresis, ataxia and severe opisthotonus, thrombosed nearly completely and after posterior fossa bony decompression she has remained well for 21 years (Fig. 13.3). The other man, 37, remained good for only a year with partial thrombosis of the sac before deteriorating with recurrence of right hemiplegia- anesthesia and bulbar paresis. He died suddenly two years later from rupture of the aneurysm (P.C. in Fig. 13.1).

Eleven patients had intracranial clip occlusion of the dominant vertebral artery intracranially above PICA. In two, only one vertebral formed the basilar artery (Fig. 13.4). Both aneurysms became completely occluded. One remains well; the other was worse after a transtentorial attempt to trap and evacuate the mass by basilar occlusion above which was abandoned when anterior-inferior cerebellar artery (AICA) was found arising from the very top of the sac and was known to fill by retrograde flow back down the basilar artery. He was "locked in" postoperatively.

Five of the nine patients with occlusion of one of two vertebral arteries had good outcomes with complete or virtually complete thrombosis in all. The four bad results had incomplete thrombosis. In one hypertensive woman, 61, with hard severely atherosclerotic arteries, the clipped right vertebral thrombosed retrogradely down to C6, causing a spinal hemiplegia on the third day. She died two years later from rupture of the open sac (L.K. in Fig. 13.1).

Three patients died. The first with severe bulbar paresis and papilledema was well for three weeks after posterior fossa decompression and left vertebral occlusion. Nine hours after only a transtentorial exploration when trapping was abandoned he suddenly became "locked in" and died two days later. Angiography revealed massive thrombosis of the sac and a long segment of the involved basilar artery, even though only one vertebral was occluded.

The second death was tragic in a severely hypertensive woman, 33, with a renal artery bypass for fibromuscular dysplasia (L.G. in Fig. 13.1). After clipping the terminal right vertebral, a tourniquet was placed on the left artery but left open. Two days later after an episode of auricular fibrillation and hypotension (80/60), she became "locked in" but recovered with artificial hypertension to systolic 160. A brief recurrence two days later was without known hypotension. Then the recovery room physician, concerned about her severe hypertension, used antihypertensive agents. On the sixth day, a third recurrence was aborted in 10 minutes by again allowing her hypertension to return but 24 hours later in spite of these experiences she lapsed into irreversible deep coma on a nitroprusside drip. She had good posterior communicating arteries (PComAs) but the left vertebral artery had been shown postoperatively to be severely stenosed intracranially. At autopsy there was a dissecting aneurysm of this artery presumably produced by practice occlusion of the snare (Fig. 6.14). She obviously needed her hypertension for brain stem perfusion. The third death was a deaf-mute bedridden with severe ataxia. Except for more dysphagia he was unchanged for four days when the aneurysm, shown to be massively thrombosed, ruptured twice.

Bilateral Vertebral Occlusion

Ordinarily, for bilateral vertebral occlusion, the terminal dominant vertebral artery was clipped at intracranial exploration. The site and method of occlusion of the other artery varied with the deemed extent of the PComA collateral determined angiographically; intracranially by clip or tourniquet beyond PICA, in the neck by Selverstone clamp or detached balloon at the atlas on or in its lower cervical segment. Selverstone clamp occlusion of the artery near its origin was used when PComA collateral was marginal or not visible. Refilling of the artery above the clamp from deep cervical collateral but with reduced flow in the aneurysm might provide for brain stem perfusion, yet promote thrombosis in the aneurysm.

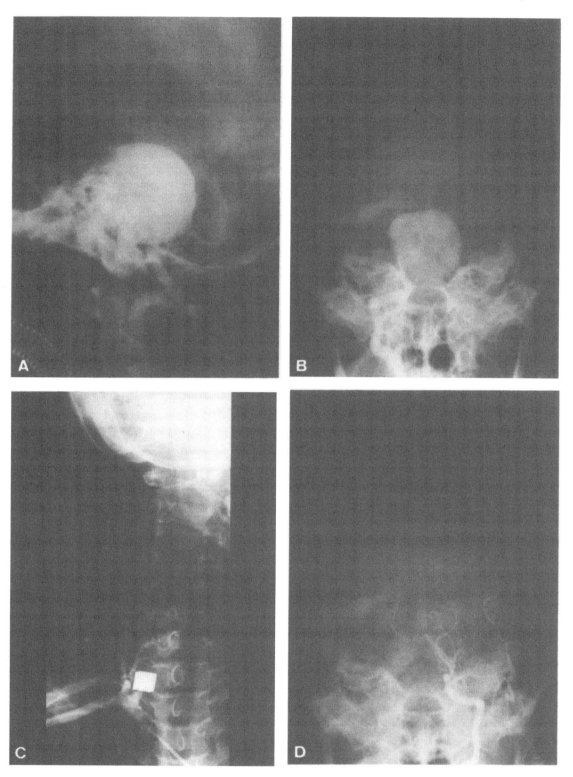

Figure 13.3 A–D. P.B., F, 14, giant vertebrobasilar junction aneurysm (**A, B**), one year headache, vomiting, bulbar palsy, ataxia and severe opisthotonus. After Selverstone clamp occlusion of the right vertebral in April 1971 (**C**), there was only a tiny portion of the thrombosed aneurysm filling from the left (**D**). Following suboccipital bony decompression to relieve the mass effect she made a complete recovery and 23 years later is raising a family. Outcome excellent

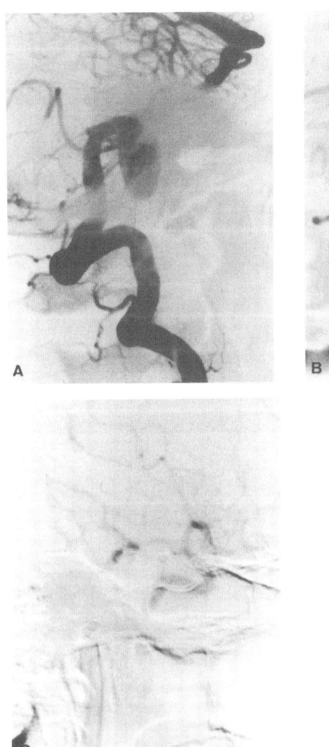
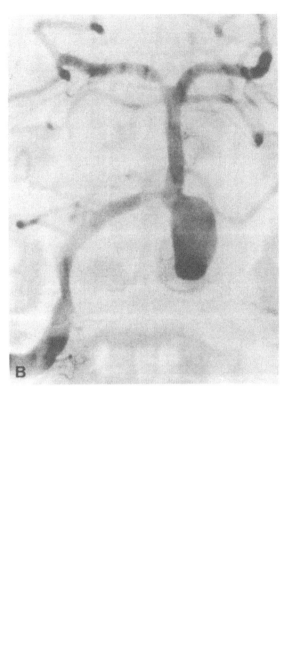

Figure 13.4 A–C. M.F., F, 56, giant vertebrobasilar junction aneurysm, only one vertebral artery (**A, B**), headache, bilateral facial numbness and paraesthesia, bulbar paresis. After terminal vertebral clipping in April 1982, aneurysm thrombosed and there was excellent basilar artery filling from the carotids (**C**). Outcome excellent

One boy, 15, had bilateral Selverstone vertebral artery occlusion four months apart. Reconstitution of the right vertebral artery from deep cervical collaterals caused continued enlargement of the aneurysm and the artery was clip occluded uneventfully at the atlas (Fig. 13.5).

Five patients, all with one or two large PComAs had simultaneous clip occlusion of both terminal vertebral arteries (Fig. 13.6); in another it was possible to place one clip just above the union of the vertebral arteries (Fig. 13.7), all had good outcomes with complete thrombosis of the aneurysm.

A woman, 50, with hemifacial spasm had clip occlusion of the left vertebral artery and the tourniquet only placed on the right artery. She was relieved of her facial spasms but the right vertebral was found to be occluded at the tourniquet site in postoperative studies, presumably by inadvertent closure in bringing the stem out the back of her neck (Fig. 13.8).

Five patients had intracranial clip occlusion of one artery followed by Selverstone clamp occlusion of the other in the neck. Four had good outcomes with complete thrombotic occlusion of the aneurysm (Fig. 13.9). In the poor result, a woman 60, with SAH and tiny PComAs the vertebral artery was refilled above the clamp by deep cervical collateral refilling the lower third of the aneurysm. She had developed some dysphagia, mild right leg weakness and ataxia after clipping the left vertebral and a medial rectus palsy after the clamp occlusion. She claims to be disabled although she leads an active life with diplopia and mild leg paresis.

Two patients had the second vertebral occluded by detached balloon at the sulcus arteriosus of the atlas. A woman, 58, had right hemiparesis, severe ataxia, and dysphagia with CNVII, CNIX, CNX and CNXII palsies. After the first vertebral clipping she required a tracheostomy for worsening of the bulbar paresis but after the balloon occlusion of the second artery the aneurysm thrombosed. At re-operation, the mass was reduced with partial evacuation of the thrombus. Her hemiparesis became mild and in spite of the dysphagia she leads an active life.

In the other severely disabled patient, the aneurysm re-ruptured 12 hours after the detached balloon occlusion of the second vertebral and she died after the family refused re-exploration and evacuation of the sac. The second death was in a 46 year old male, two and half months after clipping of the right vertebral and failed tourniquet occlusion of left vertebral artery because of respiratory arrest and temporary quadriparesis during two attempts.

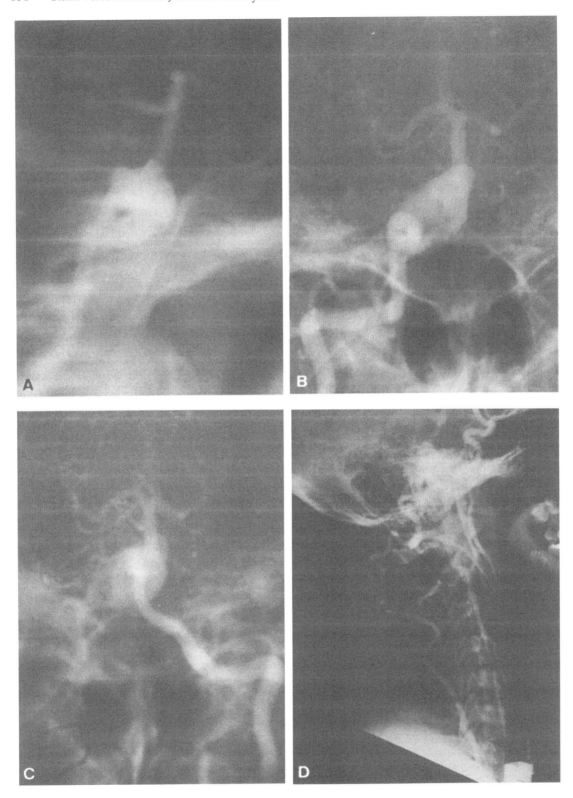

Figure 13.5 A–D

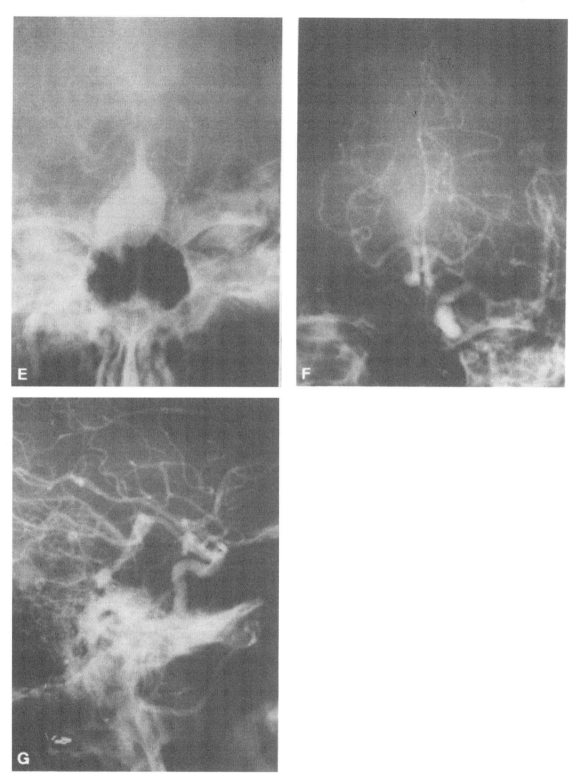

Figure 13.5 E–G

Figure 13.5 A–G. J.B., M, 15, ruptured giant vertebrobasilar junction aneurysm, three bleeds, Grade 1. Lateral (**A**) and AP (**B, C**) views of each vertebral artery filling giant aneurysm. Bilateral Selverstone clamp occlusion of the vertebral arteries in 1970 four months apart. Four months later the right vertebral artery had been reconstituted (**D**) by deep cervical collateral and was filling an enlarged aneurysm (**E**). Bilateral vertebral artery occlusion at sulcus in atlas produced complete thrombosis of aneurysm except for its apex giving rise to AICAs (**F, G**). Outcome excellent over 20 years (now an orthopedic surgeon!)

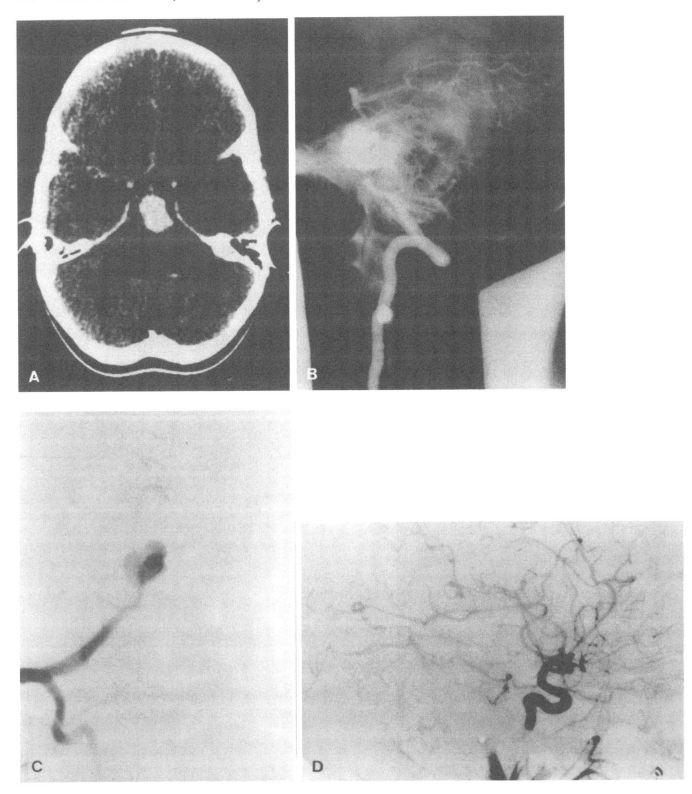

Figure 13.6 A–D. O.C., F, 57, ruptured giant vertebrobasilar junction aneurysm (**A–C**). Transmastoid transpetrosal clipping of both vertebral arteries in December 1982 seven weeks after bleed in Grade 1. The basilar artery is filled by both carotids down through AICAs to the thrombosed aneurysm (**D**). Outcome excellent

Giant Vertebrobasilar Junction Aneurysms 187

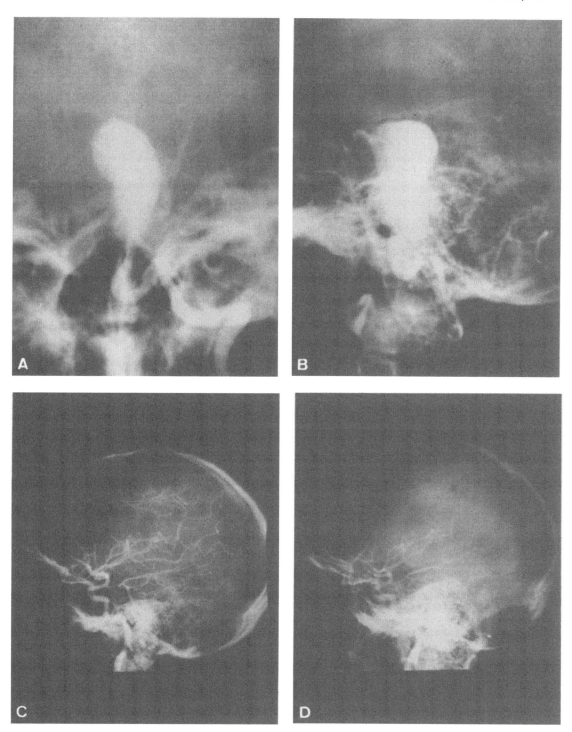

Figure 13.7 A–D. N.P., F, 25, giant vertebrobasilar junction aneurysm (**A, B**), six months headache, ataxia, left hemiparesis and dysphagia. Clip occlusion of the origin of the basilar artery in January 1973. A stormy postoperative course with immediate bulbar and quadriparesis. The left carotid fills the whole of the basilar artery down through AICAs (**C, D**). There was virtual complete recovery over several months except for a husky voice. Outcome excellent

188 Giant Vertebrobasilar Junction Aneurysms

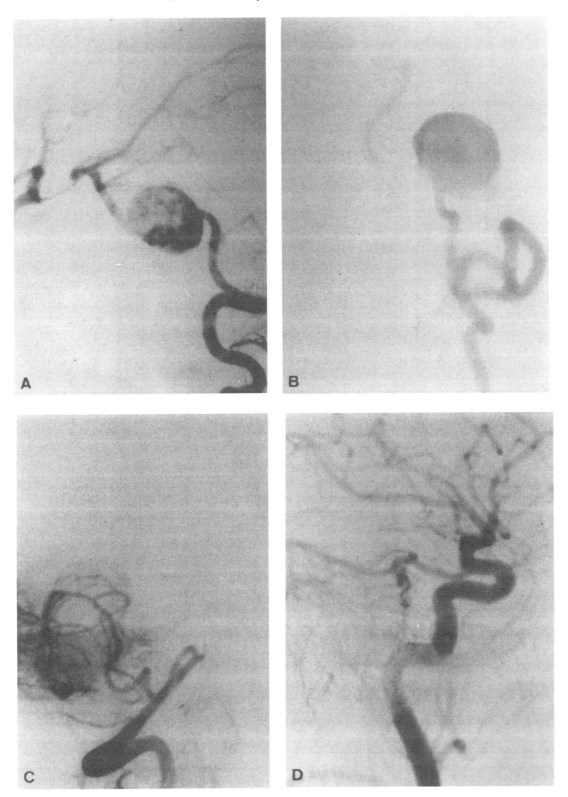

Figure 13.8 A–D. P.B., F, 50, intact giant vertebrobasilar junction aneurysm (**A, B**), two years hemifacial spasm. Clip occlusion of the terminal left vertebral, tourniquet occlusion of terminal right vertebral artery in January 1986 (**C**). Complete occlusion of aneurysm and excellent basilar artery filling down through AICAs (**D**). The hemifacial spasm diminished immediately and was relieved completely within a month and has remained so for 8 years

Giant Vertebrobasilar Junction Aneurysms   189

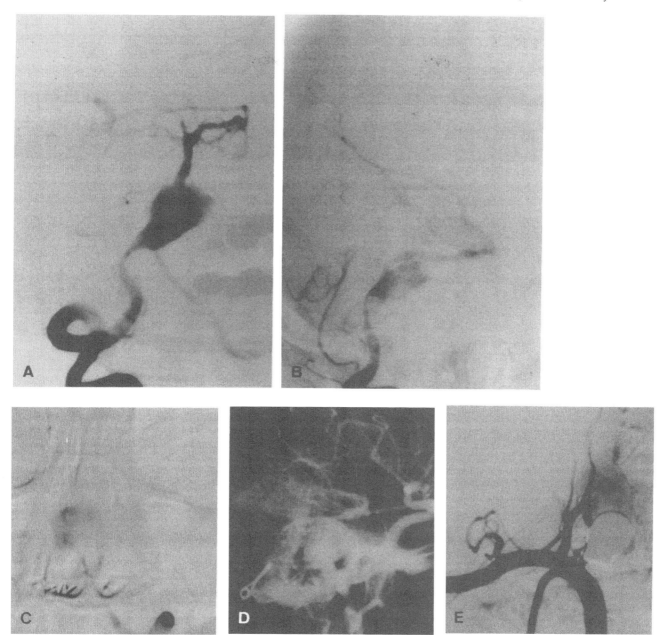

Figure 13.9 A–E. F.M.,F, 57, ruptured partially thrombosed giant vertebrobasilar junction aneurysm (**A, B**). At suboccipital craniotomy, 45 days after bleed in Grade 1, in November 1981 the left vertebral was clipped but she had respiratory arrest after 10 seconds of temporary right vertebral occlusion. Therefore the right vertebral was Selverstone clamp occluded so that its reconstitution from deep cervical collateral would provide enough flow to irrigate the medulla (**C, D**). The aneurysm underwent complete thrombosis while the right carotid artery filled the entire basilar artery (**E**). Outcome excellent

190 Giant Vertebrobasilar Junction Aneurysms

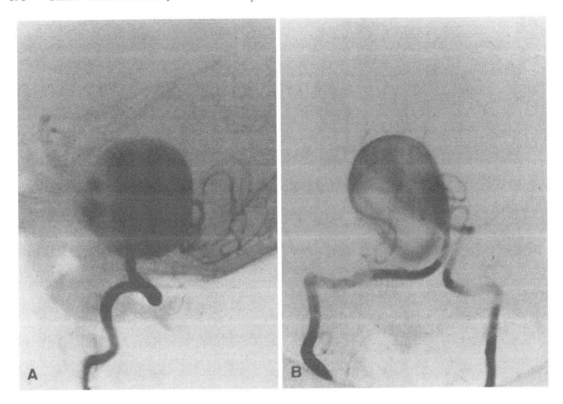

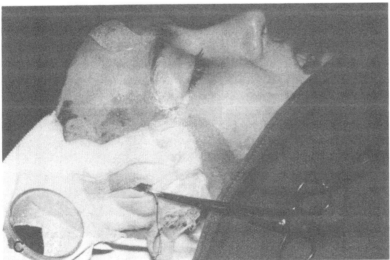

Figure 13.10 A–C

Giant Vertebrobasilar Junction Aneurysms   191

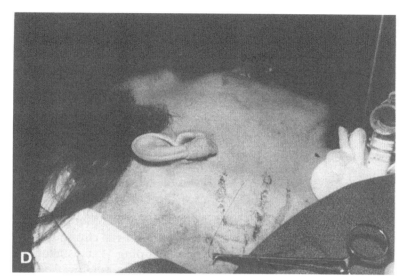

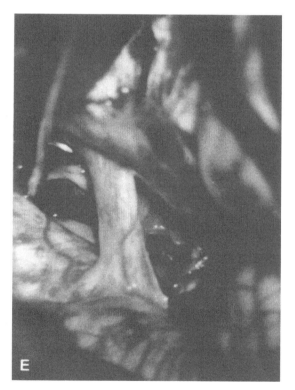

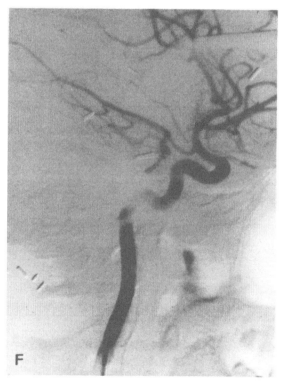

Figure 13.10 D–F

Figure 13.10 A–E. S.N., F, 23, giant vertebrobasilar junction aneurysm (**A, B**), three months progressive near complete bulbar and quadriparesis, tracheostomy. The left vertebral artery was clipped intracranially in July 1977, and the tourniquet applied to the right vertebral (**C**) near the aneurysm has been occluded for 24 hours and was buried (**D**) but there was no improvement. At transtentorial exploration for trapping one week later AICA was seen arising from apex of aneurysm. Therefore a tourniquet was placed on the basilar artery near the aneurysm and the artery was occluded without sequelae. Operative view of transtentorial exposure of sac after its evacuation with trigeminal nerve overlying (**E**). Excellent filling of basilar artery from carotid artery (**F**). Complete recovery except for right abducens nerve paresis. Outcome excellent

Trapping and Evacuation

Two patients were treated by trapping and evacuation of the thrombus from the aneurysm to reduce mass effect which had severely compromised brain stem function. In both cases, both AICAs were known to come from the aneurysm.

The first a woman 23, had had a tracheostomy and was on a respirator with severe bulbar palsy and left hemiplegia (Fig. 13.10). She tolerated clip and tourniquet occlusion of the vertebral arteries but did not improve. Subtemporal-transtentorial exposure and incising the sac produced bleeding even though the angiogram suggested complete thrombosis. The sac was sewn closed and the tourniquet placed on the basilar artery as it emerged from the huge fusiform aneurysm. Subsequent occlusion of the basilar artery produced no change and so at re-exposure the tourniquet was replaced with a clip and the aneurysm reopened and evacuated. But dramatic arterial bleeding came from the sac. It was found to be back bleeding from the orifices of each AICA. After each was plugged with muscle, the sac remained dry and collapsed. Dramatic virtual complete neurological recovery ensued over a few weeks, except for a partial sixth nerve palsy.

The second patient, 44, had a left angle syndrome with a similar mass. After right vertebral clipping, he had no gag reflexes and had a respiratory arrest after extubation. Subsequently he breathed but inadequately and there was increasing right hemiparesis. As the aneurysm was thrombosed incompletely, a clip was placed on the left vertebral intracranially. As the hemiparesis continued to worsen with a left facial nerve palsy, thrombotic swelling of the aneurysm was thought possible as the cause. After transtentorial clipping of the basilar artery above for trapping 11 days later, the sac was opened and evacuated but vigorous arterial bleeding came from the aneurysm and in spite of a prolonged search the orifices of AICAs could not be found as in the first case. The incision in the aneurysm had to be closed. He remained in coma and died two days later (Fig. 13.11). In retrospect, he might have survived had the mass of the aneurysm been greatly reduced by plication with sutures.

The results can be seen in Tables 13.1 to 13.5.

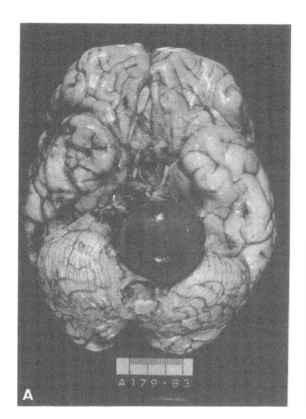 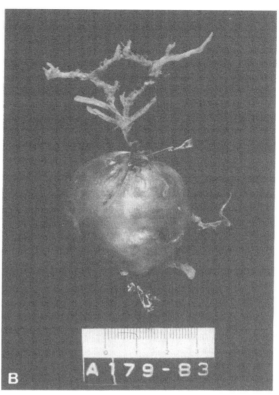

Figure 13.11 A, B. S.V., M, 44, giant vertebrobasilar junction aneurysm, one year neck pain, left facial numbness, decreased left hearing and dysphagia. Giant vertebrobasilar junction aneurysm in situ (**A**) and dissected free (**B**) to show AICAs arising from the sac. He was right hemiplegic after right vertebral clipping in September 1983 and not improved after left vertebral clipping one week later. After transtentorial basilar artery clip trapping there was uncontrollable bleeding from the interior of the aneurysm after evacuation and the sac had to be sewn closed, died two days later

194 Giant Vertebrobasilar Junction Aneurysms

Table 13.1. Preoperative Grade and outcome in 39 patients with giant VB junction aneurysms

Grade	Excellent	Good	Poor	Dead	Total
0[a]	12	5	7	7	31
0g	*8*	*3*	*1*	*3*	*15*
0p	*4*	*2*	*6*	*4*	*16*
1	5	2		1	8
Total	17	7	7	8	39
	43.6%	17.9%	17.9%	20.5%	100.0%

[a] *0* Unruptured aneurysm or remote hemorrhage (> 1 year). *0g* Good risk without major neurological deficit. *0p* Poor risk patient with major neurological deficit (severe confusion or dementia or stupor or coma, dysarthria or bulbar paralysis, severe dysphasia or severe mono-, hemi-, or tetraparesis).

Table 13.2. Age related to outcome in 39 patients with giant VB junction aneurysms

Age group (years)	Excellent	Good	Poor	Dead	Total
10–19	3				3
20–29	3	1			4
30–39	1	1	2	2	6
40–49	2	1	2	4	9
50–59	6	3	2	1	12
60–69	2	1	1	1	5
Total	17	7	7	8	39

Table 13.3. Operative method and outcome in 39 patients with giant VB junction aneurysms

Operative method	Excellent	Good	Poor	Dead	Total
Clip	3	1	2	2	8
Vertebral ligation	13	6	3	5	27
Unilateral[a]	*5*	*1*	*2*	*3*	*11*
Bilateral	*8*	*5*	*1*	*2*	*16*
Explored only			2		2
Trapping	1			1	2
Total	17	7	7	8	39

[a] Two had only one vertebral artery.

Table 13.4. Operative method and completeness of aneurysm treatment in 39 patients with giant VB junction aneurysms

Operative method	Total obliteration	Residual neck	Residual fundus	No obliteration	Unknown	Total
Clip	7		1			8
Vertebral ligation	17	1	8		1	27
Explored only				2		2
Trapping	2					2
Total	26	1	9	2	1	39

Table 13.5. Timing of surgery and outcome in 8 patients with ruptured giant VB junction aneurysms

Timing of surgery	Excellent	Good	Poor	Dead	Total
4–6 day	1				1
11–30 day	1	2		1	4
31–365 day	3				3
Total	5	2		1	8

Chapter 14
Non-Giant Aneurysms of the Vertebral Artery
181 Patients

Anatomical Features

The vertebral artery may give rise to saccular aneurysms throughout its intracranial course, but two-thirds occurred at the distal crotch of origin of posterior-inferior cerebellar artery (PICA). The notorious tortuosity of the vertebral artery and the varying level of origin of PICA have placed vertebral aneurysms anywhere from positions near the intracranial entry of the vertebral artery under the first dentate ligament, even in the upper lateral cervical canal, to that portion of the vertebral artery under the middle of the medulla. Right vertebral aneurysms have even been seen and operated on the left side of the midline. Most vertebral aneurysms project upward, lying shallowly on the medulla, either laterally or in front. A few project more posteriorly into the medulla, while others may have a dome adherent to the clivus. There is often an intimate relationship to the twelfth nerve, which usually lies across the upper side of the neck (Illustration 14.VIII, C), although it has been seen to be split in two by the growth of the sac and thus lie on both sides of the neck, but only seven patients had hypoglossal paresis and three of them were redo-aneurysms. Peculiar to vertebral aneurysms (and superior cerebellar aneurysms) is for PICA (or superior cerebellar artery (SCA)) to emerge more from the side of the neck than from the parent artery.

Classification

Classification of vertebral aneurysms has proved to be difficult: in the following the most simple and surgically important grouping has been used (Fig. 14.1).

Ten aneurysms had their origin from PICA usually within a centimeter or so from its origin, two of these were dissecting aneurysms. Thirteen were more distally located. Six, one proximal and five distal at or beyond the caudal loop, were associated with arteriovenous malformations (AVMs) (Fig. 14.2).

Rare proximal aneurysms (four cases – see Chapter 15) can arise extra- and intradurally, or both, and were in this series always of giant size except an incidental large one associated with a giant PICA aneurysm. Remarkably three saccular aneurysms arose from the inferior aspect of the origin of PICA (prePICA); six dissecting and one traumatic aneurysm had the same site. Another group of 27 aneurysms arose between the origin of PICA and the vertebrobasilar (V-B) junction usually well under the medulla, possibly, when saccular, at the site of origin of the anterior spinal artery or some smaller, unnamed perforating branch (distal vertebral artery aneurysms, Fig. 14.3). The most common vertebral aneurysm site is however at the distal side of the PICA origin, the classic PICA aneurysm. Two-thirds were located on the left (121 postPICA aneurysms, Figs. 14.4, 14.5).

Twenty-five aneurysms in the vertebral-PICA region were dissections (Fig. 14.6), two of them

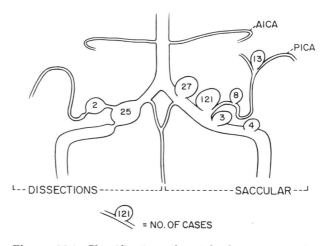

Figure 14.1. Classification of vertebral aneurysm sites, 203 patients with vertebral aneurysms of this series. Some of the aneurysms of giant size involve several sites and were excluded

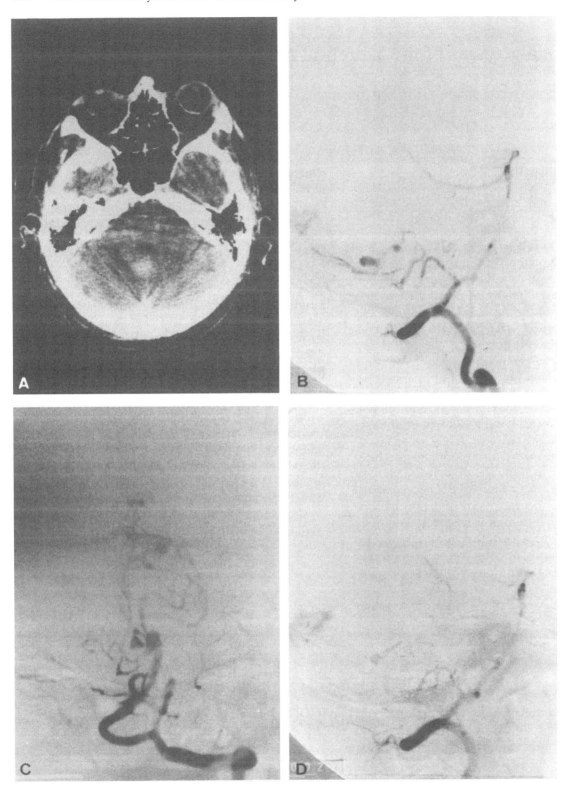

Figure 14.2 A–D. G.McN., M, 65, CT scan with central cerebellar hematoma (A). Two peripheral PICA aneurysms with accessory dural arteriovenous fistula (B, C). Operation in January 1982 10 days after bleed in Grade 1: Scoville clip to the larger and ruptured aneurysm, the smaller aneurysm was coagulated and encased in a Sundt clip graft (D). Outcome excellent

traumatic. Most commonly, dissecting aneurysms are located in the distal vertebral artery (14). Two were bland and discovered in the investigation of headache; one of these was shown to be enlarging during six months. Two of the hemorrhagic dissections occurred in PICA near its origin but confined to the artery.

Clinical Features

Of the 181 patients with small and large vertebral aneurysms, 145 (80.1%) were females. Age ranged from 17 to 70 years. Female excess was still more pronounced in saccular aneurysms (125 : 21 = 85.6%) and clear in fusiform (6 : 3) as sex distribution among dissecting aneurysms was equal (12 : 11). From the different locations mean age was highest in PICA distal aneurysms (54.1 years) and lowest in PICA proximal aneurysms (42.9 years).

It is perhaps remarkable that lower cranial nerve paresis was not more common with rupture of a vertebral aneurysm. CNIX-CNX paresis was seen in 10% of the patients but one-third of them were redo-aneurysms. Sixth nerve was the most frequent but false localizing palsy in 26 patients, bilateral in 14 of them. Remarkably, 14 patients had trigeminal nerve affected, but only one had trochlear nerve paresis. Sixteen facial pareses occurred and bilateral deafness once, unilaterally eight times. Medullary signs were uncommon too. Cardiorespiratory arrest with the bleed, requiring intubation, was recorded in at least eight patients. Hemiparesis and monoparesis of upper or lower extremity occurred seven times but rarely was persisting, dysarthria was seen in six cases. Cerebellar clot occurred three times but only from rupture of peripheral PICA aneurysms or with associated AVMs. Blood seen in the CT scan in the fourth ventricle alone, or associated with blood in the third ventricle with enlarged ventricles, visualization of a basilar trunk or vertebral aneurysm can be anticipated in the angiograms.

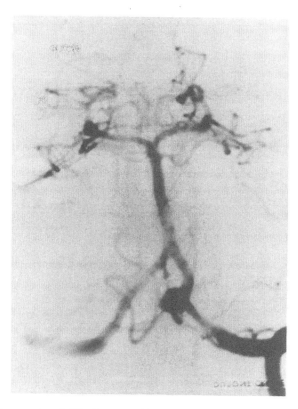

Figure 14.3. M.E., F, 55, midline ruptured distal vertebral aneurysm arising 1 cm above PICA origin was clipped in October 1985 4 days after bleed in Grade 1. Sac was aspirated and collapsed, no postoperative angiography was done. Outcome excellent

Ruptured dissections of the vertebral artery have a fairly typical story, sudden severe lateralized suboccipital pain usually in a known hypertensive, occasionally occurring with effort. Only two lateral medullary syndromes were seen with the 25 dissections. Sixth nerve palsy bilateral (2), unilateral facial paresis (2) and hearing loss (1), CNIX-CNX paresis unilateral (1) and bilateral (1), CXI unilateral (2) and CNXII bilateral (1), quadriparesis (2) and pontine gaze palsy (1) were also seen.

198   Non-Giant Aneurysms of the Vertebral Artery

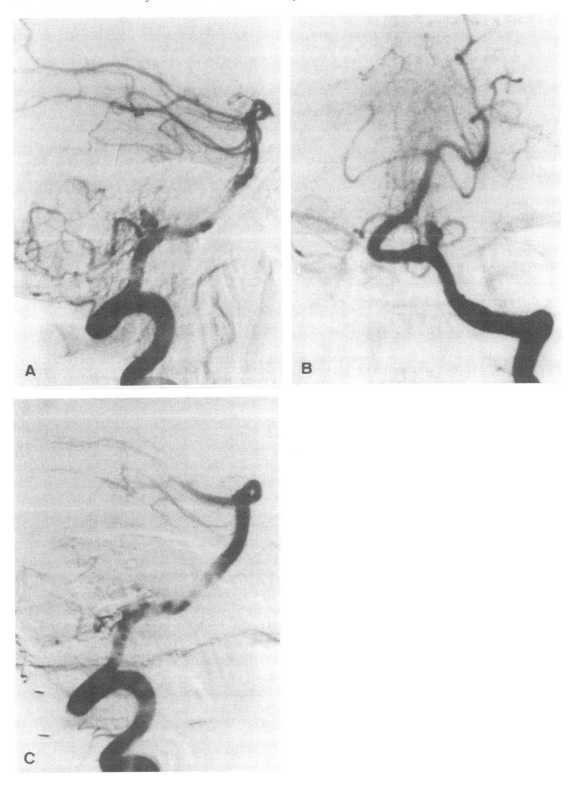

Figure 14.4 A–C. R.B., F, 49, typical ruptured vertebral-PICA aneurysm (**A, B**) was clipped in December 1982 11 days after bleed in Grade 1. Lateral view after clipping but with narrow residual sac (**C**). Outcome excellent with no recurrence after 12 years

Non-Giant Aneurysms of the Vertebral Artery 199

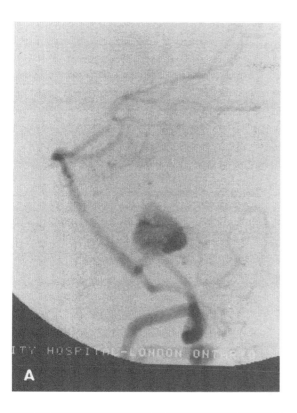
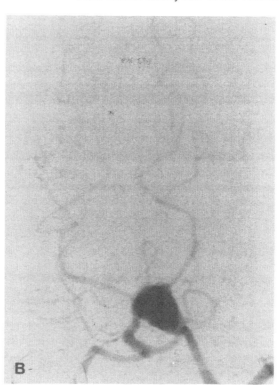
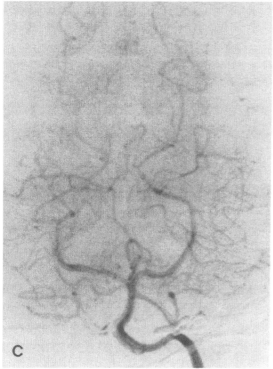

Figure 14.5 A–C. B.R., F, 49, large partially thrombosed vertebral-PICA aneurysm (**A, B**) was clipped in August 1994 (a recent case of Dr. Ferguson, not in our series). Seven months of vomiting, ataxia, right sided numbness and horizontal and vertical nystagmus with diplopia. After repeated attempts, clip finally stayed in position on neck without slipping down to occlude PICA. Outcome excellent, diplopia resolved

200   Non-Giant Aneurysms of the Vertebral Artery

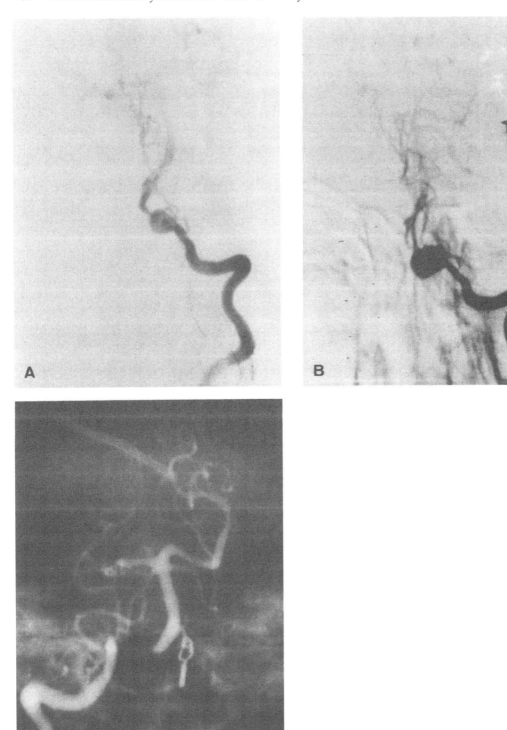

Figure 14.6 A–C. R.D., F, 53, growth of a left vertebral artery dissecting aneurysm over 12 days with two rebleedings (**A, B**). The left vertebral artery was clip occluded 10 hours after last bleed in September 1984 at the dural entrance with thrombosis of the aneurysm (**C**). The right vertebral artery shows persisting vasospasm beyond PICA. After tracheostomy and ventriculoperitoneal shunting she made an ultimate good recovery, in spite of operation in poor Grade 4!

Approaches

Originally, from a surgical viewpoint, these aneurysms were divided into three groups, depending on their relation to the medulla: lateral, paramedullary and paramedian. It was thought that the difficulties in exposure expanded dramatically for those at or near the midline under the medulla and over the lower one-third of the clivus. This area was considered a no-man's land since it was difficult to see from below because of the jugular tubercle and reluctance to retract the medulla. A transoral-transclival approach was developed for midline vertebral aneurysms. There is no question that a midline vertebral aneurysm can be done by the transclival approach but the exposure is narrow, approximately 12 mm wide by 15 mm long (Drake 1973). The first case was uneventful; however, in the second case, a fatal meningitis occurred. This small aneurysm was located just off the midline, was not seen clearly enough for clipping, and was packed in gauze. The patient was well for three days, and although there was no evidence of cerebral spinal fluid (CSF) leak into the pharynx, he rapidly became comatose and died within six hours from pneumococcal meningitis. This confirmed that, in addition to the narrow and confining nature of the transclival opening, it was also dangerous. Since that unwarranted publication of the method based on one case, several other surgeons in personal communications have encountered this dangerous complication. The senior author feels that it should be abandoned as an intradural procedure for aneurysms, although modern dural closures reinforced with thrombin glues may be more watertight.

Even so, it has been found that all non-giant, saccular aneurysms overlying the lower one-third of the clivus, even in the midline, can be exposed through the lateral suboccipital-subcerebellar approach (vide supra) (Illustration 14.VIII). A left vertebral aneurysm has even been done from the right side when the craniotomy was made on the wrong side. It was learned too that the medulla withstands a fair degree of retraction and rotation without consequence. The best indicator of excessive force has been found to be apnea while the patient is breathing spontaneously; apnea always occurred before cardiovascular aberrations.

The approach to vertebral aneurysms follows the same route as for the V-B junction (vide supra). Since PICA usually arises proximal to the sac, the vertebral artery is followed from the region of the first dentate ligament to the PICA origin which is a landmark to denote the presence of the neck just beyond (Illustration 14.VIII C). Lower or lateral aneurysms will be seen immediately at this stage, although higher aneurysms may be concealed by the filaments of CNX or the medulla. Ordinarily, the route of exposure is below the lower filaments of CNX, but between the medullary filaments of CNXI (Illustration 14.VIII D). The latter may be bundled together or be separate, tiny, tender strands. Great care must be taken when working between or around them, for they are easily injured. They arise from the nucleus ambiguus and are the motor supply to the pharynx and larynx. Dysarthria and dysphagia as a result of their injury are not only distressing but also dangerous. Repeated soiling of the upper airway may occur with choking or from spillover from an enlarged pyriform fossa. The latter occurs only with severe unilateral pharyngeal palsy, but may require repair if reinnervation does not take place.

As the neck of the aneurysm is glimpsed beyond PICA, it may be best to work medially on either side of the PICA origin and along the sides of the vertebral artery beyond to see the sides of the neck, the back of which may have to be separated from the medulla. Temporary vertebral clipping will soften the sac for this dissection if necessary. The vertebral artery should then be followed on its underside, beyond the neck so that its direction is known for the placement of the clip across the neck, truly along the axis of the artery (Illustration 14.VIII D). It may be difficult with a larger sac to see this portion of the artery, but it can be visualized by holding the neck closed with forceps, or even with coagulation of the neck. It may also be seen by allowing the blades of the clip to close slowly to narrow the neck when, with the position of the artery beyond coming into view, the blades may be realigned and positioned correctly just before the final closure.

The fact that PICA commonly emerges more from the side of the neck often makes clipping awkward since clip blades crossing from just above the PICA origin to the opposite side of the neck may leave some neck open just medial to the PICA origin, or the clip may simply slip down to kink PICA (Illustration 14.VIII E-H). Coagulation of the neck may solve this problem, as may the use of the

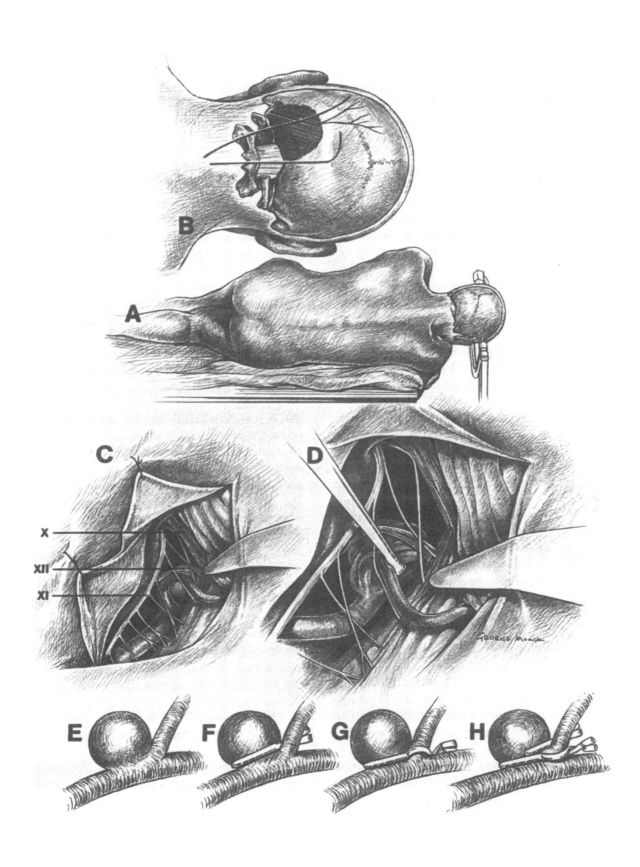

14.VIII

Drake-Sugita fenestrated clip with PICA in the aperture. With larger aneurysms, the tandem technique has been used twice with the second tandem clip occluding that portion of the neck near PICA remaining open in the aperture. Of course, the tips of any clip blade must be placed inside any perforators or filaments of CNX, CNXI or CNXII that have been separated from the neck.

Proximal vertebral clipping was used with good results for six large saccular aneurysms. Two were remarkable: one was partially fusiform in a 15 year old boy, but the other could not be seen clearly because of a swollen cerebellum in spite of removal of fresh shallow subdural and cisternal clot from a rupture during the craniotomy. Both had excellent outcomes, even though in the former the clip was proximal to PICA.

Results

The results can be seen in Tables 14.1 to 14.15. There were 7 bad outcomes in 142 good condition patients (6%) with small aneurysms. One woman with a huge clot from hemorrhage into a Dandy-Walker cyst requiring permanent tracheostomy remained disabled with ataxia and a feeding jejunostomy. Another patient developed a PICA infarction after a difficult re-operation for a midline aneurysm; the artery filled feebly in the postoperative angiogram. Coma-producing cerebellar swelling was relieved by resection of the outer third of the cerebellum but she remained disabled.

Two of the five deaths were from postoperative hemorrhage, one when an older clip slipped off the aneurysm. In the other, bleeding into the fourth ventricle occurred after clipping a ruptured peripheral PICA aneurysm and resection of a 3.5 cm anterior cerebellar AVM. PICA infarction caused another death when that artery had to be trapped to control rupture at the neck of the aneurysm which occurred spontaneously after deep hypotension with nitroprusside had been allowed to fall to 20 and then urgently was raised to 200 systolic. Another death, mentioned above, was from pneumococcal meningitis on the third day after transoral packing of a poorly visualized aneurysm. The last occurred two days after discharge from massive pulmonary embolism.

There were only 3 poor outcomes in 27 large aneurysms and no deaths. Three were fusiform and were treated by proximal vertebral occlusion distal to PICA, uneventfully and with complete thrombosis in the aneurysm. The Grade 4 patient had only partial recovery of her medullary and cerebellar deficit.

Dissecting aneurysms (2 of them traumatic) had occurred in the vertebral artery in 25 patients; 2 were bland but the remainder had ruptured into the subarachnoid space. Both bland dissections, one of which was shown to be enlarging, were treated by proximal vertebral occlusion distal to PICA with good outcomes.

One left-sided dissection below PICA, presumed to have occurred with a hemorrhage nine months before and discovered incidentally in a severely hypertensive women, was explored because there appeared to be a saccular component. It was completely fusiform and was not treated except for a dacron patch to separate it from the medulla. She remained normotensive during her hospital stay but has been lost to follow-up. One dissection was packed in cottonoid and another small dissection was encased in a clip graft. Clip grafts were used in two others to reinforce the artery below PICA.

---

14. VIII. Lateral suboccipital approach to vertebral and vertebral-basilar junction aneurysms. **A, B** The inverted hockey stick incision provides an opening satisfactory for most vertebral PICA aneurysms not buried under the medulla and spares scalp sensation. In order for the approach to be as far lateral as possible beside and under the medulla, the head is less rotated than in the full "park bench" position. The rim of the foramen magnum must also be removed anterolaterally near to the occipital condyle. **C** The retractor is elevating the cerebellar tonsil and medial hemisphere to expose the lower cerebellopontine angle with the 10th nerve at the apex. **D** The slender fragile strands of the medullary filaments of the 11th nerve always cross the field and must carefully be preserved. The 12th nerve usually crosses the neck or waist of this aneurysm. Visualization of the vertebral artery beyond the neck is essential for clip alignment and gentle retraction of the medulla is well tolerated. The origin of PICA more from the base of the neck than the artery shown here is not unusual and may complicate complete neck clipping. **E** Schematic of vertebral aneurysm with PICA emerging more from base of sac. **F** A single clip placed across the neck and flush with the origin of PICA will leave an elipse of neck open for subsequent enlargement to another aneurysm. **G** This elipse may be eradicated by using a fenestrated clip leaving the orifice of PICA open at the aperture or **H** by using the tandem technique

In the remaining 20 dissections, the vertebral artery was clip occluded in 19, balloon occluded in 1 at the atlas. Seven of the clip and the balloon occlusions were proximal to PICA and no lateral medullary infarctions occurred in the five good condition patients. AICA-PICA anastomoses were seen in most of these in postoperative angiograms. Two patients were in Grade 4 states with medullary and cerebellar injury presumed to be from the hemorrhage. In one, the vertebral artery ended or was occluded beyond PICA. Their recovery was incomplete, but one is self-sufficient.

Lateral medullary infarction occurred in one patient when, after recurrent bleeding, the aneurysm was trapped. The rebleeding had occurred on the fifth day after a vertebral clip distal to PICA. At re-operation, the dissection was shown to extend to the V-B junction, but could be trapped with a clip on the termination of the vertebral artery to prevent dissection up into the basilar artery. She awoke with a Wallenberg syndrome but over several months made a virtually complete recovery.

Both proximal PICA dissections were treated by encasement in clip grafts, using two in one; both made excellent recoveries.

Table 14.1. Preoperative Grade and outcome in 154 patients with small vertebral aneurysms

Grade	Excellent	Good	Poor	Dead	Total
0	10	1			11
1	101	5	1	4	111
2	15	3	1	1	20
3	3	4		2	9
4			2	1	3
Total	129	13	4	8	154
	83.8%	8.4%	2.6%	5.2%	100.0%

Table 14.2. Aneurysm site and outcome in 154 patients with small vertebral aneurysms

Site	Excellent	Good	Poor	Dead	Total
Vertebral prePICA	5		1	1	7
Vertebral postPICA	89	11	3	6	109
PICA proximal	9				9
PICA distal	11	1		1	13
Vertebral distal	15	1			16
Total	129	13	4	8	154

Table 14.3. Age related to outcome in 154 patients with small vertebral aneurysms

Age group (years)	Excellent	Good	Poor	Dead	Total
20–29	4			1	5
30–39	21	1	1		23
40–49	45	2	1		48
50–59	39	4		4	47
60–69	20	6	1	3	30
70 or more			1		1
Total	129	13	4	8	154

Table 14.4. Operative method and outcome in 154 patients with small vertebral aneurysms

Operative method	Excellent	Good	Poor	Dead	Total
Clip[a]	108	10	3	6	127
Silk ligature	1				1
Wrapping	3	1		1	5
Hunterian ligation	17	2	1	1	21
Total	129	13	4	8	154

[a] Includes 6 clip grafts.

Table 14.5. Operative method and completeness of aneurysm treatment in 154 patients with small vertebral aneurysms

Operative method	Total obliteration	Residual neck	Residual fundus	No obliteration	Not known	Total
Clip[a]	119	7			1	127
Silk ligature	1					1
Wrapping				5		5
Hunterian ligation	17		3		1	21
Total	137	7	3	5	2	154

[a] Includes 6 clip grafts.

Table 14.6. Timing of surgery and outcome in 143 patients with small vertebral aneurysms

Timing of surgery	Excellent	Good	Poor	Dead	Total
0–1 day	7	2	1	1	11
2–3 day	4	1		1	6
4–6 day	4	2	1	1	8
7–10 day	22				22
11–30 day	59	4	2	5	70
31–365 day	23	3			26
Total	119	12	4	8	143

Table 14.7. Preoperative Grade and outcome in 27 patients with large vertebral aneurysms

Grade	Excellent	Good	Poor	Total
0	3	1		4
1	13			13
2	5			5
3		2	1	3
4		1	1	2
Total	21	4	2	27

Table 14.8. Aneurysm site and outcome in 27 patients with large vertebral aneurysms

Site	Excellent	Good	Poor	Total
Vertebral prePICA	2	1		3
Vertebral postPICA	9	1	2	12
PICA proximal	1			1
Vertebral distal	9	2		11
Total	21	4	2	27

Table 14.9. Age related to outcome in 27 patients with large vertebral aneurysms

Age group (years)	Excellent	Good	Poor	Total
10–19	1			1
30–39	2			2
40–49	5	2	1	8
50–59	7	2	1	10
60–69	6			6
Total	21	4	2	27

Table 14.10. Operative method and outcome in 27 patients with large vertebral aneurysms

Operative method	Excellent	Good	Poor	Total
Clip	11		2	13
Silk ligature	1			1
Wrapping	1			1
Hunterian ligation	7	4		11
Dacron patch[a]	1			1
Total	21	4	2	27

[a] Dissecting, asymptomatic.

Table 14.11. Operative method and result of aneurysm treatment in 27 patients with large vertebral aneurysms

Operative method	Total obliteration	No obliteration	Total
Clip	13		13
Silk ligature	1		1
Wrapping		1	1
Hunterian ligation	11		11
Dacron patch		1	1
Total	25	2	27

Table 14.12. Timing of surgery and outcome in 23 patients with large vertebral aneurysms

Timing of surgery	Excellent	Good	Poor	Total
0–1 day		1		1
2–3 day	1			1
7–10 day	4		1	5
11–30 day	12	1	1	14
31–365 day	1	1		2
Total	18	3	2	23

Table 14.13. Operative method and type of the aneurysm in 181 patients with small and large vertebral or PICA aneurysms

Operative method	Saccular	Fusiform	Dissecting	Atherosclerotic	Total
Clip[a]	134	3	3		140
Wrapping	4	1	1		6
Silk ligature	2				2
Hunterian ligation	5	5	20	1	31
Trapping	1				1
Dacron patch			1		1
Total	146	9	25	1	181
	80.7%	5.0%	13.8%	0.6%	100.0%

[a] Includes 6 clip grafts.

Table 14.14. Peri- and postoperative complicating factors in 181 patients with small and large vertebral aneurysms

Variable	Patients	Poor result	Dead
Intraoperative aneurysm rupture	15	1	3
Perforator injury	2	1	1
Deep hypotension during surgery	1	0	1
Inadvertent arterial occlusion (vertebral or PICA)	8	2	1
Postoperative significant spasm	6	1	2
Postoperative hematoma	9	1	3
Rebleeding from treated aneurysm	3	1	2
Sepsis	11	2	0
Meningitis	7	0	1
Respiratory	6	0	2
Bleeding diathesis	1	0	1
Pulmonary embolus	2	0	1
Combined medical complications (Infection, cardiorespiratory, etc)	9	3	3
Total	54	6	8

Table 14.15. Type of the aneurysm and outcome in 181 patients with small and large vertebral or PICA aneurysms

Type of the aneurysm	Excellent	Good	Poor	Dead	Total
Saccular	121	12	5	8	146
Fusiform	9				9
Dissecting	19	5	1		25
Atheroscl.	1				1
Total	150	17	6	8	181

Chapter 15
Giant Vertebral Aneurysms
40 Patients

Forty giant aneurysms arose from and were isolated to the intracranial segment of the vertebral artery; eight were illustrated and described previously (Fig. 15.1).

Anatomical Features

Their size often obscures their exact site of origin. Presumably many of these aneurysms arise from smaller sacs at the distal crotch of origin of posterior-inferior cerebellar artery (PICA) from the vertebral artery. Four clearly arose from the artery below PICA and 14 distal to PICA. One-third were clearly fusiform taking up most of the artery; three were atherosclerotic. While most of these giant aneurysms have been centered beside and just under the medulla with the ninth, tenth and eleventh cranial nerves draped over their sides, others were more centrally placed under a posteriorly displaced and flattened medulla. Such compression of the IVth ventricle and its outlets may give rise to hydrocephalus and papilledema, however a shunt operation was seldom needed (3).

Clinical Features

Fourteen patients presented with recent subarachnoid hemorrhage (SAH) usually with mild mass effect except one who was solidly hemiplegic from a small clot in the pons. Two had a remote history of bleeding when the aneurysm presumably was smaller. The majority had mass effect only, featuring varying degrees of bulbar paresis and ataxia (18), often with mild (14) hemiparesis, hemisensory loss and limb dysmetria. Three had severe quadriparesis and two were admitted with tracheostomies. Ipsilateral trigeminal hypalgesia was common (12), and was once bilateral. Paresis of CNVI (5), CNVII (9) and CNVIII (5) were also more frequent than occasional. Further CNIX-X palsies were common (13), and in five instances were bilateral. Two patients had eleventh and four, fwelfth nerve palsies, the latter even once bilaterally. Lateral and even upward gaze palsies were each seen once. Two patients had frank papilledema with hydrocephalus.

Treatment

One recent case, a man, 54, had no definitive surgical treatment for his huge 5 cm atherosclerotic aneurysm. After trial with endovascular Guglielmi detachable coils (GDC) with incomplete occlusion, the posterior fossa was explored. The aneurysm was hard with atheroma and none of the saccules could be clipped. He was transferred, with tracheostomy in poor condition one month later to another hospital.

Only in four patients could the aneurysm be clipped, in two of these after temporary trapping and evacuation of clot from the sac (Fig. 15.2). Two patients had no deficit but the other two were classified only as good results, one because of dysarthria and the other from dysphagia which had existed preoperatively though to a lesser degree. In all four, the vertebral artery was occluded in the postoperative angiograms from slipped or kinking clips.

Proximal vertebral artery occlusion was used in the remainder, eight of which were additionally trapped and evacuated.

Vertebral artery occlusion was extracranial in six patients, but only in the lower neck by Selverstone clamp in one early case. About two-thirds of this aneurysm thrombosed, but it enlarged after one year with more mass effect from retrograde filling from the other vertebral and reconstitution of the ipsilateral vertebral from deep cervical collateral. An attempt at trapping in another institution failed and he refused bilateral vertebral occlusion. Sudden death from rebleeding occurred two years after the first procedure. A ruptured aneurysm in a man,

208 Giant Vertebral Aneurysms

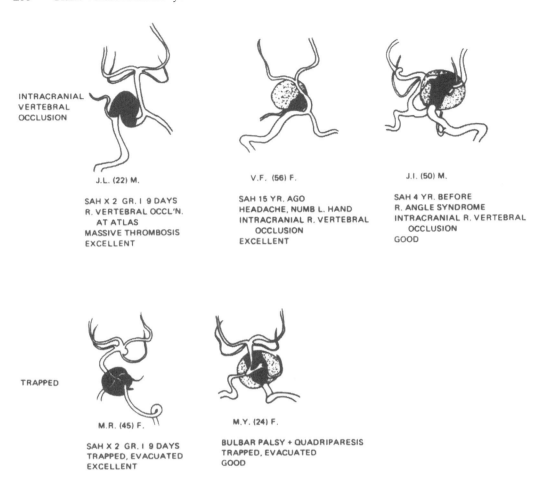

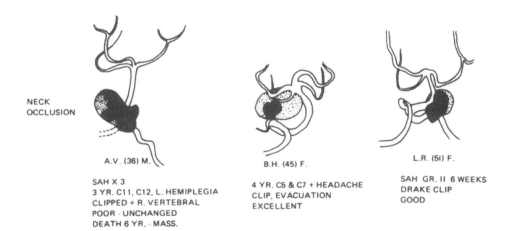

Figure 15.1. The origin, size and shape of giant vertebral aneurysms and the extent of their mural thrombosis described and illustrated by tracings in the early experience. (Reprinted from Clin Neurosurg 26, 1979, p. 90 by courtesy of Williams and Wilkins)

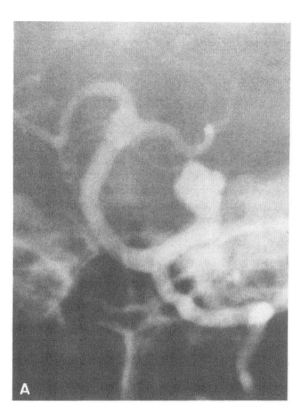 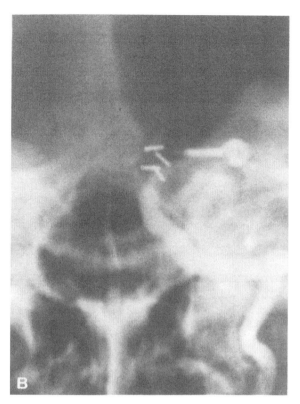

Figure 15.2 A, B. B.H., F, 46, giant partially thrombosed left vertebral-PICA aneurysm (**A**), headache and left facial palsy and loss of hearing left. Operation in March 1976, Scoville clip occluding neck also virtually occludes the vertebral artery with only a trickle getting through (**B**). Outcome excellent

22, was fusiform and retrogradely extended to the dural entrance. It was obliterated by proximal clip occlusion of the vertebral artery in the sulcus arteriosus of the atlas. The aneurysm in another woman, 58 and morbidly obese, extended extracranially with a proximal saccule on the vertebral artery in the sulcus arteriosus (Fig. 15.4). This artery was clipped after exposure between the transverse processes of C1 and C2 and the aneurysm became completely thrombosed.

The other three patients were treated by detached balloon occlusion of the artery at and/or just before the sulcus arteriosus of the atlas (Fig. 15.3).

All but the first patient with lower cervical clamp occlusion had complete thrombosis of their aneurysms and good long-term outcomes, although in three there was incomplete but non-disabling recovery from pre-existing ataxia and bulbar paresis.

Intracranial vertebral artery occlusion was used in 21 patients with 13 satisfactory outcomes and in all but 7, the aneurysms were completely occluded by thrombosis or nearly so (Figs. 15.5, 15.6, 15.7). The apex of a few still filled for a few millimeters from the opposite vertebral artery. In four, the sac continued to fill and enlarge requiring trapping and evacuation. The aneurysm arose from a single vertebral artery in one patient (Fig. 15.8).

Of the six poor results, three were in poor condition preoperatively and two even had slight improvement. Two other patients in poor condition were worse, one with more bulbar palsy and respiratory failure requiring a respirator, and the other with the addition of an opposite hemiparesis to the one existing with spastic legs. The last poor result was tragic, a hemiplegia from a plunging burr during the craniotomy.

The first death occurred in a girl, 8, who was well for three days after the occlusion even though PICA arose from the side of the non-thrombosed aneurysm (Fig. 15.9). Then the aneurysm ruptured

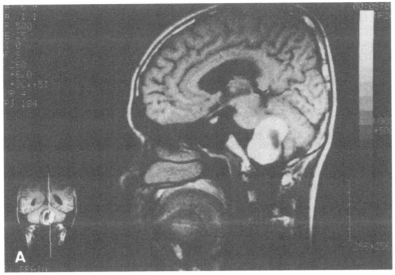
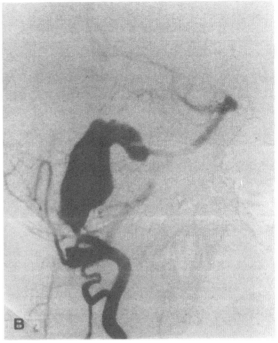
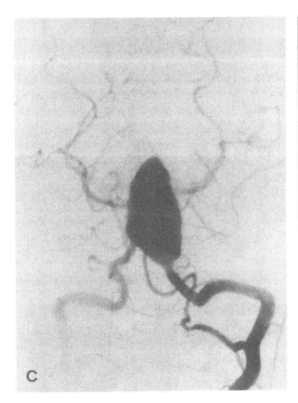
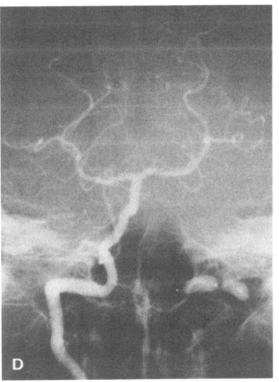

Figure 15.3 A–D. L.H., M, 16, giant fusiform left vertebral aneurysm (**A**), three months severe ataxia and bulbar palsy. PICA arose from the left vertebral artery below C1-C2 (**B, C**). After double detached balloon occlusion of the vertebral artery at the atlas in July 1991, the aneurysm became occluded (**D**) and the boy made a dramatic recovery with mild ataxia and horseness. Good outcome

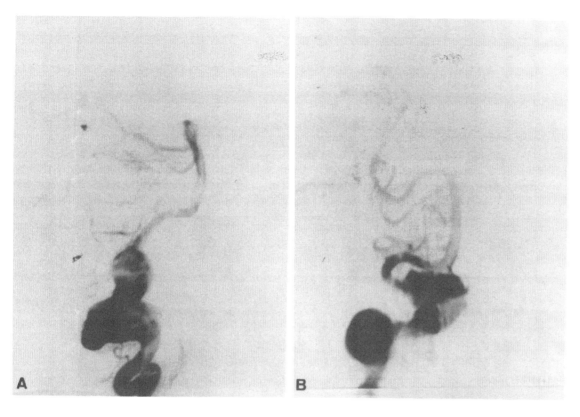

Figure 15.4 A, B. S.W., F, 58, giant partially thrombosed extracranial and intracranial fusiform aneurysm of right vertebral artery (**A, B**), five months vertigo, ataxia, dysphagia and diplopia. There was complete thrombosis of both aneurysms following clipping of right vertebral artery between foramina transversaria of C1 and C2 in June 1986. Outcome excellent

in spite of the vertebral occlusion and all but the upper centimeter was thrombosed. She recovered even to extubation but death occurred the next day from an unexplained cardiac arrest. Autopsy was refused. The other death was in a man, 57, with diffuse atherosclerosis, although his fusiform aneurysm was not obviously diseased. He was unchanged for 12 days after vertebral clipping when he suddenly became "locked in". At autopsy, the aneurysm was thrombosed but there was a hemorrhagic infarct in the pontine tegmentum.

In eight patients, trapping by distal vertebral artery clipping with evacuation of the aneurysm was added to the proximal vertebral artery occlusion. In four, the trapping procedure was used initially because of severe brain stem compression; all had remarkably good results. In four patients, the trapping was delayed for 14 days, 1 month, 8 months and 7 years respectively, in each case to relieve severe mass effect developing after the vertebral artery clipping (Fig. 15.10). In each, the aneurysm continued to fill and enlarge, massively in two, from the flow from the opposite vertebral artery. Remarkably each has had gratifying outcomes from major brain stem compression after evacuation of the sac, even from respiratory dependency in one. One of these patients redeveloped quadriparesis and respiratory arrest nine days after the evacuation but recovered nicely after re-opening and removal of bulging fresh clot in the aneurysm (Fig. 15.11). The bleeding source was not discovered.

There was only one vertebral clamp occlusion low in the neck but this and other experience suggest that any control of the aneurysm is temporary because of reconstitution of the artery from deep cervical collateral which prevents or retards thrombosis in the sac. There was no notable difference in outcome whether the vertebral was occluded just extracranially or intracranially since the intervening collateral branches if any are small and the artery is not reconstituted.

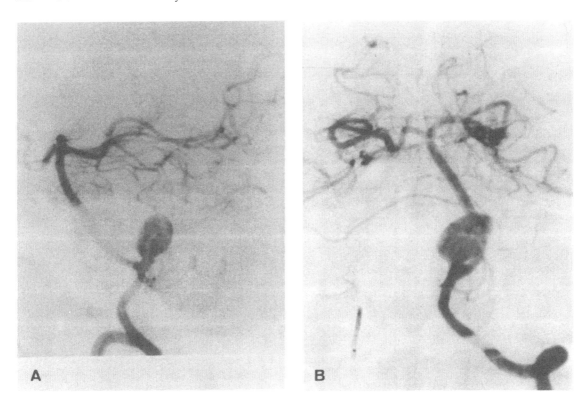
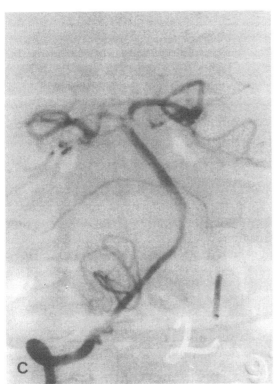

Figure 15.5 A–C. I.L., F, 32, giant partially thrombosed left vertebral-PICA aneurysm with remote SAH 8 years ago (**A, B**), one year quadriparesis more on left and dysarthria. After left vertebral artery clip occlusion proximal to PICA in January 1972, there was no filling of aneurysm from right vertebral artery (**C**). Outcome excellent

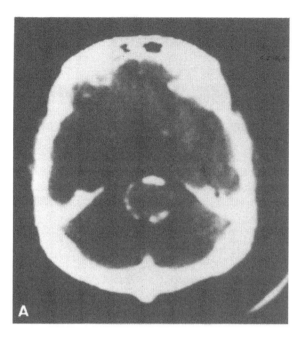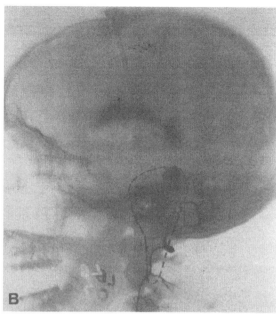

Figure 15.6 A, B. T.B., M, 21, huge left vertebral aneurysm (**A, B**), five months quadriparesis more on left. First explored transtentorially in September 1979 as a basilar aneurysm. One week later, at suboccipital exploration, the sac was found to extend down to C2 but the left vertebral artery could be clipped distal to PICA. After evacuating the aneurysm he made an excellent recovery

A huge aneurysmal varix was completely obliterated after clipping of PICA and a second branch arising from the vertebral artery (Fig. 15.12).

Only the posterior cerebral artery (PCA) giant aneurysms had a better outcome but the number of poor results in these patients is disturbing since all had the other vertebral to provide basilar artery flow. Four were in poor condition preoperatively and survived but little changed by the procedure. Brain stem infarction occurred rarely presumably from occlusion of perforating vessels arising from the thrombosed aneurysm. Even though the mass is restricted to the one vertebral artery, a few will continue to fill retrogradely from the opposite vertebral which continues their enlargement and rarely causes rupture. Trapping proved to be very successful whether immediate or delayed and should be considered more often perhaps when there is refilling. Concern over the exclusion of PICA was unfounded in most; even the majority of single vertebral occlusions were proximal to the origin of PICA which often could be seen filling from the anterior-inferior cerebellar artery (AICA) collateral.

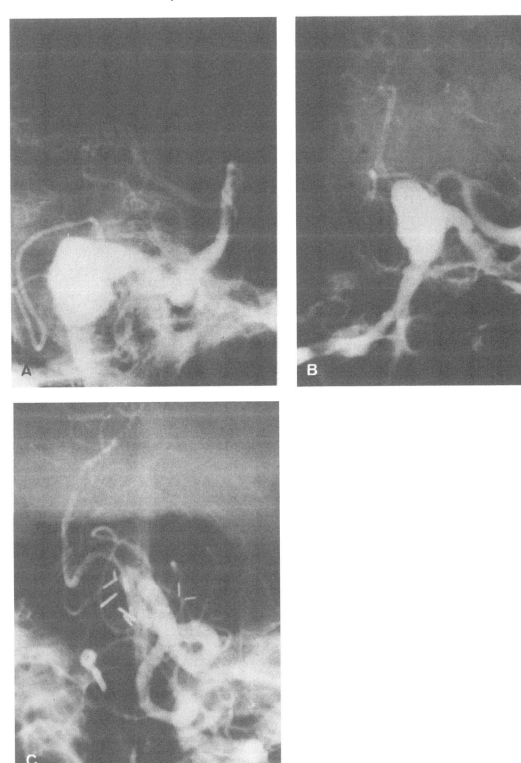

Figure 15.7 A–C. A.L., M, 58, giant fusiform right vertebral aneurysm with PICA arising from the sac (**A, B**), 11 years remote SAH, one year ataxia and bulbar palsy. After right vertebral artery clipping in May 1978 there was no filling of the aneurysm from the left vertebral artery (**C**). Persistent dysarthria and dysphagia, good outcome

Giant Vertebral Aneurysms 215

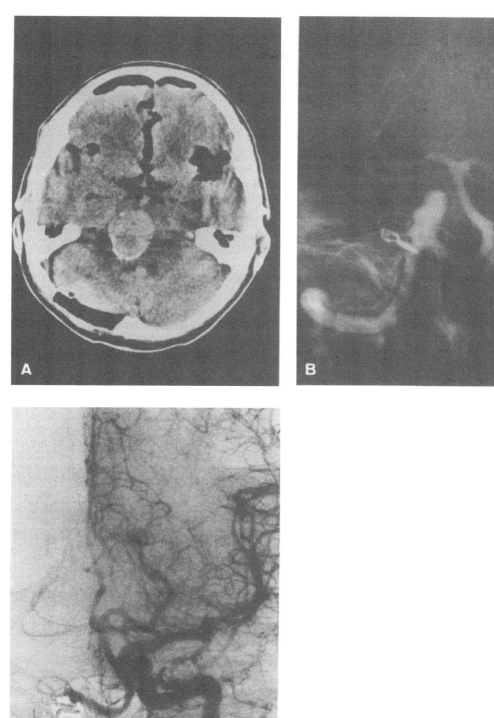

Figure 15.8 A–C. D.C., F, 61, giant vertebral aneurysm on single vertebral artery, 6 months headache, right deafness, hemiparesis and ataxia. CT of giant aneurysm arising from single right vertebral artery; the left ended in PICA. (**A**) First clip incompletely occludes vertebral artery in March 1988 (**B**). Bayonet clip applied below the first clip, the left carotid angiogram showed retrofilling of the whole basilar artery, the distal right vertebral artery and PICA underneath the neck of the thrombosed aneurysm. Good outcome, hoarseness

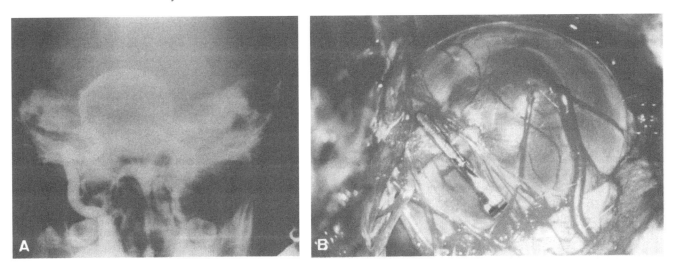

Figure 15.9 A, B. S.V., F, 8, giant fusiform left vertebral aneurysm (**A**), headache and vomiting four months. Operative exposure in June 1985 with clip on vertebral artery as it entered aneurysm (**B**). PICA arises separately from the sac. Postoperatively well until day 4: sudden coma and cardiorespiratory arrest. CT revealed posterior fossa bleeding, even though angiography showed virtual complete thrombosis of the aneurysm. On the following day recovered, was alert and moving limbs. Left lung consolidation with low pO$_2$. Death after series of cardiac arrests thought to be due to hypoxemia. PM refused

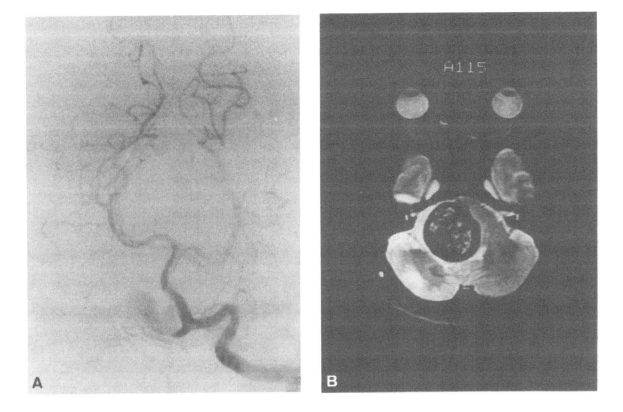

Figure 15.10 A, B. R.T., M, 50, giant right vertebral aneurysm, six months right facial numbness and palsy. Giant aneurysm still filling from left after right vertebral artery clipping in September 1986 (**A**) MRI 9 months later (**B**). He had continued to decline with severe ataxia, dysphagia and dysarthria with massive enlargement of aneurysm. After a trapping clip on the distal right vertebral artery and evacuation of the aneurysm he made virtual complete recovery over several months. Excellent outcome

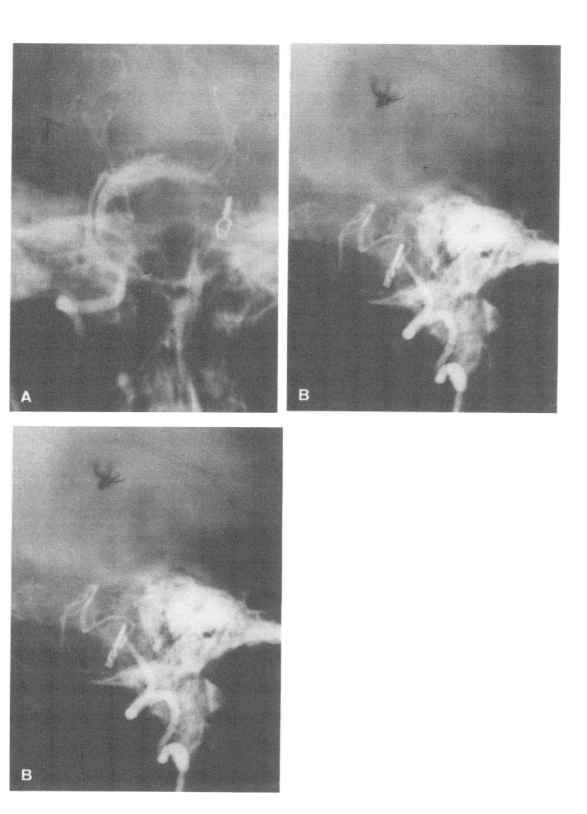

Figure 15.11 A–C. E.S., F, 49, giant left vertebral aneurysm, four months ataxia. Right vertebral angiogram (**A**) showing crescentic filling of dome of giant left vertebral aneurysm, (**B**) after left vertebral artery clipped beyond PICA in December 1985. Through a transtentorial approach it was not possible to clip the distal left vertebral artery. A tourniquet was placed on the terminal right vertebral artery and replaced by a clip when its occlusion was uneventful (**C**). However as it was not possible to wean her from the respirator the aneurysm was reexplored, opened and evacuated. She declined again and the aneurysm was found by transcutaneous ultrasound to have refilled with clot. After the second evacuation she finally had a good outcome

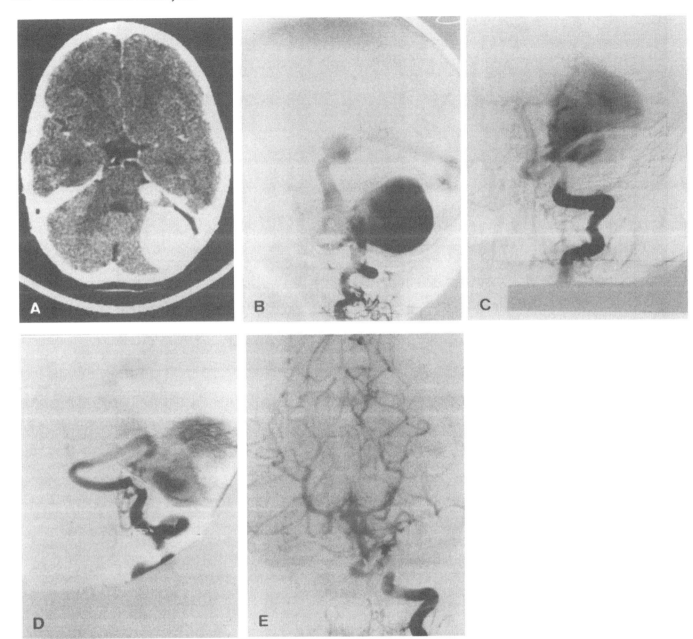

Figure 15.12 A–E. S.R., M, 4, huge aneurysmal varix of a A–V fistula arising from left PICA – lateral mesencephal vein (**A–C**), increasing head size noted by the family. After clipping PICA in July 1982, the varix still filled through another large vertebral artery branch (**D**). Complete obliteration of the fistula after clipping of the second branch (**E**)

Table 15.1. Preoperative grade and outcome in 40 patients with giant vertebral aneurysms

Grade	Excellent	Good	Poor	Dead	Total
0[a]	14	6	6	2	28
0g	9	1	2	1	13
0p	5	5	4	1	15
1	5				5
2	2	2	1		5
3		2			2
Total	21	10	7	2	40
	52.5%	25.0%	17.5%	5.0%	100.0%

[a] *0* Unruptured aneurysm or remote hemorrhage (> 1 year). *0g* Good risk without major neurological deficit. *0p* Poor risk patient with major neurological deficit (severe confusion or dementia or stupor or coma, dysarthria or bulbar paralysis, severe dysphasia or severe mono-, hemi-, or tetraparesis).

Table 15.2. Aneurysm site and outcome in 40 patients with giant vertebral aneurysms

Site	Excellent	Good	Poor	Dead	Total
Vertebral proximal	2	1	1		4
Vertebral-origin of PICA	10	6	1	2	19
PICA distal[a]	3				3
Vertebral distal	6	3	5		14
Total	21	10	7	2	40

[a] All 3 were giant aneurysmal varices associated with single arteriovenous fistulae.

Table 15.3. Age related to outcome in 40 patients with giant vertebral aneurysms

Age group (years)	Excellent	Good	Poor	Dead	Total
0–9	1			1	2
10–19	1	1			2
20–29	4	1			5
30–39		1			1
40–49	2		3		5
50–59	7	3	1	1	12
60–69	5	4	3		12
70 or more	1				1
Total	21	10	7	2	40

Table 15.4. Operative method and outcome in 40 patients with giant vertebral aneurysms

Operative method	Excellent	Good	Poor	Dead	Total
Clip	2	2			4
Hunterian ligation	14	5	6	2	27
Extracranial	3	3			6
Intracranial	11	2	6	2	21
Trapping	5	3			8
Exploration only			1		1
Total	21	10	7	2	40

Table 15.5. Operative method and result of aneurysm treatment in 40 patients with giant vertebral aneurysms

Operative method	Total obliteration	Residual neck	Residual fundus	No obliteration	Unknown
Neck clipping	4				
Hunterian ligation	17	2	7		1
Trapping	8				
Exploration only				1	
Total	29	2	7	1	1

Table 15.6. Timing of surgery and outcome in 12 patients with giant vertebral aneurysms

Timing of surgery	Excellent	Good	Poor	Dead	Total
2–3 day			1		1
4–6 day		1			1
7–10 day	2				2
11–30 day	4	1			5
31–365 day	1	2			3
Total	7	4	1		12

Chapter 16
Non-Giant Aneurysms of the Posterior Cerebral Artery
59 Patients

Anatomical Features

The posterior cerebral artery (PCA) has been divided into P1, P2, P3 and P4 segments; P1 includes the artery from its origin to and including the P1-P2-posterior communicating artery (PComA) confluence. P2 extends to and includes the first major branching on the side of the midbrain – usually the anterior temporal artery. The next segment up to the origin of the parieto-occipital and calcarine arteries is called P3 and the most distal part P4.

These aneurysms arise either on the P1 segment, presumably at the origin of P1 thalamoperforating branches or circumflex arteries, at the P1-P2 PComA junction, or more peripherally, especially at the first major branching on the side of the midbrain (P2) (Table 16.3). Seven small peripheral aneurysms arose on tertiary branches P3-P4; one was mycotic. Another tiny aneurysm arose on a mesencephalic branch of P1, lying on the root of CNIII, perhaps the lesser circumflex and its rupture had caused an oculomotor paresis.

Ten small and one large aneurysm arose on the artery feeding an arteriovenous malformation (AVM), four on P1 and two on P2 and five on P4. The aneurysm had ruptured in 7 of these 11 patients. Multiple aneurysms were seen frequently in this group, in 37%.

Clinical Features

Remarkably, no significant temporal lobe hemorrhage occurred in the series and there was only one trochlear paresis from a P2 aneurysm. One patient had bilateral sixth nerve palsy. A transient homonymous field defect occurred with the hemorrhage in two patients. Eight patients had preoperative severe hemiparesis: two had hemianesthesia as well, presumably from lateral thalamoperforating artery involvement from the hemorrhage. The hemorrhage from a large left P2 aneurysm left the patient stuporous with severe quadriparesis and hydrocephalus. Repeat preoperative angiography revealed complete spontaneous thrombosis of the aneurysm and P2. Shunting was followed by remarkable but incomplete recovery.

Ten patients presented with CNIII paresis, one bilaterally, but six had P1 aneurysms projecting posteriorly, two had large aneurysms located at the P1-P2 junction or on the P2 segment respectively, and one small at the P2. The tiny aneurysm on a mesencephalic branch has already been mentioned.

Subtemporal Approach

Those arising from P1 are approached in the same fashion as for the basilar bifurcation, with the same precautions because of their common, intimate involvement with one or more thalamoperforating arteries (Fig. 16.1). Since the oculomotor nerve has an inferior relationship to the artery, it is seldom a concern unless the sac projects inferiorly, or into the interpeduncular cistern. Most P1 aneurysms are located very high in the relation to the posterior clinoid process and some may have to be approached through a frontotemporal craniotomy: in one giant aneurysm, it was necessary to abandon a subtemporal and proceed through a transsylvian exposure. In fact, in P1 and P1-P2 aneurysms the proportion of highly located necks is greatest of all aneurysms in close vicinity of the basilar tip. Otherwise, the main indication for a frontotemporal approach were associated anterior circulation aneurysms.

Larger P1-P2 junction aneurysms can be tricky in that P1, P2 and PComAs may splay out into a common base for the sac, which will require ingenuity in clipping to preserve the integrity of all three vessels (Figs. 16.2, 16.3).

The P2 segment is hidden under the parahippocampal gyrus as it winds around the side of the midbrain. Usually as P2 is followed back from

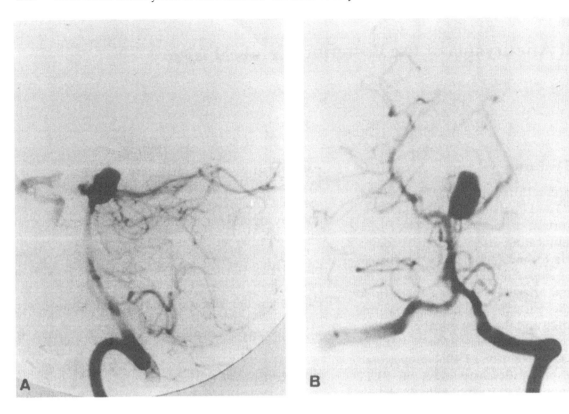

Figure 16.1 A, B. J.F., M, 45, large P1 aneurysm (**A, B**), which was opened and evacuated 11 days after bleed in Grade 1 in May 1981. No control studies, outcome excellent

its anterior extremity, it is possible to elevate this gyrus gently with the tip of the retractor to come upon the branching and the neck of the aneurysm (Fig. 16.4). Occasionally, it is necessary to remove a centimeter or so of the gyrus in order to expose a highly placed or more complex aneurysm lying on the upper midbrain in the choroidal fissure. A number of unusual aneurysms of large size have been seen at this site whose necks involve the origin in a fusiform way and require some ingenuity with clip selection and placement to preserve branch continuity, e.g. tandem clips or clip grafts. Perforators are not ordinarily a problem, but one must search for midbrain branches. The PCA may be followed nearly to the midline behind the quadrigeminal plate, through a temporal bone flap, if necessary (Figs. 16.5, 16.6). For aneurysms beyond this (P4 aneurysms), an occipital flap should be used so that the occipital pole, usually not tethered by draining veins, may be retracted laterally and upward from the falx-tentorial junction, using the semiprone "park bench" position.

Methods other than neck clipping have been used in an unusual number of these patients (Table 16.5). A tiny aneurysm on an ascending branch of P2 was found intact and thus not responsible for a ganglionic hemorrhage and was packed in cottonoid. Five of the 11 aneurysms associated with AVM were clipped, 5 were excised with an AVM and 1 was treated by proximal occlusion. Clip grafts were used in three patients – one was placed over the P1-P2 junction to occlude a small aneurysm which had been torn at the neck. Two P2 fusiform aneurysms, one small, one large, were treated similarly, the latter with two clips in tandem. All had good outcomes with preservation of the parent artery.

Occlusion of the PCA for small or even large aneurysms is seldom a consideration except for fusiform or unusually complex saccular aneurysms. From experience with deliberate occlusion for giant P1 or P2 aneurysms, it has been found that this artery has remarkable leptomeningeal collateral from A2 and M2 branches, such that occipi-

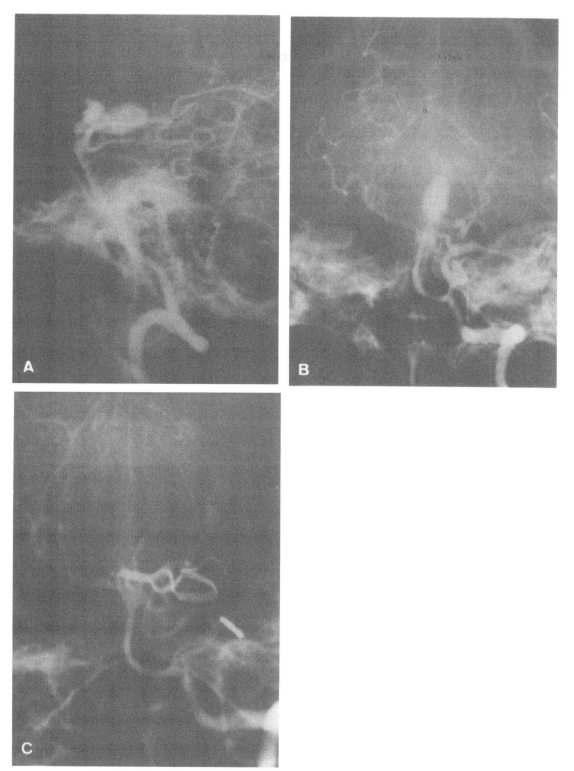

Figure 16.2 A–C. V.S., F, 52, large posteriorly projecting P1-P2-PComA aneurysm (**A, B**), six weeks complete left oculomotor palsy and confusion. Neck clipping in November 1976 preserving the union of the three arteries (**C**). Outcome excellent

224 Non-Giant Aneurysms of the Posterior Cerebral Artery

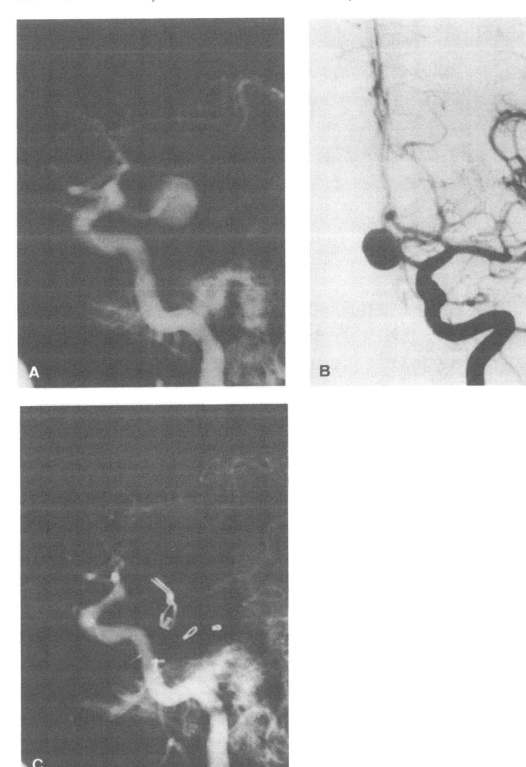

Figure 16.3 A–C. K.M., F, 58, large intact P1-P2-PComA aneurysm (**A, B**), six months headache and peculiar attacks of streak of light inside of head, "like firecracker with noise". Neck clipping in May 1979 preserving the parent vessels (**C**). Outcome excellent

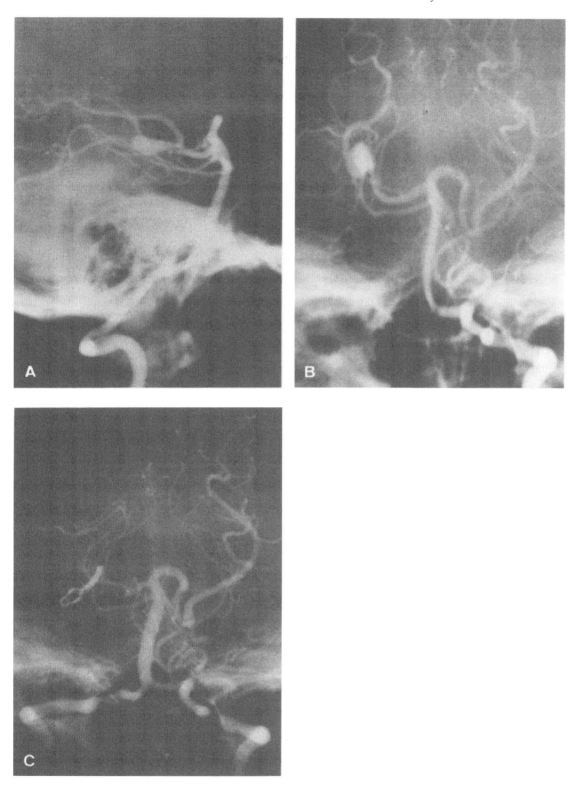

Figure 16.4 A–C. J.S., F, 49, ruptured large P2 aneurysm (**A, B**), neck clipping two days after bleed in Grade 1 in August 1987. Preservation of parent branching (**C**). Outcome excellent

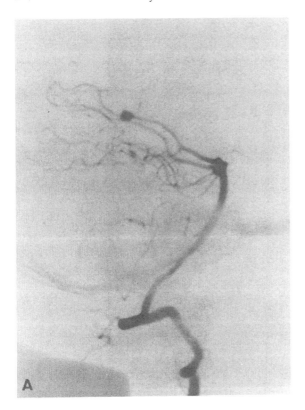 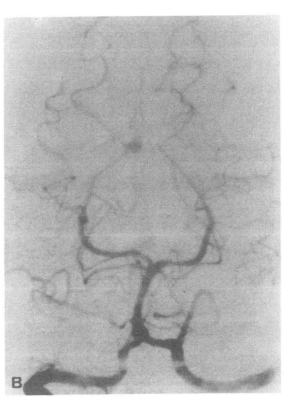

Figure 16.5 A, B. C.H., F, 49, small intact P3 aneurysm lying on quadrigeminal plate, discovered during investigation of Wallenberg syndrome from right vertebral occlusion probably from a bland dissection (**A, B**). The aneurysm was clipped and aspirated through a subtemporal approach in March 1986. No control studies, outcome excellent

tal infarction is rare after either P1 or P2 occlusion or trapping. Advantage has been taken of this collateral when a tear occurred at the neck or an unclippable aneurysm was exposed. Adequacy of collateral can be anticipated by the amount of back bleeding, after temporary proximal occlusion, from a tear or through a needle puncture. The P1 segment can be occluded if a good PComA exists, but even in its absence or where the integrity of the P1-PCom junction cannot be maintained. If doubt exists and the sac is not bleeding, then a tourniquet can be placed for occlusion after the patient wakens. Trapping aneurysms on the P1 segment must be done with great caution, lest hidden thalamoperforating vessels be trapped too, with devastating infarction.

P1 clipping was used for a small bilocular sac which was torn at its base and for a large partially fusiform aneurysm, with good outcomes.

P2 occlusion was used for one small and two large aneurysms which were partially fusiform with good results and no field defects, although two had temporary hemiparesis. In one of these, the tourniquet occlusion was used one week after further enlargement of the artery under the clip occluding the saccular portion of the aneurysm.

Two large P2 bulbous aneurysms were trapped; both were poor preoperative grades and did not survive. One further large P2 aneurysm with an excellent outcome was excised to be certain that it was not mycotic. The five distal aneurysms associated with AVMs had excellent outcomes as well.

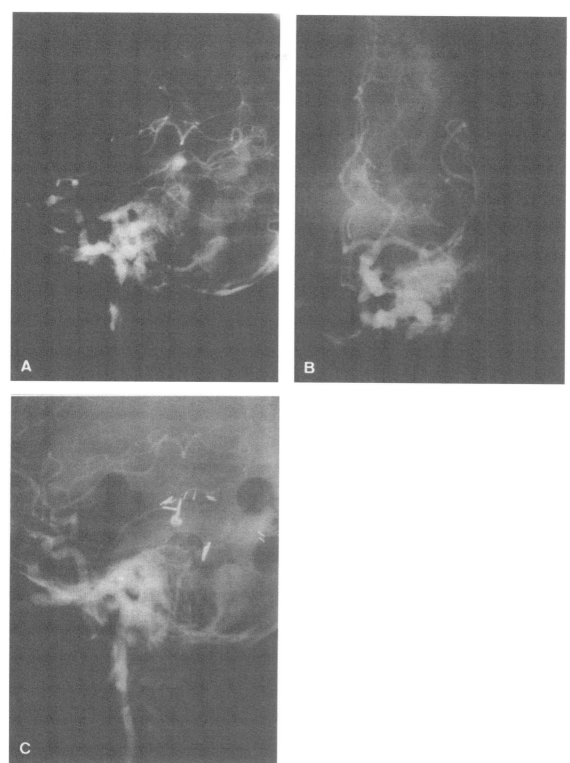

Figure 16.6 A–C. W.J., F, 39, intact left P3 aneurysm fed by foetal PComA (**A, B**). Operation in December 1975, P3 integrity after clipping (**C**). No field defect, outcome excellent

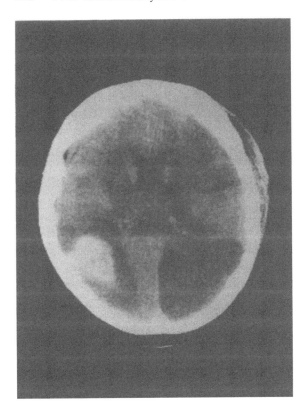

Figure 16.7. B.Y., F, 59, left eye pain, glaucoma? CT then angiography revealed intact left carotid-posterior communicating and left P1-P2 aneurysms. Massive bilateral cerebral infarction from diffuse vasospasm followed clipping of both aneurysms in July 1986, died ten days after operation

Results

The origin of the P1 and P1-P2 junction aneurysms did not appear to influence the outcome as there were no ischemic calamities from inadvertent branch or perforator occlusion. In two P1-P2 cases it was necessary to clip either P1 or the PComA. The former made excellent recovery but the latter died as a result of multiple ischemic lesions from vasospasm. Three good risk patients had minor disabilities from resolving postoperative hemiparesis. There were three bad outcomes among the small P1 and P1-P2 aneurysms. In two Grade 3 patients, major preoperative deficits existed from vasospasm; one was hemiplegic and the other dysphasic with hemisensory loss and hemianopia. The death was in a patient whose P1-P2 aneurysm was intact and who had an intact carotid communicating aneurysm, both incidental. Incredibly, severe diffuse vasospasm developed postoperatively with massive, bihemispheric hemorrhagic infarctions (Fig. 16.7). There had been no misadventure except for a little bleeding from the PComA when it had to be sharply dissected from the sellar margin; the rent and the vessel were occluded with a small Sugita clip. It is only the second example in the authors experience of severe vasospasm in dealing with intact aneurysms.

One large P1 aneurysm was clipped without difficulty in a Grade 3 patient. But an associated intact carotid communicating aneurysm ruptured at the far side of the neck during coagulation and in spite of clipping, massive rebleeding occurred during closure. She did not survive the brain swelling.

For the P2 aneurysms, the single poor result was the result of a spontaneous preoperative ganglionic hemorrhage, the tiny branch P2 aneurysm being found intact and remote from the clot cavity. Two of the three deaths were in Grade 4 and 5 patients in whom the aneurysm was trapped. The other death was in a Grade 3 patient who died from pulmonary embolism on the eleventh day when recovery seemed assured. Two of three patients operated on the day or next after recurrent subarachnoid hemorrhage died, both were Grade 5. Remarkably, all non-giant aneurysms of the PCA were totally obliterated.

Table 16.1. Preoperative grade and outcome in 59 patients with small and large posterior cerebral artery aneurysms

Grade	Excellent	Good	Poor	Dead	Total
0	15		1	1	17
1	25	5			30
2	1	1			2
3	1	2	3	1	7
4				1	1
5				2	2
Total	42	8	4	5	59
	71.2%	13.6%	6.8%	8.5%	100.0%

Table 16.2. Aneurysm size and outcome in 59 patients with small and large posterior cerebral artery aneurysms

Size	Excellent	Good	Poor	Dead	Total
Small	28	6	3	2	39
Large	14	2	1	3	20
Total	42	8	4	5	59

Table 16.3. Aneurysm site and outcome in 59 patients with small and large posterior cerebral artery aneurysms

Site	Excellent	Good	Poor	Dead	Total
P1	12	4	3	1	20
P1 Mesencephalic artery	1				1
P1–P2	9	1		1	11
P2	13	3	1	3	20
P3–P4	7				7
Total	42	8	4	5	59

Table 16.4. Age related to outcome in 59 patients with small and large posterior cerebral aneurysms

Age group (years)	Excellent	Good	Poor	Dead	Total
10–19	2				2
20–29	8	1			9
30–39	5	1	1	1	8
40–49	12	3	2	3	20
50–59	11	1	1	1	14
60–69	3	2			5
70 or more	1				1
Total	42	8	4	5	59

Table 16.5. Operative method and outcome in 59 patients with small and large posterior cerebral artery aneurysms

Operative method	Excellent	Good	Poor	Dead	Total
Neck clipping[a]	32	7	3	3	45
Silk ligature	1				1
Hunterian ligation	3	1			4
Trapping				2	2
Excision	6				6
Shunt only			1		1
Total	42	8	4	5	59

[a] Includes 3 clip grafts.

Table 16.6. Timing of surgery and outcome in 42 patients with small or large posterior cerebral artery aneurysms

Timing of surgery	Excellent	Good	Poor	Dead	Total
0–1 day	1			2	3
2–3 day	1				1
4–6 day	1	2		1	4
7–10 day	3	2			5
11–30 day	12	4	1	1	18
31–365 day	9		2		11
Total	27	8	3	4	42

Chapter 17
Giant Posterior Cerebral Aneurysms
66 Patients

Since the illustration and description of the first 13 aneurysms (Fig. 17.1), another 53 have been operated upon. Altogether 39 have arisen from the P1 or the P1-P2 junction, 20 from the P2, and 7 from the P3 or P4 portion of the artery (Table 17.2).

Anatomical Features

P1 Aneurysms

The position of the P1 segment in the interpeduncular fossa and in front of the peduncle readily explains the frequency of oculomotor and pyramidal tract disorder as P1 aneurysms reach giant size (Weber's syndrome). Admittedly, the distinction between giant aneurysms of saccular and fusiform origin is blurred because of the size of the necks but 12 of the 26 aneurysms arising from P1 itself seemed to be fusiform from some unknown arteriopathy. Again, one-fifth of these giant aneurysms occurred in ages below 20. None appeared to have an atherosclerotic origin. The remainder must result from enlargement of small saccular aneurysms which arise at perforator origins or the P1-posterior communicating artery (PComA) junction.

P1 gives rise to numerous perforating vessels supplying the mammillary bodies, medial thalamus and midbrain. Two other branches, the short and long circumflex arteries arising more laterally, supply the peduncle, lateral geniculate body and colliculi.

As at the basilar bifurcation, these perforators assume great importance during treatment of P1 aneurysms. Their integrity must be preserved in the few aneurysms that can be clipped, but the origins of one or more may have to be left to thrombose with the aneurysm beyond a proximal P1 clip.

P1-P2 Junction Aneurysms

Thirteen aneurysms arose at the P1-P2 junction at the origin of the PComA and all but four were obviously saccular.

P2 and P3-P4 Aneurysms

Most P2 aneurysms seemed to arise at the first major branching of P2 on the side of the midbrain (anterior temporal artery). Five distal aneurysms arose from the artery just behind the quadrigeminal plate at the beginning of P3, one of which had produced a trochlear palsy. They presented beside or over the edge of the tentorium, a relationship probably responsible for the headache. Often P2 entered the sac on its medial side making awkward its identification and separation of its insertion into the sac; 12 aneurysms had to be opened and evacuated first.

Clinical Features

P1 and P1-P2 Junction Aneurysms (39 Patients)

Eleven of the 39 patients presented with recent subarachnoid hemorrhage (SAH), one of whom was in Grade 4 condition with a large temporal lobe clot. Three were incidental findings. Otherwise intractable headache was the most common complaint probably related to pressure of the sac on the sensitive tentorial edge as it expanded. Diplopia with CNIII paresis occurred in 14 and this was associated with hemiparesis in 6 (Weber's syndrome). Hemiplegia existed without oculomotor palsy in one further patient. Four patients had pre-existing field defects, two quadrantic and two hemianopia. Ataxia with limb clumsiness was present in two patients with huge aneurysms.

P2-P4 Aneurysms (27 Patients)

An even higher number presented with SAH, 13 patients, 3 of whom were in Grade 3 condition, 1

Giant Posterior Cerebral Aneurysms 231

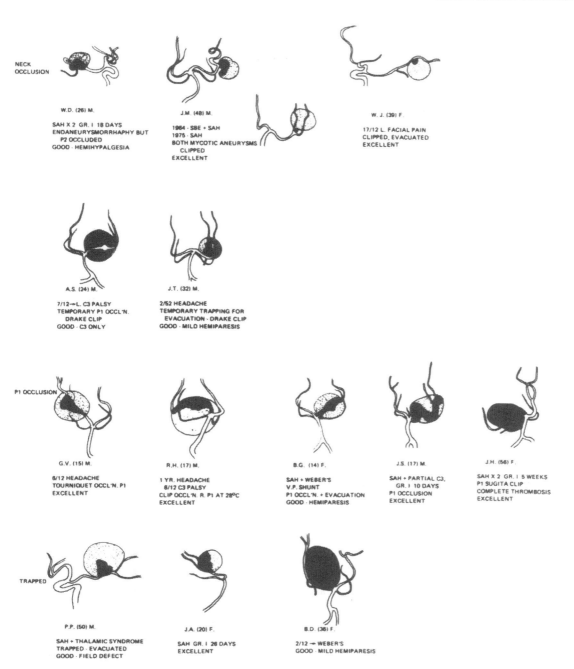

Figure 17.1. The origin, size and shape of giant posterior cerebral artery aneurysms and the extent of their mural thrombosis described and illustrated by tracings in the early experience. (Reprinted from Clin Neurosurg 26, 1979, p. 57 by courtesy of Williams and Wilkins)

with a temporal lobe hematoma. Two were incidental findings. Headache was as much a feature as with P1 aneurysms, probably for the same reason. Third nerve paresis occurred only in two proximal P2 aneurysms but a more distal one produced a CNIV palsy. Preoperative hemianopia existed in four patients, one with a huge mass, one after a hemorrhage and two which seemed clearly related to an embolus from the partially thrombosed aneurysm. Hemiplegia was present only in four with huge masses.

Treatment

The treatment of giant posterior cerebral aneurysms has been divided between those arising from P1 and P1-P2 junction and P2-P4 segments.

P1 Aneurysms

Giant P1 aneurysms are considered separately because of the origin of the medial thalamoperforating and circumflex vessels from this segment which are potentially the cause of most of the surgical morbidity, as the former were for aneurysms at the basilar bifurcation. As it happened, all five of the poor P1 results occurred because of brain stem infarction from injury or occlusion of these vessels.

Neck clipping. Only 6 of 26 P1 aneurysms could be clipped (Figs. 17.2, 17.3, 17.4). Perforators had to be separated from the necks of each aneurysm before clipping using a temporary P1 clip in two, and four had good results with continuity of P1 preserved. One poor result occurred when, during separation of a perforator, the proximal neck was torn into the origin of P1, which could be repaired with a narrow clip graft. Unfortunately, the basilar bifurcation became occluded and extensive bilateral brain stem infarction occurred from which she has made only a partial recovery. In the other, vasospasm caused hemiplegia after uneventful reoperation for a still filling aneurysm 17 days post third bleed.

P1 occlusion was used in 13 P1 aneurysms with good outcomes in 11, only 1 of which developed an occipital infarction with quadrantanopia. Postoperative angiograms showed magnificent leptomeningeal collateral in each often filling P2 retrogradely to near the P1-P2 junction. Two of the aneurysms were evacuated and all became completely thrombosed. Although several appeared to arise at the basilar bifurcation itself in the angiograms, in each there was 1 or 2 mm of P1 remaining over which a narrow clip could be placed (Fig. 17.5). But it may be very difficult to place even a very small narrow clip on P1 between the aneurysm and the medial thalamic perforating arteries which usually arise from the first mm or so of the P1 origin; one or more may have to be left to the mercy of collateral flow to their territory. It is remarkable how often this appears to exist, although it cannot be determined beforehand.

The two poor results both occurred from perforator infarction. In the first, a woman, 29, where P1 almost immediately expanded into the aneurysm, it was just possible to place a small curved clip across its origin. Although it narrowed the termination of the basilar artery and the opposite left P1, there seemed to be enough channel to irrigate the left P1. She awakened with bilateral oculomotor palsies, left hemiparesis and amnesia from bilateral thalamic infarcts, no doubt due to occlusion of the medial thalamic perforating vessels. She recovered to a mild hemiparesis and vertical gaze palsy but with a profound amnestic syndrome. The other had a large perforator arising from the back of P1 at the neck which could not be spared and midbrain and medial occipital infarcts occurred. She recovered remarkably but has been left with a mild hemiparesis, upper quadrantanopsia and anomic dysphasia.

Two patients classified as good had preoperative fully developed Weber's syndromes from which recovery has been gratifying to the extent of returning to their usual occupation with mild disability. Each, however, had small midbrain or thalamic low densities postoperatively.

Trapping after P1 clipping and evacuation of giant aneurysms restricted to P1 was used in five patients, two at the time (Fig. 17.6) and three with a delayed procedure. The indications were to relieve mass effect and/or refilling of the sac through the PComA in most; three had severe hemiparesis. In two, it was necessary to divide the tentorium and use temporary trapping with a temporary clip on the basilar artery to slacken the sac enough to be able to see the origin of P1 for clipping. In another, it was necessary to partially evacuate the sac of thrombus before visualizing P1 and he was the only poor result from massive midbrain infarction from presumed perforator occlusion on the hidden portion of the aneurysm base (Fig. 17.7).

The delayed trappings were because of unrelieved mass effect in two and a rebleeding in the other 12 days later in spite of upper basilar artery tourniquet occlusion when P1 could not be visualized from the opposite side. All three had good outcomes although two are functioning with mild residual hemiparesis.

Endovascular *embolization* was used in one patient who had refused treatment two years before. He was severely disabled with severe right hemiparesis, ataxia, dysphagia, dysarthria and emotion-

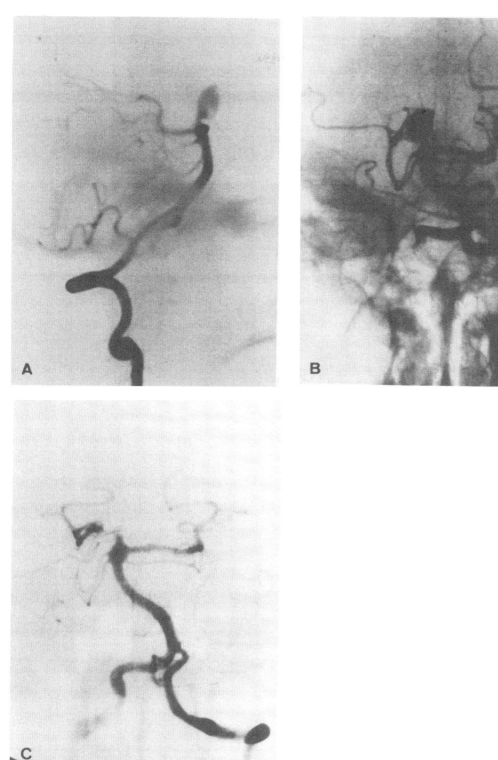

Figure 17.2 A–C. L.B., F, 38, giant partially thrombosed right P1 aneurysm (**A, B**), 8 months headache. Clip occlusion of neck with preservation of P1 after temporary P1 occlusion and evacuation of the sac in May 1983 (**C**). Outcome excellent

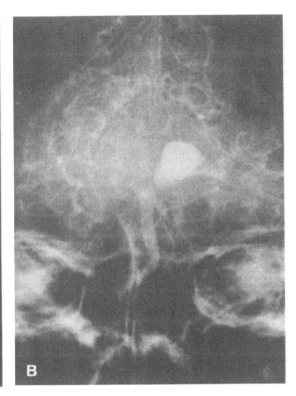
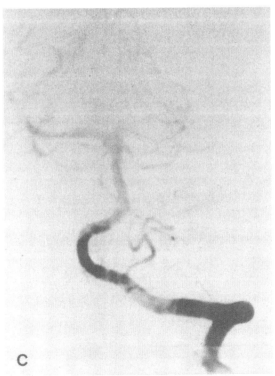

Figure 17.3 A–C. M.A., F, 59, giant partially thrombosed left P1 aneurysm (**A, B**), three months early Weber's syndrome. Neck clipping in April 1984 produced stenosis of P1 without sequelae (**C**). Outcome excellent

Giant Posterior Cerebral Aneurysms 235

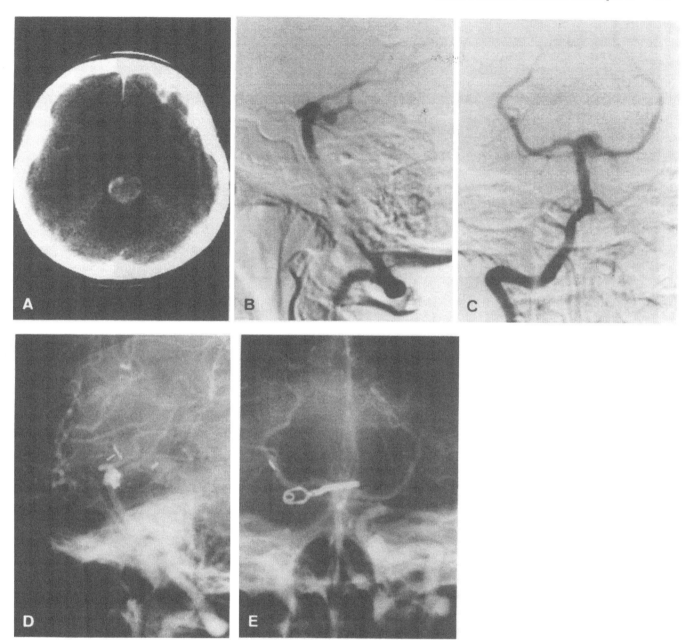

Figure 17.4 A–E. L.B., M, 60, intact giant proximal P1 aneurysm appearing to arise at basilar bifurcation (**A–C**), rheumatoid arthritis with gaze paresis and ataxia. Clipping in February 1984 revealed P1 origin (**D, E**). Outcome excellent

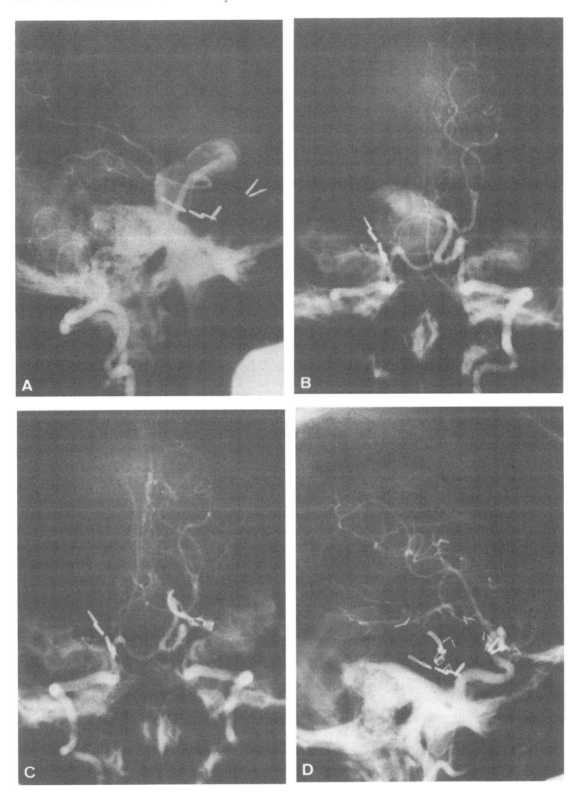

Figure 17.5 A–D. J.H., F, 56, ruptured giant right P1 saccular aneurysm which had been explored elsewhere (**A, B**). Operation in September 1978 five weeks after bleed (Grade 1); clipping of P1 was done from left approach due to displacement of basilar bifurcation (**C**). Lateral carotid showing tiny portion of sac filling at insertion of small posterior communicating artery into the sac. No field defect (**D**). Outcome excellent

Giant Posterior Cerebral Aneurysms   237

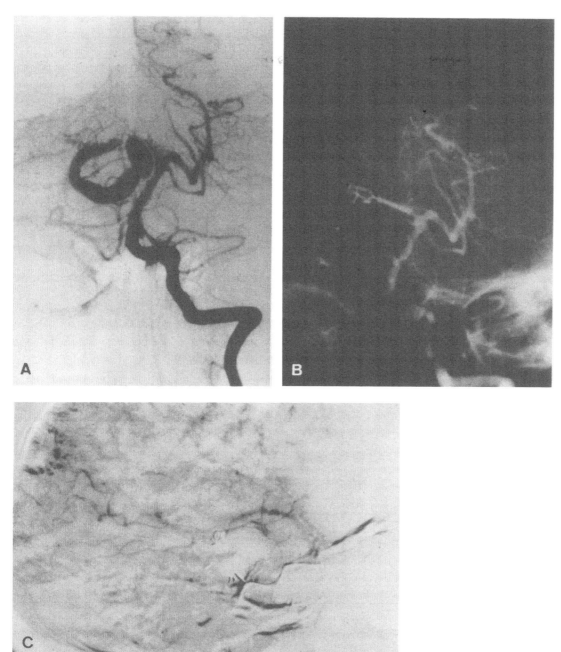

Figure 17.6 A–C. S.W., M, 42, intact giant P1 aneurysm, partially thrombosed, with serpentine channel through it (**A**), headache and right oculomotor palsy. Aneurysmal mass obscured basilar bifurcation even after evacuation with five temporary basilar occlusions in March 1981. Division of P2 allowed sac to be displaced forward so clip could be placed on P1 origin free of perforators (**B**). Excellent leptomeningeal collateral filling posterior cerebral artery territory even back to near aneurysm site (**C**). Outcome excellent

238 Giant Posterior Cerebral Aneurysms

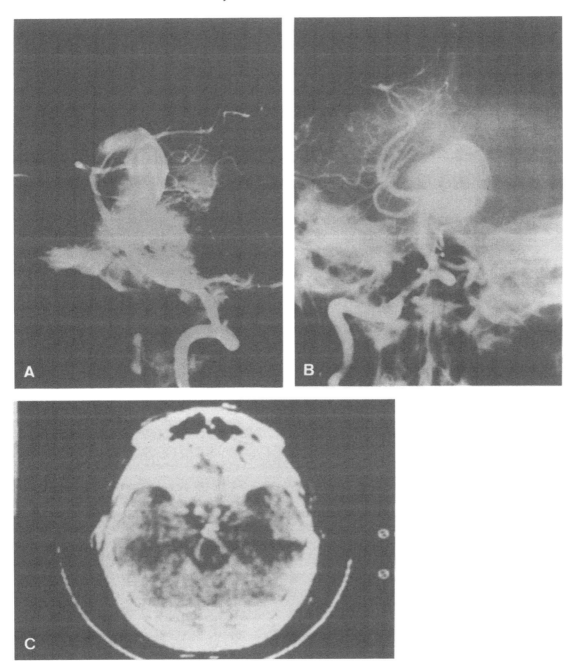

Figure 17.7 A–C. K.N., M, 44, intact giant P1 aneurysm (**A, B**), five months headache, left arm paresis and severe ataxia. CT after trapping in May 1980 shows large infarction central midbrain. It was not possible to place a clip on P1 origin without stenosing basilar bifurcation until aneurysm had been trapped with a P2 clip and evacuated (**C**). Outcome poor with MLF syndrome and severe ataxia but with normal mentation

al lability. The mass was huge and P1 could not be separated either by subtemporal or transsylvian exploration. An attempt at endovascular detached balloon occlusion of P1 failed when it could not be detached without occluding the basilar bifurcation. A 1 cc bolus of fast polymerizing isobutyl-2-cyano acrylate (IBCA) was injected while P1 was still balloon occluded but it did not polymerize immediately and when the catheter was withdrawn a shower of IBCA occluded the basilar artery and several perforators. In CT, there was some IBCA in the aneurysm and both posterior cerebral arteries (PCAs). Deep unresponsive coma was immediate and he survived the massive infarction less than 24 hours (Fig. 24.2, Case 2 in Table 24.1).

P1-P2 Posterior Communicating Aneurysms (12 Patients)

Neck clipping was accomplished only in four patients, all after temporary trapping and evacuation of the sac (Fig. 17.8). All had good outcomes, one in spite of the clip occluding P1, even though the aneurysm had been evacuated before clip application. An arm paresis recovered so that he is working.

P1 occlusion was used in four patients using the tourniquet in the first. PComA occlusion was added in one to prevent inflow into the aneurysm (Figs. 17.9, 17.10). All except one with hemiplegia had good results, although two had small brain stem infarcts from which they made virtually complete recoveries.

PComA occlusion alone at its entrance into the aneurysm was used in one patient where the aneurysm appeared to arise from the distal portion of this vessel (Fig. 17.11). Good outcome resulted with complete thrombosis in the aneurysm.

Trapping was used in four, all *acutely*. One became necessary when P2 had to be divided in order to see P1 medial to the huge mass. The other two needed PComA occlusion as well.

The death was tragic in a woman, 59, with Weber's syndrome and there was a giant arteriovenous malformation (AMV) beyond on P2. Clips were placed on the PCom, P1 and P2 although visualization of P1 was difficult. After initial slackening, the aneurysm refilled but it was thought due to retrograde perforator flow; unfortunately the clip position on P1 was not verified. She was much the same in the recovery room for two hours when sudden coma occurred leading to her demise. At autopsy, the clip had slipped off the large P1 so that unrestrained P1 flow entered the blind sac without outflow, rupturing this previously intact aneurysm.

The outcome from the interruption of posterior temporal and occipital lobe blood supply by P1 and P2 clipping and trapping will be discussed after the P2 series.

P2-P4 Aneurysms (27 Patients)

Neck clipping was accomplished in six patients, although in three the aneurysm had to be evacuated first after temporary P2 clipping. In one of these an endoaneurysmorrhaphy was done, closing the ostium with fine silk, but P2 was occluded in the control angiograms. He made a virtually complete recovery from a hemianesthesia from a small preoperative clot in the thalamus. Another man had a second giant left middle cerebral aneurysm on the same side. Both were mycotic from subacute bacterial endocarditis one year before and their small necks were easily clipped during the same craniotomy. His left parietal dural AVM was left in place. In a woman, 44, P1 was stenosed at the clip site, and although the CT showed no low density, she developed a partial right upper quadrantanopsia, dyslexia and dysnomia. Her speech improved so that she was not disabled for ordinary life.

Proximal occlusion of P2 was used in 17 patients and all had good outcomes, all with complete thrombotic occlusion of the aneurysm. In three, the sac was largely evacuated of clot without trapping. In one, tourniquet occlusion of P1 was used because a large perforator arose at the neck. No deficit occurred over 24 hours and the snare was permanently occluded and buried.

Three patients were classified as good. One in Grade 3 recovered to "70%" from hemiplegia after evacuation of a temporal hematoma; the other improved from a partial left hemianesthesia and clumsiness but is also working. The third man, aged 50, was confused and drowsy with a left hemiplegia and periodic breathing from a 6 cm aneurysm, massively thrombosed with a tortuous channel through it. It was realized from previous experience when P1 and its origin were buried in the brain

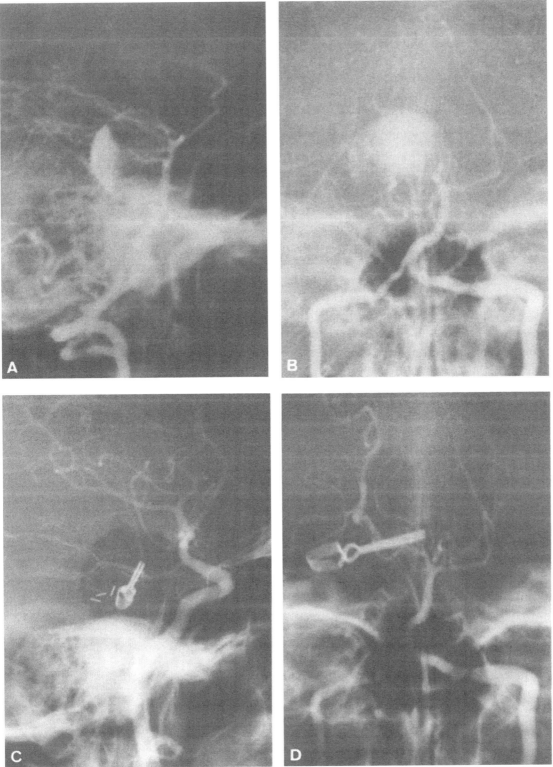

Figure 17.8 A–D. A.S., M, 24, intact giant right P1-P2 aneurysm (**A, B**), 7 months headache and complete oculomotor palsy. Neck clipping in February 1978 after temporary P1 clip and evacuation (**C, D**). Outcome excellent

Giant Posterior Cerebral Aneurysms 241

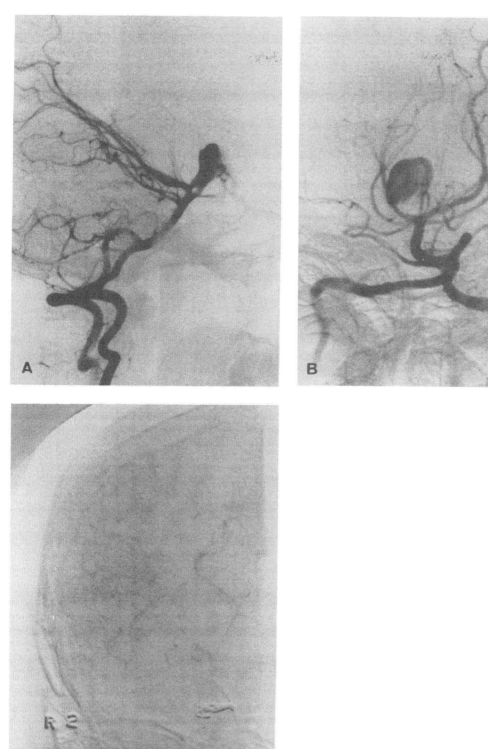

Figure 17.9 A–C. E.F., M, 22, ruptured giant partially thrombosed P1-P2 aneurysm, explored elsewhere (**A, B**). Complete thrombosis of aneurysm after clipping P1 and posterior communicating arteries in June 1988, three months after bleed in Grade 1. Luxuriant leptomeningeal collateral even fills P2 retrogradely to aneurysm site (**C**). No field defect. Outcome excellent

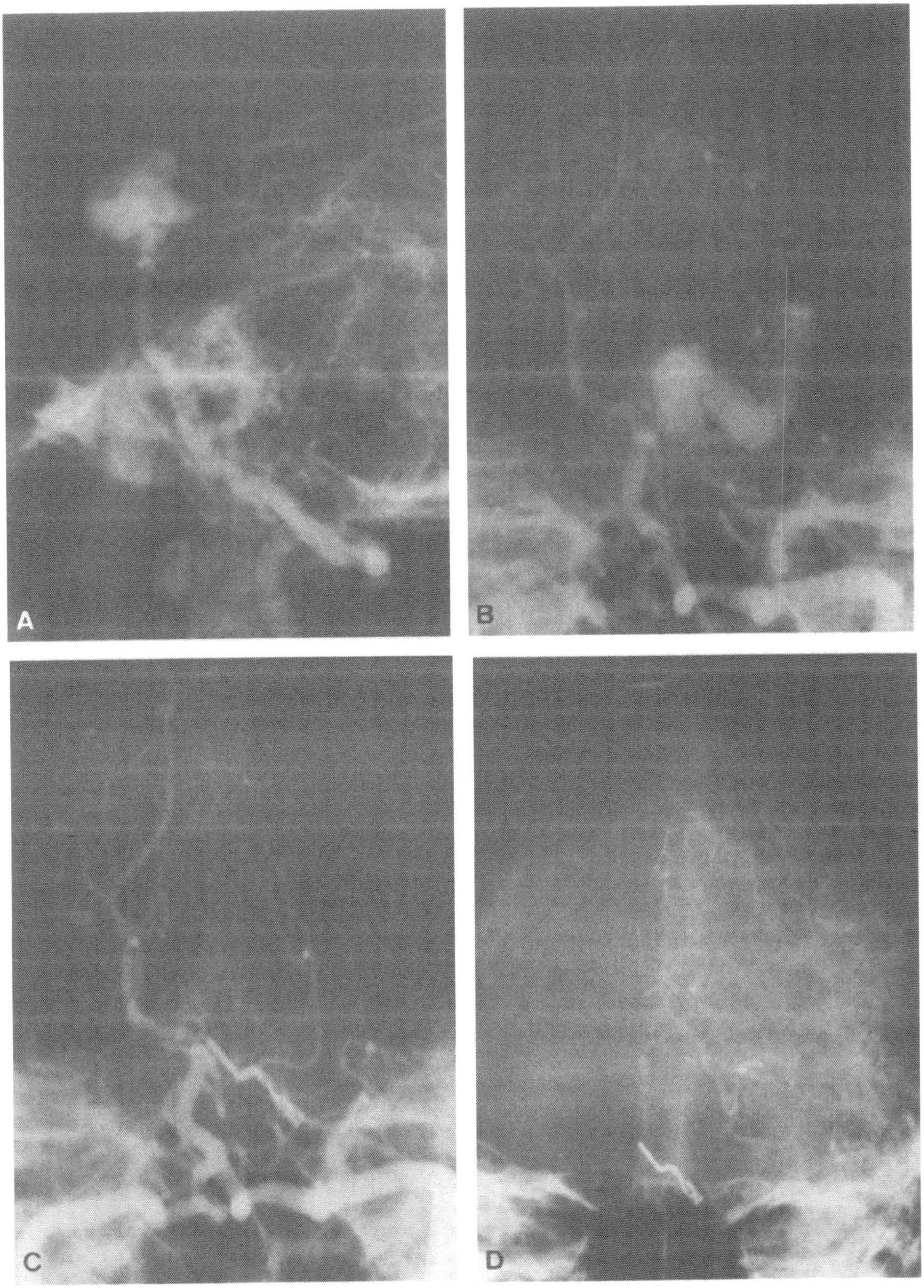

Figure 17.10 A–D. J.S., M, 18, ruptured giant left fusiform P1-P2 (**A, B**), three months of headache, one bleed 10 days earlier with partial oculomotor palsy, Grade I. Clipping of P1 origin in September 1977 (**C**). Luxuriant leptomeningeal collateral filling of posterior cerebral branches retrogradely to end of thrombosed aneurysm. No field defect (**D**). Outcome excellent

Giant Posterior Cerebral Aneurysms   243

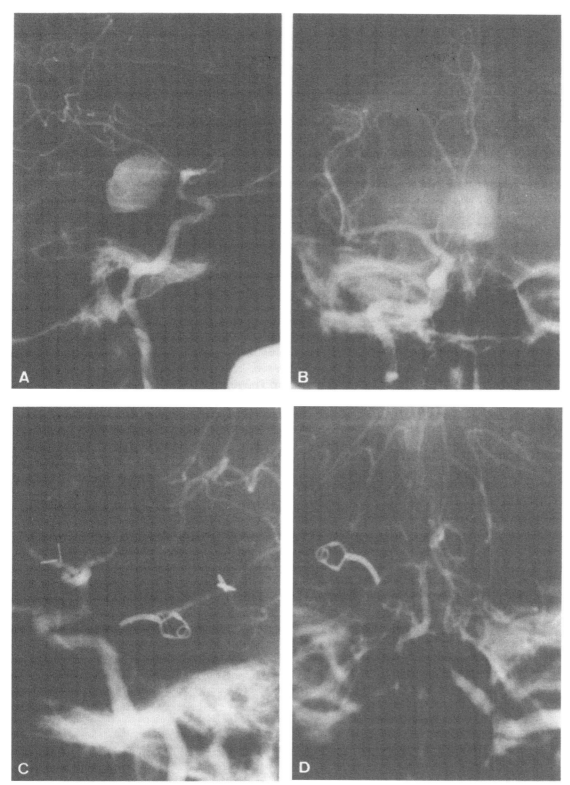

Figure 17.11 A–D. M.L., F, 53, giant aneurysm of posterior communicating artery (**A, B**), psychotic, three years of headache. After clipping of posterior communicating artery in November 1978 the aneurysm thrombosed and there was no retrograde filling from the right P1 (**C, D**). No field defect. Outcome excellent

stem under the mass, that P1 could not be seen for clipping without injuring the peduncle. As detached balloon occlusion in P1 might occlude perforators, it was decided to occlude the origin of the sac with detached wire coils. Fortunately, at the beginning of the channel there was a small loculus into which could be detached six platinum coils. These produced complete thrombosis of the channel so that two days later at craniotomy, the aneurysm was opened and nearly completely evacuated of thrombus. At discharge he was still hemiplegic but two months later he had made a "dramatic" recovery in the use of his left limbs (Fig. 17.12, Case 5 in Table 24.1).

Trapping was used in five patients to decrease mass effect and all had satisfactory results (Fig. 17.13). One man, 50, in Grade 3, was left with a right homonymous hemianopia and mild dyslexia. Another, 55, had a postoperative hemiplegia with a full field defect after trapping and evacuating a 5 cm aneurysm. In addition to an occipital infarction there were small low densities in the left thalamus and posteriorly in the posterior limb of the capsule. Remarkably what was to become functional recovery of limb function began in hospital but although he is active on the farm with mild hemiparesis, there is dyslexia and word-finding difficulty.

Proximal parent artery occlusion or trapping for obliteration of giant aneurysms has an effect on two collateral circulations, that of the perforating branches arising from or very near the aneurysm and that of the main branches of the artery arising beyond the aneurysm. The effect will depend on the collateral circulation to these two territories. Unfortunately, the extent of the former awaits thrombosis of the aneurysm and therefore cannot be tested prior to the occlusion, even by tourniquet. The outcome related to perforator occlusion in P1 and P2 giant aneurysms has been discussed. It is remarkable how often sufficient collateral to this small deep brain stem circulation must exist to explain the absence of brain stem infarction when visualized as well as presumed perforators were occluded by the aneurysm thrombosis.

The outcome after removing antegrade flow in the P2 and P3 branches is even more remarkable (Table 17.7). When the preoperative hemianopias (3) and those unknown because of the condition of the patient (2) are excluded, there remain 47 patients in whom the outcome re. occipital infarction could be determined. Only 5 of the 47 cases developed hemianopias postoperatively and 1 of these was only superior quadrantic. Two patients died and in two cases the fate of visual fields was not known. The reason for the preservation of occipital function was luxuriant leptomeningeal collateral from terminal anterior and middle cerebral branchings which often filled P3 retrogradely and even P2 back to near the site of the aneurysm. Its frequency and extent is such as to question surgical bypass to P2 when it is to be occluded, at least for a giant aneurysm of the posterior cerebral artery (PCA). The number of PCA occlusions in non-giant aneurysms was only four, but none of these developed visual field deficits.

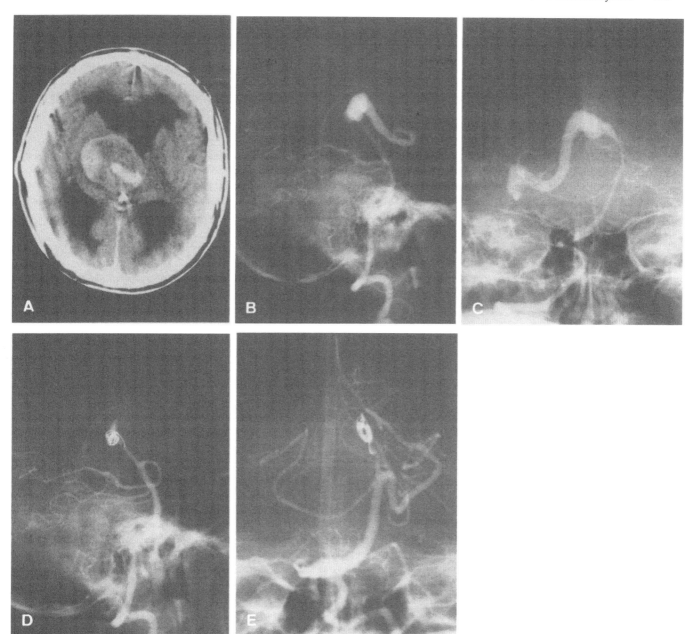

Figure 17.12 A–E. R.S., M, 50, huge P2 aneurysm (**A–C**), headache 1 1/2 years with left hemiparesis progressing to solid hemiplegia. The aneurysm is massively thrombosed except for serpentine channel running through it irrigating the posterior cerebral artery. Embedding of such a large mass in the brain stem made unlikely an attempt to clip the right P1 but smaller saccular enlargement at beginning of channel offered possibility of its endovascular occlusion. Six wire coils have been deposited in proximal saccular channel in June 1990, occluding P2 (**D, E**). Declining consciousness with respiratory arrhythmia led to subtemporal Cavitron evacuation of the aneurysm two days later. After four months dramatic recovery from paralysis had occurred. Good outcome

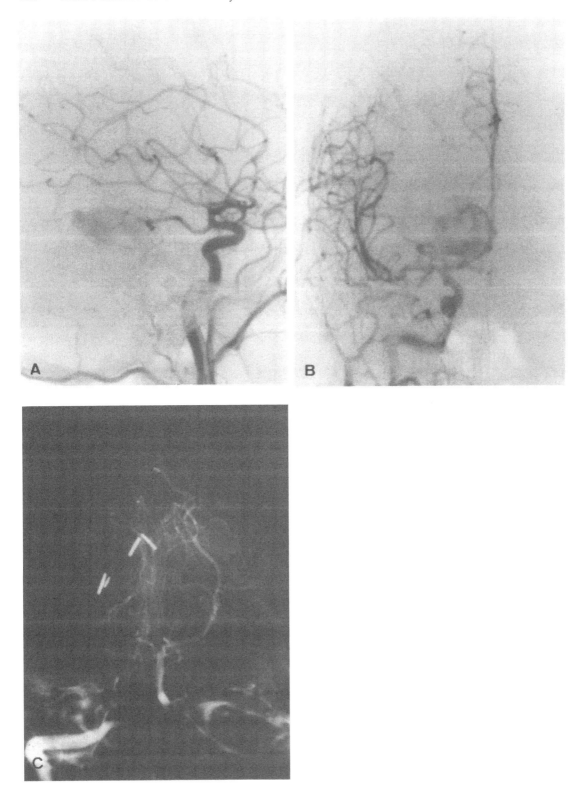

Figure 17.13 A–C. S.R., F, 15, ruptured giant distal P2 aneurysm, faintly filling (**A, B**), one bleed two weeks after 6 weeks of headache and a seizure, Grade 1. After trapping and evacuation in June 1980 there was no field defect (**C**). Outcome excellent

Table 17.1. Preoperative Grade and outcome in 66 patients with giant posterior cerebral artery aneurysms

Grade	Excellent	Good	Poor	Dead	Total
0[a]	31	7	3	2	43
0g	28	4	2	0	34
0p	3	3	1	2	9
1	15	1	2		18
3	1	3	1		5
Total	47	11	6	2	66
	71.2%	16.7%	9.1%	3.0%	100.0%

[a] *0* Unruptured aneurysm or remote hemorrhage (> 1 year). *0g* Good risk without major neurological deficit. *0p* Poor risk patient with major neurological deficit (severe confusion or dementia or stupor or coma, dysarthria or bulbar paralysis, severe dysphasia or severe mono-, hemi-, or tetraparesis).

Table 17.2. Aneurysm site and outcome in 66 patients with giant posterior cerebral artery aneurysms

Site	Excellent	Good	Poor	Dead	Total
P1	17	3	5	1	26
P1–P2	10	1	1	1	13
P2	14	6			20
P3–P4	6	1			7
Total	47	11	6	2	66

Table 17.3. Age related to outcome in 66 patients with giant posterior cerebral artery aneurysms

Age group (years)	Excellent	Good	Poor	Dead	Total
0–9	1				1
10–19	10	1			11
20–29	8	1	1		10
30–39	5	3		1	9
40–49	10	2	2		14
50–59	9	4	2	1	16
60–69	4		1		5
Total	47	11	6	2	66

Table 17.4. Operative method and outcome in 66 patients with giant posterior cerebral artery aneurysms

Operative method	Excellent	Good	Poor	Dead	Total
Clip	11	2	2		15
Hunterian ligation	28	5	3		36
Trapping	7	4	1	1	13
Endosaccular glue			1		1
Exploration only	1				1
Total	47	11	6	2	66

Table 17.5. Operative method and result of aneurysm treatment in 66 patients with giant posterior cerebral artery aneurysms

Operative method	Total obliteration	Residual neck	Residual fundus	No obliteration	Total
Clip	15				15
Hunterian ligation	33	1	2		36
Trapping	12			1[a]	13
Endovascular glue	1				1
Exploration				1	1
Total	61	1	2	2	66

[a] Proximal P1 clip slipped and aneurysm ruptured.

Table 17.6. Timing of surgery and outcome in 23 patients with giant posterior cerebral artery aneurysms

Timing of surgery	Excellent	Good	Poor	Dead	Total
4–6 day	1				1
7–10 day	2	1			3
11–30 day	7	1	3		11
31–365 day	6	2			8
Total	16	4	3		23

Table 17.7. The outcome of visual fields after removing antegrade flow in the P1 and P2 branches in 52 patients with posterior cerebral artery aneurysms (non-giant and giant)

	Pre-op. No.	Defect	Post-op. No defect	Acquired defect	Unknown
P1 occlusion	17[a]		15	1[b]	1
P1 trapped	8		6	0	2
P2 occlusion	20	3	16	1	0
P2 trapped	7		3	3	1
Total	52	3	40	5	4

[a] PCom artery clipped in one patient.
[b] Right upper quadrantic only.

Chapter 18
Multiple Aneurysms
462 Patients

The number of associated aneurysms in this series is high as most patients had both vertebral and carotid trees studied. The incidence of multiple aneurysms (26.2%) therefore probably approximates the actual figure. The female sex predominated (73%). Hypertension was not more frequent (20%) and the mean age of these patients was three years higher than with single aneurysms.

Two-thirds of the patients presented with subarachnoid hemorrhage (SAH). In 45 patients, the bleeding aneurysm was in the anterior circulation (Table 18.1). Multiple SAHs were not more common than in single aneurysms.

Ten percent of the aneurysms were found in examinations for other reasons as cranial nerve palsies or headache. Less than 10% presented as mass lesions. Third nerve paralysis was rather frequent (12.5%), otherwise this group did not differ from clinical signs of single aneurysms. Site of the vertebro-basilar artery (VBA) aneurysm with multiple aneurysms did not differ from the usual distribution in single aneurysm cases (Table 18.2).

Seventeen and a half percent (17.5%) of multiple aneurysms were on the vertebrobasilar circulation and 82.5% were on the anterior circulation where over half were internal carotid aneurysms (Tables 18.1 and 18.2).

A large number of patients had three or more aneurysms. A few patients had six or even eight aneurysms. More than 100 patients with multiple aneurysms had additional aneurysms on the posterior circulation; even four vertebrobasilar aneurysms were seen in six patients. Posterior cerebral artery (PCA) aneurysms were least likely to bleed (Tables 18.4 and 18.5).

Of the non-giant posterior circulation aneurysms, superior cerebellar artery (SCA) and PCA aneurysms were most often associated with multiple aneurysms followed by small basilar bifurcation aneurysms. Giant aneurysms were less frequently associated with other aneurysms.

Nearly half of the arteriovenous malformations (AVMs) in the total series (59) were associated with multiple aneurysms (26 cases). AVMs were associated with a large number of aneurysms: 10 with 2, 9 with 3, 6 with 4 and 1 with 5 aneurysms.

Treatment

In dealing with multiple aneurysms, a principle has been to deal with the ruptured aneurysm first and that going well, proceed to the largest intact sac and then the next. If there is concern about any, the pursuit of the intact sac(s) is abandoned. Usually the deepest aneurysm was exposed and clipped first to avoid clip blades and handles obstructing the approach.

The symptomatic and the additional aneurysms influenced the selection of the approach. Eighty percent of the symptomatic aneurysms in this series were located at the basilar tip. As carotid aneurysms, most frequently at the posterior communicating artery (PComA), dominate as an associated aneurysm, a subtemporal approach was used in most cases for ipsilateral carotid aneurysms below the bifurcation which can be exposed satisfactorily for clipping. The subtemporal approach has also been used for dealing with combined upper and lower basilar aneurysms or even a vertebral aneurysm through a divided tentorium.

Carotid bifurcation, middle cerebral artery (MCA) and anterior communicating artery (AComA) aneurysms require a frontotemporal transsylvian approach and this was used in one-third of the 462 multiple aneurysm cases in this series, 80% of frontotemporal approaches for basilar aneurysms were done in multiple aneurysm cases. Usually an intact MCA aneurysm would be covered and bypassed after its exposure to approach the basilar aneurysm beside the carotid over the posterior clinoid. But an intact carotid aneurysm had to be clipped and collapsed to provide exposure. In many cases, due to the confining nature of this exposure, it was changed to the subtemporal or half and half approach (vide supra). As well many of the basilar aneurysms were low behind the clivus or backward pointing. The intact aneurysm(s) was dealt with on the way out if appropriate.

After introduction of the microscope, some aneurysms of the *contralateral* lower carotid artery or proximal MCA were done from the transsylvian approach; AComA aneurysms regularly. But in most cases where the first aneurysm was found to be intact a second flap was turned to discover a contralateral ruptured sac. Depending on patient condition, a few weeks interval was allowed if the intact aneurysms could not be approached from the same opening (Fig. 18.1). Where a posterior fossa approach had to be used for a ruptured lower basilar or vertebral aneurysm, a supratentorial aneurysm was left for a delayed procedure. It can be combined with the subtemporal approach which was used on a few occasions.

More than half of the additional aneurysms were clipped; several were left for observation as they were small, for technical, somatic, or geographic reasons, or the patients refused additional operations (Tables 18.5 and 18.6). If unruptured or in Grade 1, the treatment of additional aneurysm(s) did not seem to influence the results; in Grade 2, the combined mortality and morbidity was higher than in the patients with single aneurysms (Table 18.7). Early surgery on days 2 and 3 after bleeding carried a high mortality, and maybe was influenced by the additional manipulation of the vessels and brain required in multiple aneurysms as the results were significantly better in single aneurysms (Table 18.8).

Although it could not be determined exactly, the additional morbidity due to the repair of an additional aneurysm was low (Table 18.9). However, two fatal outcomes were due to the repair of the additional aneurysm. The additional manipulation in poor grade patients or soon after SAH cannot be discounted and a delayed procedure for the asymptomatic aneurysms should often be considered (Fig. 18.1). However in our series of intact vertebrobasilar aneurysms, the morbidity from operative causes alone was only 2.4%.

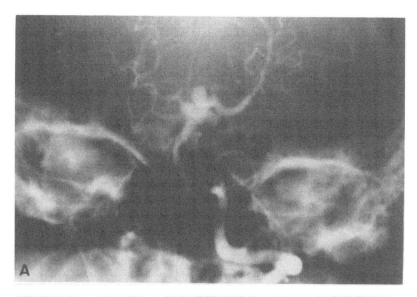

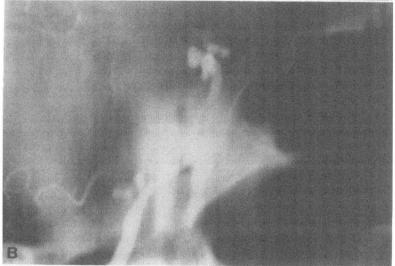

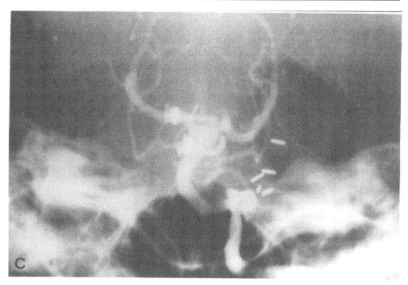

Figure 18.1 A–C. H.M., F, 61, AP and autotomogram lateral view of multiple aneurysms confined to vertebrobasilar circulation (**A, B**). Ruptured left SCA aneurysm and intact basilar bifurcation aneurysm were ligated seven days after second bleed in Grade 3 in October 1976. Right subtemporal approach was selected because of left hemiparesis. Left vertebral-PICA aneurysm was clipped two weeks after the upper basilar artery aneurysms (**C**). Outcome excellent

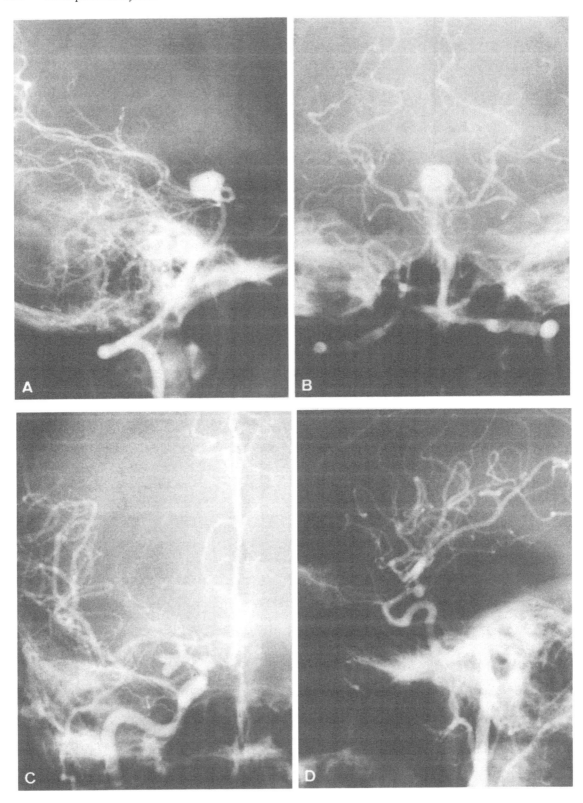

Figure 18.2 A–D

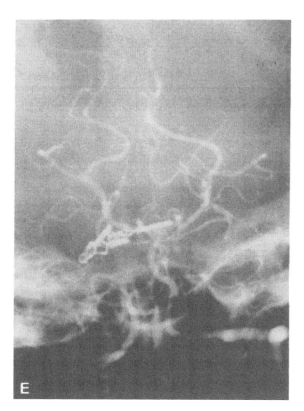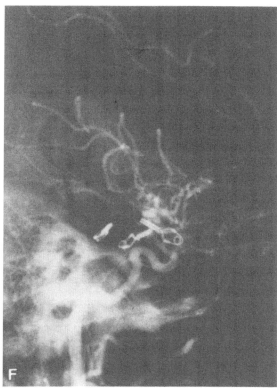

Figure 18.2 E, F

Figure 18.2 A–F. B.M., F, 38, multiple aneurysms on posterior and anterior circulations (**A–D**). Ruptured basilar bifurcation aneurysm, right carotid communicating and anterior choroidal and left carotid communicating aneurysms. Operation in October 1987 was delayed to 12th day after single bleed because of mild carotid vasospasm, she was in Grade I. Frontotemporal flap with subtemporal clipping of basilar bifurcation aneurysm and transsylvian clipping of right carotid aneurysms. Well for 36 hours then decline with vasospasm and irreversible ischemia leading to massive right middle cerebral infarction and death. We were concerned that the additional manipulation through the Sylvian fissure may have worsened the course of the vasospasm

Multiple Aneurysms

Table 18.1. Anterior circulation aneurysms in 462 patients with multiple aneurysms. Number of ruptured aneurysms in parenthesis

Site	Total	Percent
Carotid	343 (28)	52%
MCA	223 (12)	34%
ACA	93 (5)	14%
Total	659 (45)	

Table 18.2. Posterior circulation aneurysms in 462 patients with multiple aneurysms

Site	Aneurysms	Percent
Basilar bifurcation	291	48%
SCA	136	23%
Midbasilar trunk	12	2%
AICA	14	2%
Vertebrobasilar junction	16	3%
Vertebral	60	10%
PCA	70	12%
Total	599	

Table 18.3. Site of multiple aneurysms on vertebrobasilar tree in 113 patients

Site	No.	Percent
Basilar bifurcation	73	30%
SCA	65	27%
Midbasilar trunk	4	1.5%
AICA	9	4%
Vertebrobasilar junction	4	1.5%
Vertebral	34	14%
PCA	55	23%
Total no. aneurysms	244	

Table 18.4. 86 patients with SAH and multiple vertebrobasilar aneurysms

Site	Aneurysms	Ruptured
Basilar bifurcation	58	66%
SCA	46	41%
Midbasilar trunk	2	100%
AICA	8	50%
Vertebrobasilar junction	4	50%
Vertebral	26	50%
PCA	39	20%
Total no. aneurysms	183	

Table 18.5. Frequency of aneurysms treated

Second aneurysm treated	64%
Third aneurysm treated	55%
Fourth aneurysm treated	45%
Fifth aneurysm treated	30%
Sixth aneurysm treated	18%

Table 18.6. Treatment of associated aneurysms

Treatment	Percent
Same operation	43%
Other operation	18%
Not treated	39%

Table 18.7. Preoperative Grade and outcome in 462 patients with multiple aneurysms

Grade	Excellent	Good	Poor	Dead	Total
0	106	17	16	9	148
1	156	22	11	8	197
2	38	20	11	10	79
3	10	9	11	3	33
4			1	3	4
5				1	1
Total	310	68	50	34	462
	67.1%	14.7%	10.8%	7.4%	100.0%

Table 18.8. Timing of surgery and outcome in 314 patients with multiple aneurysms

Timing of surgery	Excellent	Good	Poor	Dead	Total
0–1 day	3	2	1	1	7
2–3 day	7	4	3	6	20
4–6 day	11	6	2	1	20
7–10 day	28	6	3	4	41
11–30 day	112	21	19	12	164
31–365 day	43	12	6	1	62
Total	204	51	34	25	314

Table 18.9. Outcome comparing single and multiple aneurysms in good grade non-giant vertebrobasilar aneurysms

Aneurysms	Poor	Dead
Single	4.5%	3.3%
Multiple	7.2%	4.8%
2 aneurysms	6.7%	4.8%
3 aneurysms	10.6%	8.5%
4 or more aneurysms	14.9%	4.1%

Chapter 19

Vertebrobasilar Aneurysms and Associated Arteriovenous Malformations

54 Patients

With a Contribution of **J. Rinne**

One or two percent of patients with intracranial aneurysms also have an intracranial arteriovenous malformation (AVM) and 5–8% of the patients with an AVM also have an associated aneurysm. In the senior author's earlier (until 1979) experience with 166 cerebral AVMs, 27 (16%) were associated with cerebral aneurysms. This high number of aneurysms might be due to selection of the patients. Recently endovascular surgeons using selective microcatheter injections find more intranidal aneurysms, and the frequency of aneurysms with AVMs has increased up to 30–40% (personal communication P. Lasjaunias). Their role in AVM bleeding is still uncertain, but they might be the site of potential rupture, and consequently this combination should possibly be treated more aggressively. These intranidal aneurysms may be arterial or venous (varices) and sometimes it is difficult to be sure which is which (personal communication A. Fox).

Posterior circulation aneurysms seem, in our experience, to be more often associated with AVMs than those of the anterior circulation, but in J.L. Fox's analysis of literature on 109 patients with a combination of cerebral AVM and aneurysm (9 patients of Suzuki counted twice were excluded), 10 patients had both a posterior fossa AVM and a posterior circulation aneurysm (3 of them were cases of the London Ontario series). This frequency is not different from general frequency of posterior circulation aneurysms.

In our most recent series of 125 patients with posterior fossa AVMs (116 having open surgery for their lesion), 27 (22%) had associated intracranial aneurysms. Many times, the aneurysms will arise from vessels feeding the AVM, and presumably develop from the high flow through the feeding artery accelerating the hemodynamic stress to the vessel wall.

The most accurate figures on frequency of different lesions can be drawn from a series where all the patients in a defined area are treated by the same neurosurgical unit. In an unselected and consecutive series from a defined catchment area (Kuopio, Eastern Finland), without any admission biases, only 10 AVMs were found among 1314 patients with cerebral aneurysms (106 of them in the posterior circulation). In the same time period, a total of 130 intracranial AVMs (12 in the posterior fossa) were treated. The aneurysms associated with the 10 AVMs were as follows: 7 in the anterior circulation (2 ICA, 2 MCA and 3 AComA) and 3 in the posterior circulation (1 vertebral-posterior-inferior cerebellar artery (PICA), 1 basilar superior cerebellar artery (SCA), 1 P3). Two of the 10 AVMs were infratentorial.

General Principles of Treatment

If both an AVM and an aneurysm exist in one patient, the risk of hemorrhage is increased, how much is still unknown. If a patient with both an AVM and an aneurysm presents with a subarachnoid hemorrhage (SAH), in two-thirds the aneurysm has ruptured.

The ruptured aneurysm should be treated according to the principles detailed in other chapters. Generally, the aneurysm should be treated before the AVM, as 1) it is most frequently ruptured, 2) the natural history of an aneurysm is worse, 3) alterations of the flow by removing the AVM first might cause the aneurysm to rupture, 4) the aneurysms are usually located proximal to the AVM and these proximal vessels are often the first exposed, 5) it is usually easier to secure, and 6) many times AVMs are of very large or giant size and too risky for single stage removal.

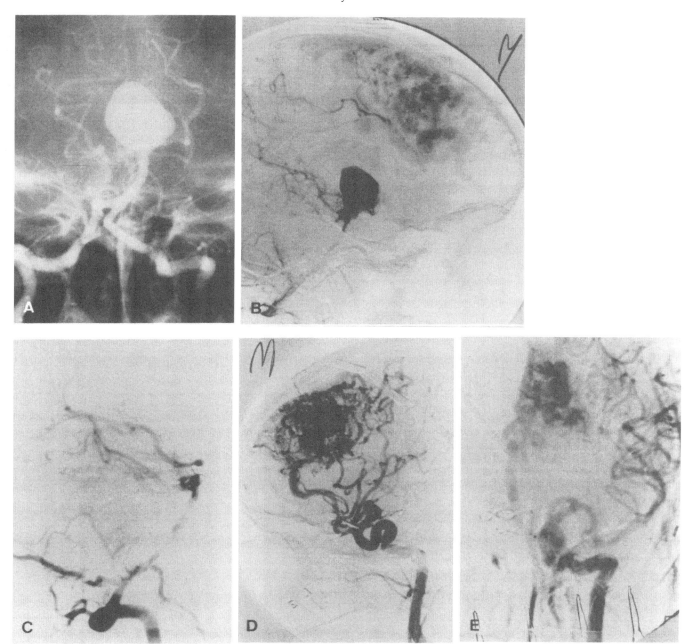

Figure 19.1 A–E. A.C., M, 51, hydrocephalus discovered after 10 years intellectual decline, probably due to giant unruptured basilar bifurcation aneurysm (**A, B**). Modest improvement after ventriculoperitoneal shunt in October 1982. In addition there were an anterior communicating and small bilateral middle cerebral artery aneurysms and a large left frontal AVM (**B, D, E**). The giant basilar aneurysm was clipped uneventfully (**C**) as well as the anterior communicating and right middle cerebral artery aneurysms in January 1983 (**D, E**). The fenestrated clip is on the basilar aneurysm (**E**). Subsequently, the A2 feeders of the AVM were embolized transfemorally, but with little effect. The patient refused further treatment and had a fair outcome from shunt improvement until death from an AVM rupture eight months later

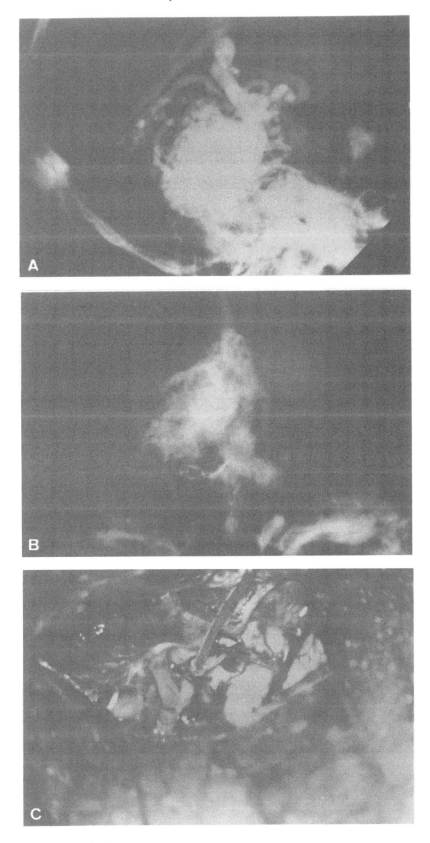

Figure 19.2 A–C

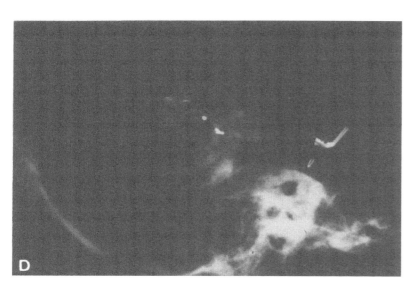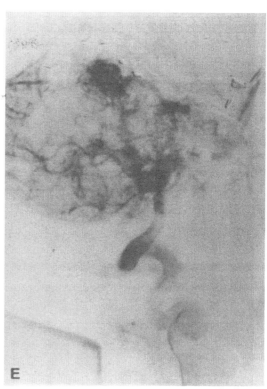

Figure 19.2 D, E

Figure 19.2 A–E. M.K., F, 52, lateral view of ruptured right basilar SCA aneurysm (**A**) and AP (**B**) after aneurysm clipping in November 1980 in Grade 1 19 days after single bleed; a giant right cerebellar AVM is intact. Reopening one week after aneurysm clipping showing cannulation of right superior cerebellar artery for direct selective embolization of AVM (**C**). Plain X-ray shows distribution of 1.2 cc of Bucrylate in AVM (**D**). Lateral postoperative angiogram showing complete clipping of aneurysm and near complete obliteration of AVM (**E**). Outcome good over 14 years with mild ataxia and left hemihypalgesia

Where the approach to the AVM is *remote* from that to the associated *intact* aneurysm(s), the aneurysm is done first to preclude its rupture. This is based on two cases of the senior author where intact aneurysms ruptured after AVM removal. This is in contrast to some radiological experience (personal communication J. Picard) that aneurysms regress after AVM embolization (which we have not seen). With the embolization of the AVM, a few distal aneurysms (and of course those intranidal) can be wiped out.

The natural history of untreated AVMs is unfavorable, a bleed or rebleed rate of about 4%/year. The decision of whether or not to treat and the form of treatment is complex, and one must take into consideration: (1) the presentation and natural history of the lesion; (2) the known results of the available therapeutic alternatives; (3) the patient's age, general medical and neurologic condition; (4) the presenting symptoms (hemorrhage, epilepsy, headache, or asymptomatic); (5) the physical parameters of the AVM including its location, size, the number and flow pattern of the feeding vessels, venous drainage; (6) the presence of a recent or remote hematoma; and (7) the site of the lesion – the precise anatomical relationship of the malformation to surrounding brain and cranial nerves. Some AVMs are easily and safely treated by one method, and are quite unsuitable for others. Finally, the surgeon's own record of success or failure with these treatment modalities needs to be factored into the decision tree.

The risk of surgical removal increases drastically with the larger AVM, particularly those with a nidus over 5 cm. As well, the site of the malformation is critical. A small, even tiny, malformation within the brain stem will be surgically inaccessible. Simple ligation of the feeding vessels of the

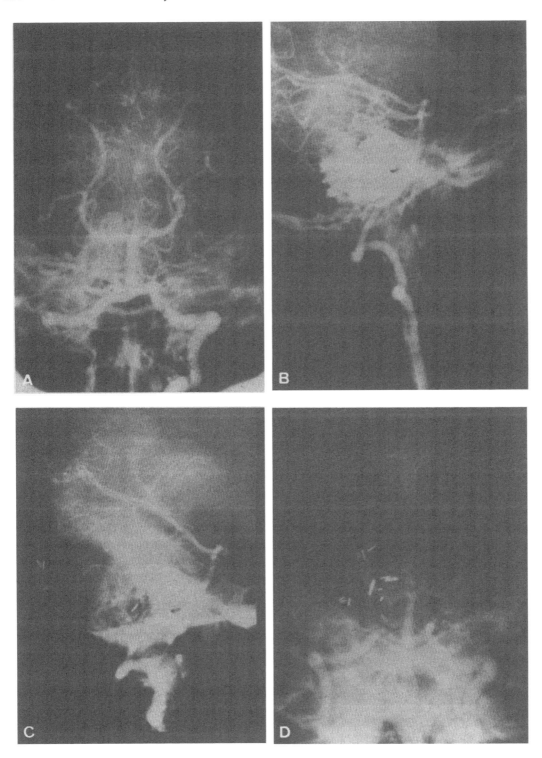

Figure 19.3 A–D. F.S., F, 28, lateral right cerebellopontine angle AVM with ruptured peripheral AICA aneurysm (**A, B**). Both bleeds, in 1971 and 1972, produced respiratory arrest and prolonged ICU care with severe neurological deficits (CNV-CNX paralysis right, severe trunk and limb ataxia). Excision of aneurysm and AVM was done in April 1972 in Grade 3 one month after the second bleed (**C, D**). Outcome was good after prolonged recovery to mild ataxia with right deafness and synkinetic facial function. (Courtesy J Neurosurg 43: 661–670, 1975)

Vertebrobasilar Aneurysms and Associated Arteriovenous Malformations 261

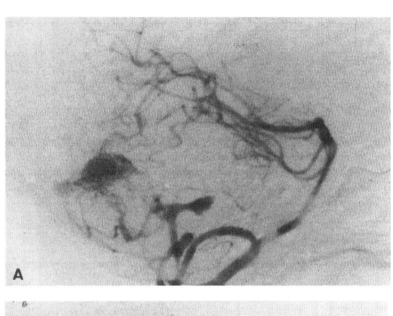

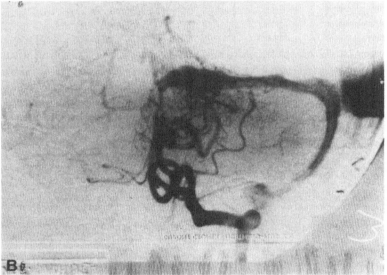

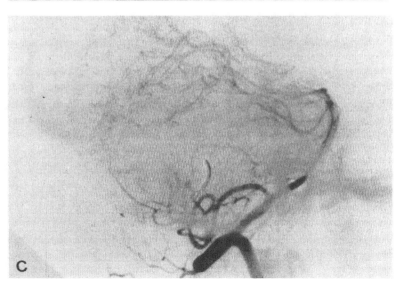

Figure 19.4 A–C. N.B., M, 45, lateral and AP view of ruptured distal left PICA aneurysm and feeding intact paravermian AVM (**A, B**). In March 1987 one month after bleed in Grade 1 lower vermis was split to follow PICA to ruptured aneurysm, which was clipped and the intact AVM was removed. During dural closure bleeding occurred in cavity, after reopening dry field. Postoperative lateral angiogram demonstrates complete excision of AVM and occlusion of aneurysm and PICA beyond (**C**). Outcome excellent after rapid recovery of postoperative ataxia

malformation is completely ineffectual. The fistulous connection between arteries and veins in the nidus of the lesion will rapidly recruit surrounding vessels and rapidly make them as prominent as those that have been ligated.

Postoperative clots are more frequent than in supratentorial AVMs, and were the cause of most of the morbidity and mortality in our series of posterior fossa AVMs. Hemostasis of tiny and fragile feeders and drainers to the deepest portion of the lesion most cumbersome in close proximity to the ventricle, remain the most difficult part of the procedure. Bleeding is difficult to control as these vessels have very little tissue for coagulation to be effective. Unfortunately, the bleeding from these vessels usually occurs at the end of the procedure when the surgeon may also becoming tired. The new microclips by Sundt and Sugita are useful to control bleeding from these troublesome vessels. Preoperative embolization and use of postoperative hypotension to prevent postoperative hematomas has proved to be important. We did attempt to maintain the MAP 20% below the norm by restricting fluid and using hypotensive medication for 3–7 days.

Patients

In this series of 1767 patients with vertebrobasilar artery aneurysm (VBAA), 59 patients also harbored an AVM, a frequency of close to 3%. From final analysis five patients were excluded: two of them with dural malformations and three with extracranial vertebral artery fistulas (one after direct puncture for vertebral angiography, one after open surgery for ligating both vertebral arteries and one after head injury). Out of the remaining 54, 29 were females. Mean age was in both genders 45 years (range 3 – 70 years). There was no excess of young patients: only 5 patients were less than 20 years of age.

In 30 patients, the aneurysm had ruptured (56%), in 17 patients the aneurysm was unruptured, and in 7 patients the aneurysm was unruptured but symptomatic with mass effect. In nine patients, the AVM was the cause for rupture. Fifteen patients had intact aneurysms and AVMs. These 24 cases with intact aneurysms are classified as Grade 0 patients in Table 19.1. Fourteen patients (11 with ruptured aneurysm and 3 with ruptured AVM) had recurrent SAH.

Basilar bifurcation aneurysms associated with AVMs were unusual in this group (Tables 19.3, 19.4). Nine aneurysms were giant and six large, the rest being small (Table 19.5). Two aneurysms were fusiform, three were huge fistulous aneurysmal varices, and the remainder being saccular. Ten of 12 large or giant saccular aneurysms were located proximally at the origin of the feeder, 2 giant saccular aneurysms were not associated with an AVM (Table 19.6). A high number of associated aneurysms were found: these patients harbored more than 100 aneurysms which are listed in Table 19.3. Ten patients harbored 2 aneurysms, nine patients 3, six patients 4 and one patient 5 aneurysms.

Many of the additional asymptomatic aneurysms were small and a few were fusiform.

Half of the AVMs were located infratentorially (Tables 19.6, 19.7). Sixteen AVMs were small (1 of them cryptic), 21 were large (2.5–5.0 cm in diameter) and 16 giant (> 5 cm in diameter) (Table 19.9).

Treatment

Twenty patients were operated on under deep hypotension (< mean 55 mm HG) and 8 patients had temporary clipping of proximal vessel for occlusion of their aneurysms. Two patients were operated under hypothermia and one under cardiac bypass. The modes of treatment for aneurysms and AVMs are seen in Tables 19.10 and 19.11. Only two patients were operated on during the first week after SAH (Table 19.12).

Three postoperative clots were removed with no survivals and three times the wound explored for swelling with one surviving. Two patients had postoperative ischemia from vasospasm, both without major deficit. Aneurysm size or AVM size did not influence the results, admittedly many unruptured giant AVMs were left alone considering the patients' age and the small risk of bleeding as compared to the technical difficulties obvious in the removal of these huge lesions (Tables 19.5 and 19.9).

The presence of an AVM significantly alters the outcome, especially if it is removed at the same stage. All poor results but one occurred in patients with ruptured aneurysms; one had a giant intact P1-P2 aneurysm causing Weber's syndrome (Table

19.4). One poor result and two deaths were related directly to the aneurysm repair, while one poor outcome and three deaths were undoubtedly due to resection of the associated AVM, three from postoperative clots and one from rupture of a small previously intact AVM. All poor results occurred in patients with unruptured AVMs (Table 19.8).

Summary of Poor Results

Two patients remained poor and five died; they are summarized here:

A 43 year old male with hemiparesis had his P2 aneurysm clipped in 1966 five weeks after a second hemorrhage under profound hypotension (45 mm of HG for 25 minutes). His large occipital AVM was left alone. Two hours following operation, the patient became decerebrate. Urgent reopening revealed only temporal lobe swelling and the bone flap was removed for decompression. Two months later he was mentally bright, but had a left hemiparesis and right CNIII palsy.

The other poor result occurred in a Grade 1 patient when the ruptured proximal anterior-inferior cerebellar artery (AICA) aneurysm was clipped and two peripheral AICA aneurysms were excised with a 3 cm malformation. Next morning he was very well, but then soon deteriorated to stuporous state. CT scan showed a huge intracerebellar postoperative clot which was urgently removed. Bleeding source was a normal appearing artery in the superior cerebellar artery (SCA) region, one inch away from the AVM region. Control angiography after reoperation showed the proximal AICA aneurysm well clipped, and the AVM with the two distal aneurysms excised. He remained unconscious with right hemiplegia, and was transferred to his home country.

A small midbasilar aneurysm was ligated successfully with a McKenzie clip on July 12th, 1963 (Case 8, J. S.) under deep hypothermia. An associated small pontine AVM fed by SCA was packed with hammered muscle on its surface, but bled fatally five hours after operation. At autopsy, there was a massive pontine hemorrhage which was considered to have arisen from the AVM, possibly related to the use of Heparin.

In a 55 year old male, a huge postoperative bleed into the fourth ventricle occurred the same evening after clipping a ruptured distal posterior-inferior cerebellar artery (PICA) aneurysm and resection of a 3.5 cm anterior cerebellar AVM. Several hours were spent trying to stop slow ooze from many points. Finally it was decided to leave the wound open overnight in the intensive care unit (ICU). Postoperatively in the night, he was awake but soon became worse, and died from cerebellar swelling; in the postoperative angiogram clips on the aneurysm were well down in the neck at about the C2-3 level!

The death was tragic in a woman, 59, with Weber's syndrome from a giant P1-P2 aneurysm and there was a giant AVM beyond on P2. Clips for trapping the aneurysm were placed on the posterior communicating (PCom), P1 and P2 arteries although visualization of the P1 was difficult. After initial slackening, the aneurysm refilled but it was thought due to retrograde perforator flow; unfortunately the clip position on P1 was not verified. She was much the same in the recovery room for two hours when sudden coma occurred leading to her demise. At autopsy, the clip had slipped off the large P1 so that unrestrained P1 flow entered the blind sac without outflow, rupturing this previously intact aneurysm.

One large P1 aneurysm was clipped without difficulty in a Grade 3 patient also harboring a large occipital AVM. But an associated intact carotid communicating aneurysm ruptured at the far side of the neck during coagulation and in spite of clipping and the use of a piece of hammered muscle, massive rebleeding occurred during closure. She did not survive the brain swelling, and died five days later.

The fifth death occurred in a woman already demented and paraparetic from rupture of a small aneurysm arising from a midbasilar branch feeding a small AVM. The artery was clipped proximally but the trigeminal and brain stem AVM was only partially excised. She was unconscious after operation; a CT scan revealed a huge hemorrhage into the pons, the central left midbrain and the left thalamus. Angiography showed no filling of the AVM or aneurysm. She died 10 days later from bronchopneumonia.

Table 19.1. Preoperative Grade of the aneurysm rupture and outcome in 54 patients with a combination of arteriovenous malformation and vertebrobasilar aneurysm(s)

Grade	Excellent	Good	Poor	Dead	Total
0	19	4		1	24
1	11	7	1	2	21
2	1	1		1	3
3		3	1		4
4		1		1	2
Total	31	16	2	5	54
	57%	30%	4%	9%	100%

Table 19.2. Age related to outcome in 54 patients with a combination of arteriovenous malformation and vertebrobasilar aneurysm(s)

Age group (years)	Excellent	Good	Poor	Dead	Total
0–9	1				1
10–19	1	1			2
20–29	5	2			7
30–39	5	1			6
40–49	10	4	2	1	17
50–59	5	3		2	10
60–69	3	5		2	10
70 or more	1				1
Total	31	16	2	5	54

Table 19.3. Location of 77 posterior circulation aneurysms in 54 patients with a combination of arteriovenous malformation and vertebrobasilar aneurysm(s). These 54 patients had additionally 28 anterior circulation aneurysms (15 ICA, 8 MCA, 5 ACA)

Aneurysm site	Total	Percent
Basilar artery		
Bifurcation	10	13
SCA	12	15.5
SCA distal	5	6.5
AICA	2	3
AICA proximal	1	1
AICA distal	5	6.5
Trunk	3	4
Vertebrobasilar junction	1	1
Vertebral artery		
Vertebral PICA	3	4
PICA distal	10	13
Posterior cerebral artery		
P1	9	12
PCom junction P1–P2	5	6.5
P2	5	6.5
P3–P4	6	8
Total	77	100.0

Table 19.4. Aneurysm site and outcome in 54 patients with a combination of arteriovenous malformation and vertebrobasilar aneurysm(s)

Site	Excellent	Good	Poor	Dead	Total
Basilar bifurcation	6	3			9
BA-SCA	8	6			14
Basilar artery (AICA or midbasilar)	3	3	1	2	9
VB junction		1			1
Vertebral artery	7	1		1	9
PCA	7	2	1	2	12
Total	31	16	2	5	54

Table 19.5. Aneurysm size and outcome in 54 patients with a combination of arteriovenous malformation and vertebrobasilar aneurysm(s)

Size	Excellent	Good	Poor	Dead	Total
Small	25	9	2	3	39
Large	1	4		1	6
Giant	5	3		1	9
Total	31	16	2	5	54

Table 19.6. Aneurysm site, as related to the AVM, and outcome in 54 patients with a combination of arteriovenous malformation and vertebrobasilar aneurysm(s)

Aneurysm site	Excellent	Good	Poor	Dead	Total (AVM infratentorial)
Not associated with AVM	6	3		1	10 (5)
Proximal at origin of feeder	15	9	1	3	28 (9)
Distal on feeder	6	3	1	1	11 (10)
Intranidal	4	1			5 (3)
Total	31	16	2	5	54 (27)

Table 19.7. Site of the AVM and outcome in 54 patients with a combination of arteriovenous malformation and vertebrobasilar aneurysm(s)

Site of AVM	Excellent	Good	Poor	Dead	Total
Supratentorial	19	5	1	2	27
Infratentorial	12	11	1	3	27
Total	31	16	2	5	54

Table 19.8. Rupture of the AVM and outcome in 54 patients with a combination of arteriovenous malformation and vertebrobasilar aneurysm(s)

AVM	Excellent	Good	Poor	Dead	Total
Nonruptured	23	15	2	5	45
Ruptured	8	1			9
Total	31	16	2	5	54

Table 19.9. AVM size and outcome in 54 patients with a combination of arteriovenous malformation and vertebrobasilar aneurysm(s)

Size	Excellent	Good	Poor	Dead	Total
Small	9	4	1	2	16
Large	11	8	1	1	21
Giant	11	4		2	17
Total	31	16	2	5	54

Table 19.10. Operative method for the aneurysm and outcome in 54 patients with a combination of arteriovenous malformation and vertebrobasilar aneurysm(s)

Operative method	Excellent	Good	Poor	Dead	Total
Neck clipping	19	11	2	3	35
Coagulated only	1				1
Silk ligature	1				1
Hunterian ligation					
PCA occlusion		1			1
Vertebral occlusion	1				1
Trapping	3			2	5
Excision	5	3			8
Endovascular		1			1
Exploration only	1				1
Total	31	16	2	5	54

Table 19.11. Operative method of the AVM and outcome in 54 patients with a combination of arteriovenous malformation and vertebrobasilar aneurysm(s)

Operative method	Excellent	Good	Poor	Dead	Total
No treatment	14	7	1	3	25
Total excision	11	4	1	2	18
Partial excision	1				1
Transfemoral embolization, total	1				1
Transfemoral embolization, partial		2			2
Open intraoperative embolization, total	2				2
Open intraoperative embolization, partial	2	3			5
Total	31	16	2	5	54

Table 19.12. Timing of surgery for aneurysm rupture and outcome in 30 patients with a combination of arteriovenous malformation and vertebrobasilar aneurysm(s)

Timing of surgery	Excellent	Good	Poor	Dead	Total
4–6 day	1			1	2
7–10 day	1	2			3
11–30 day	5	6	1	2	14
31–365 day	5	4	1	1	11
Total	12	12	2	4	30

Chapter 20
Solitary Incidental Vertebrobasilar Aneurysms
70 Patients

With the ever-increasing number of intact aneurysms revealed by modern imaging, the options for managing these lesions are assuming great importance. As a significant lifetime risk of potentially catastrophic rupture exists with a yearly rupture rate of 1–3%, we have recommended surgery in a considerable number of cases, especially in those whose aneurysms have been 6–7 mm or more in diameter. In a recent analysis of all non-giant unruptured posterior circulation aneurysms, we recommended surgery for these lesions as the actual surgical morbidity was as low as 2.4%. In the total series of 1767 vertebral-basilar artery aneurysms (VBAA) there were 70 neurologically completely intact patients with single aneurysms which were unruptured and without mass effect, had no arteriovenous malformation (AVM) or other intracranial aneurysm. As these patients were asymptomatic and in good condition, any possible complications were related only to the surgery of this *single* lesion.

The reason for the first neuroradiological examination in most cases were prolonged headache or vertigo. Usually, an aneurysm was seen on CT and subsequent angiographies revealed the presence of a vertebrobasilar aneurysm. One small basilar bifurcation aneurysm in a female aged 38 was found during examinations for a visual loss. Eight months after resection of the detected giant bioccipital meningioma, the aneurysm was treated without incident.

In the younger age group (less than 40), all had excellent results: nine were basilar bifurcation, two superior cerebellar artery (SCA), four posterior cerebral artery (PCA) and two basilar trunk aneurysms. Three aneurysms were giant size (all posterior cerebral and one of them fistulous), seven were small and seven large. Giant aneurysms were detected due to a seizure in one, long-lasting headache and episode of flashes of light in one, and facial pain with bruit in one. There were no operations on patients aged 70 or more because of surgical risk and more sedentary lifestyle.

All patients with small aneurysms had excellent results except one female aged 50 with hemifacial spasm who developed ataxia and a Wallenberg syndrome after vertebral ligation for her distal vertebral aneurysm (Tables 20.1 to 20.5). She is self-sufficient now. A male aged 44 was found to have a large, likely dissecting, aneurysm on the basilar trunk, after exploration he had epileptic fits and dysarthria. A 48 year old female had investigations for vertigo, and a large posterior projecting basilar bifurcation aneurysm was found. Her postoperative condition was poor, with bilateral oculomotor palsies, and postoperative CTs revealed small, low densities involving midbrain and thalamus, due to perforator injury. The death was in a 40 year old male with a large SCA aneurysm, who was confused after operation but died suddenly 10 days after discharge home of suspected pulmonary embolus.

Surgical morbidity and mortality were low, about the same as yearly bleeding rates. The only death was due to pulmonary embolus, a rare occurrence in the total series of VBAA (four patients). Surgery in *experienced* hands is recommended for these lesions to prevent fatal or disabling ruptures.

Table 20.1. Cause of neuroradiological examinations in 70 patients with single incidental VBAA

Symptoms	No.	Percent
Visual loss (meningioma found)	1	1
TIA or PRIND	16	23
Seizures	2	3
Headache, vertigo, diplopia, facial pain	51	73
Total	70	100

Table 20.2. Age related to outcome in 70 patients with single incidental VBAA

Age group (years)	Excellent	Good	Poor	Dead	Total
10–19	1				1
20–29	4				4
30–39	12				12
40–49	19	1	1	1	22
50–59	18	1			19
60–69	12				12
Total	66	2	1	1	70

Table 20.3. Aneurysm size and outcome in 70 patients with single incidental VBAA

Size	Excellent	Good	Poor	Dead	Total
Small	35	1			36
Large	28	1	1	1	31
Giant	3				3
Total	66	2	1	1	70

Table 20.4. Location and outcome in 70 patients with single incidental VBAA

Location	Excellent	Good	Poor	Dead	Total
Basilar bifurcation	46		1		47
Basilar SCA	9			1	10
Midbasilar trunk	2	1			3
Basilar AICA	1				1
Vertebral artery	2	1			3
PCA	6				6
Total	66	2	1	1	70

Table 20.5. Operative method and outcome in 70 patients with single incidental VBAA

Operative method	Excellent	Good	Poor	Dead	Total
Clip	55		1	1	57
Wrapping	1				1
Hunterian ligation	7	1			8
Explored only[a]	3	1			4
Total	66	2	1	1	70

[a] Pursuit of clipping abandoned because of unreasonable risk.

Chapter 21
Vertebrobasilar Artery Aneurysms in Children
49 Patients

Intracranial aneurysms in children are unusual. Less than 1% incidence in unselected series has been found, and vertebrobasilar aneurysms in children (7%) are as rare as in adults. In this series, 49 patients were less than 18 years old, and in this group males dominated (27), as is the case also in pediatric anterior circulation aneurysms. Half of the cases presented with bleeding. Most, even those with ruptured aneurysms, had mass effect as three-fourths of the aneurysms were of giant size; only five aneurysms were small. More than half of the aneurysms were fusiform. This unknown arteriopathy was local on that intracranial arterial segment, usually on basilar or posterior cerebral arteries (PCAs), and no special general vasculopathies or system diseases were observed. (Mid)basilar trunk and PCA aneurysms were most common and in giant form in most cases. Multiple aneurysms were seldom found (5); interestingly three of them were giant extradural internal carotid aneurysms associated with one large and two giant (mid-) basilar trunk aneurysms. Three patients had arteriovenous malformations (AVMs).

Clinical Features

Twenty-four patients presented with unheralded subarachnoid hemorrhage (SAH) alone, but which occasionally precipitated focal findings such as a hemiparesis and sixth nerve palsy (4). Six patients had multiple bleeds. Eight patients had a third nerve palsy, half of them with P1 aneurysms. Dysarthria (6), often associated with quadriparesis and bulbar palsy, was usual with the largest aneurysms – five patients had severe limb paresis and six patients demonstrated a mild paresis.

Treatment (Table 21.5)

Only four patients required a shunt.

In one, no treatment was possible after exploration. This boy, aged 17, with quadriparesis, severe ataxia and pathological laughter had his giant basilar bifurcation aneurysm explored in 1975, and remained in poor condition.

Two early cases were wrapped. In 1965, a girl aged 14, had a giant basilar trunk aneurysm wrapped with plastic. One year later it became completely thrombosed, as well as the associated untreated large petrous carotid aneurysm! In 1971, a boy aged 10 had his large anterior-inferior cerebellar artery (AICA) aneurysm wrapped. Both had excellent results and are still alive and well.

A young male of 18 years had his giant ruptured basilar trunk aneurysm mostly occluded in 1973 with a silk ligature and clip. In 1984, angiograms revealed that the residual neck had become a giant aneurysm with the clip at its apex; it was treated successfully by vertebral ligation.

Nine of the 15 basilar trunk aneurysms were treated by basilar ligation (Fig. 21.1), twice with the tourniquet. Both superior cerebellar artery (SCA) and half of the basilar bifurcation aneurysms had clip ligation of the basilar artery. The fatality was a girl, $4^1/_2$, who was alert and in her preoperative condition, 24 hours later when angiography revealed that the basilar artery was occluded at the site of the open tourniquet and the aneurysm was thrombosed. Closure of the tourniquet to prevent recanalization resulted in a tear of the basilar artery presumably from rupture of a dissecting aneurysm at the site of tourniquet application (see Chapter 11 on giant basilar trunk aneurysms). A boy aged 12, with x-linked lymphoproliferative disease, was perfectly well after clip occlusion of the basilar artery for his large basilar bifurcation aneurysm. A severe hemiparesis developed but subsided. Later an unknown arteriopathy suspected to be due to a fungal infection with development of bilateral carotid and several distal middle cerebral fusiform aneurysms led to a poor result with rebleeding and

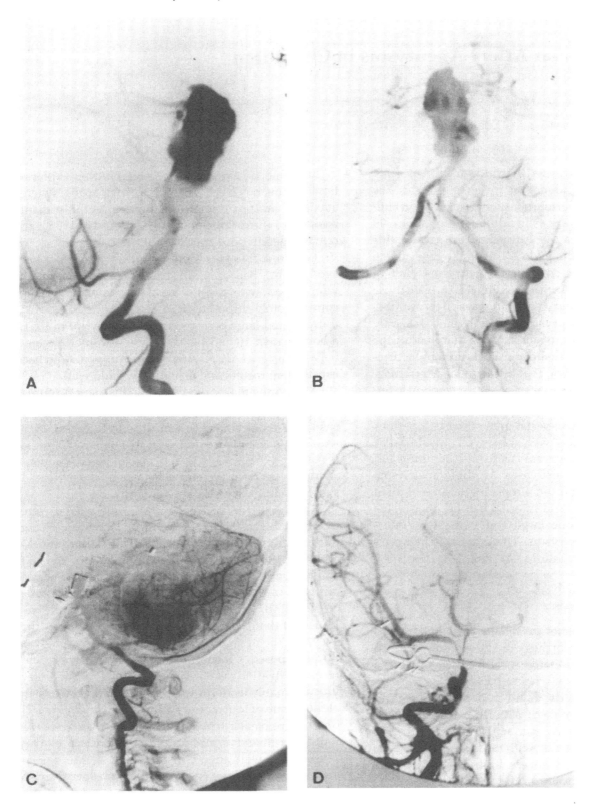

Figure 21.1 A–D. R.D., F, 4, giant midbasilar aneurysm (**A, B**). Sudden vomiting, right leg weakness followed by coma, after intubation recovery to Grade 1, no L.P. Eight days after bleed in March 1984 only long Drake clip blades could be placed across the basilar artery above the origin of AICAs which were under the overhang of the lower base of the aneurysm. The jaws of clip appliers carrying smaller clips obscured this portion of the artery. Good PICA-AICA collateral filling of superior cerebellar branches (**C**). A small posterior communicating artery was sufficient to supply the posterior cerebral circulation (**D**). Outcome excellent

late death. A girl aged 15 had preoperative right hemiplegia, and developed left hemiplegia after clip occlusion of the basilar artery. Two years later, she was ambulatory with a walker using both arms, mouthing words, but mute.

Nine patients with giant posterior cerebral aneurysms had the proximal PCA occluded, twice with the tourniquet. All had excellent results except one girl aged 14 whose preoperative hemiparesis changed to right arm tremor.

Vertebral occlusion was used in eight patients (one basilar trunk, three vertebrobasilar junction and four vertebral aneurysms). A girl aged 8 was well for four days after intracranial left vertebral clip occlusion for her huge vertebral posterior-inferior cerebellar artery (PICA) aneurysm. Then she suddenly screamed with head pain and elapsed into a deep coma and died. A post mortem examination was refused, but CT showed a posterior fossa bleed even though the aneurysm was mostly thrombosed. Recently, one girl aged 16 from overseas had a balloon occlusion of a vertebral artery for her giant distal vertebral artery aneurysm. She was improved from gait ataxia, dysarthria, dysphagia and was discharged in good condition. The remaining patients made excellent recoveries.

Three distal giant aneurysms, two on the PCA and one massive fistulous aneurysmal varix on the distal PICA, had clip occlusion of the artery proximally to the aneurysm. One small distal PCA aneurysm was excised. All had excellent results. Two giant basilar trunk aneurysms were trappped with excellent results.

A girl aged 10 had her small distal SCA and PICA aneurysms associated with a huge cerebellar AVM occluded by endovascular plastic used for the AVM with a good result. After one year, the AVM had recanalized in spite of re-embolization. A fatal hemorrhage recurred. A 16 year old boy had his small distal PCA aneurysm excised and made excellent recovery.

Six non-giant aneurysms were clipped, three at the basilar bifurcation (Fig. 21.2), and one on AICA, midbasilar trunk and vertebrobasilar junction each. All had excellent results.

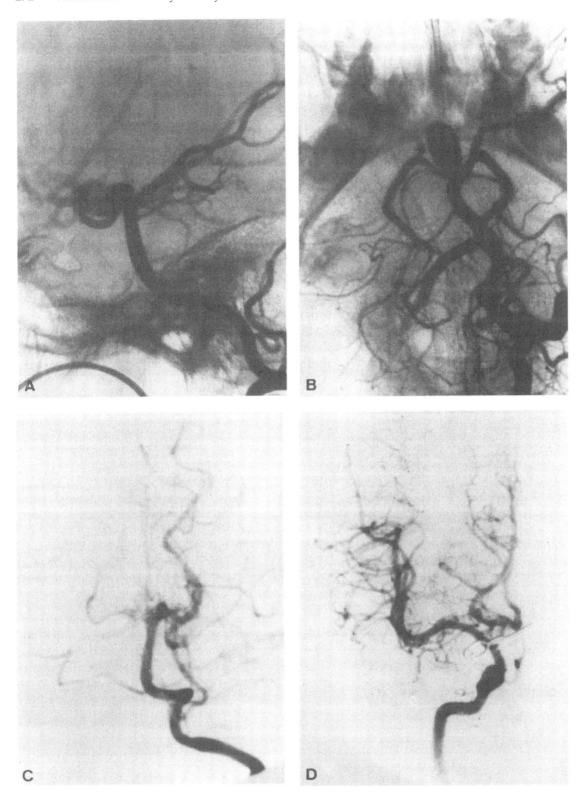

Figure 21.2 A–D. H.L., F, 5, ruptured (?) large basilar bifurcation aneurysm (**A, B**). Shunted for communicating hydrocephalus at the age of seven months. Suspected "encephalitis" age $2^1/_2$ years, result of L P unknown. CT check of hydrocephalus at age 5 revealed suprasellar calcification. In July 1980 calcification prevented clip staying out on neck and P1 was kinked and occluded also (**C**). Large right posterior communicating artery filled posterior cerebral circulation (**D**). Outcome excellent

Table 21.1. Preoperative Grade and outcome in 49 children (18 years or less) with vertebrobasilar aneurysms

Grade	Excellent	Good	Poor	Dead	Total
0[a]	20	4	2	2	28
0g	18	2	0	2	22
0p	2	2	2	0	6
1	16	1	1		18
2	1				1
3	2				2
Total	39	5	3	2	49

[a] *0* Unruptured aneurysm or remote hemorrhage (> 1 year). *0g* Good risk without major neurological deficit. *0p* Poor risk patient with major neurological deficit (severe confusion or dementia or stupor or coma, dysarthria or bulbar paralysis, severe dysphasia or severe mono-, hemi-, or tetraparesis).

Table 21.2. Type of aneurysm in 49 children (18 years or less) with vertebrobasilar aneurysms

Type of aneurysm	No.
Saccular	21
Fusiform	27
Fistulous	1
Total	49

Table 21.3. Aneurysm site and outcome in 49 children (18 years or less) with vertebrobasilar aneurysms

Site	Excellent	Good	Poor	Dead	Total
Basilar bifurcation	6		2		8
BA-SCA	2				2
Distal SCA		1			1
AICA	2				2
Midbasilar trunk	11	2	1	1	15
VB junction	4				4
Vertebral PICA			1		1
PICA distal	1				1
Vertebral distal	2	1			3
P1	4	1			5
P1–P2	2				2
P2	2				2
P3–P4	3				3
Total	39	5	3	2	49

Table 21.4. Aneurysm size and outcome in 49 children (18 years or less) with vertebrobasilar aneurysms

Size	Excellent	Good	Poor	Dead	Total
Small	4	1			5
Large	6	1	1		8
Giant	29	3	2	2	36
Total	39	5	3	2	49

Table 21.5. Operative method and outcome in 49 children (18 years or less) with vertebrobasilar aneurysms

Operative method	Excellent	Good	Poor	Dead	Total
Neck clipping	6				6
Silk ligature	1				1
Wrapping	2				2
Hunterian ligation	27	4	2	2	35
Basilar occlusion	*10*	*2*	*2*	*1*	*15*
PCA occlusion	*11*	*1*			*12*
Vertebral occlusion	*6*	*1*		*1*	*8*
Trapping	2				2
Excision	1				1
Endovascular		1			1
Exploration only			1		1
Total	39	5	3	2	49

Table 21.6. Operative method and result of aneurysm treatment in 49 children (18 years or less) with vertebrobasilar aneurysms

Operative method	Total obliteration	Residual neck	Residual fundus	No obliteration	Total
Neck clipping	6				6
Silk ligature			1		1
Wrapping				2	2
Hunterian ligation	24	2	7		33
Trapping	4				4
Excision	1				1
Endovascular	1				1
Exploration only				1	1
Total	36	2	8	3	49

Table 21.7. Timing of surgery and outcome in 21 children (18 years or less) with vertebrobasilar aneurysms

Timing of surgery	Excellent	Good	Poor	Total
4–6 day	2			2
7–10 day	6			6
11–30 day	8		1	9
31–365 day	3	1		4
Total	19	1	1	21

Chapter 22
Timing of Surgery

Early surgery for posterior circulation aneurysms was attempted in the earliest experience of the senior author. Two of the first four patients died, one with a cardiac arrest following poorly controlled hypotension and hypothermia. Due to this early experience, and due to our referral pattern, most of the more than 1300 patients with surgery of their ruptured vertebral-basilar artery aneurysm (VBAA) were operated on 14 days or more following their last subarachnoid hemorrhage (SAH) and after the immediate effects of the hemorrhage and the consequences of the hemorrhage had passed.

Rebleeding: Transfer of Patients

We are continually haunted by the deterioration and often death of patients because of recurrent hemorrhage before the aneurysm could be secured. Because of the nature of this patient referral from a wide geographic area and large number of units, we can only estimate that the overall incidence of rebleeding in this series was 10%. Analyzed, half of the patients suffering a recurrent bleed in our hospital did not survive. Eighty-four patients did survive a second (or more) hemorrhage in our unit while waiting for surgery. Twenty-one patients rebled on the day of admission and 19, the day after admission. Although the majority of the patients were transferred great distances, only one bled in an aircraft coming from overseas and another bled getting off the plane. At least three patients bled again while being moved from hospital bed to ambulance or from ambulance to the aircraft. Rebleeding with survival during the hospital stay were most frequent in aneurysms arising from vertebral artery (19 pts) and basilar trunk (12 pts). The posterior fossa aneurysms seem to rebleed easily and more fatally (48–83%) – one point for acute surgery.

Early versus Late Surgery

Since 1970, 206 patients with VBAAs have been operated on within 7 days following their last SAH (day of SAH counted as 0). This group was compared with 1040 late surgery cases with VBAA in the same time period. Three patients with acute endovascular surgery (one excellent outcome and two deaths) were included, as acute open surgery was considered in these cases. The distribution of VBAAs in this early operative group is very similar to our overall larger series (Tables 22.2 and 22.5).

The overall morbidity was 19%; it was lowest for the small aneurysms 16.7%, for large aneurysms 20.2% and for giant aneurysms 28.5% (Table 22.6). It was also clearly related to patient grade (Table 22.4). All except one (treated endovascularly) of the Grade 5 patients died and 70% of the Grade 4 patients were ultimately significantly disabled or dead. Grade 3 patients operated on early resulted in one-third of the cases with poor outcome. When examining only the Grade 1 and 2 patients and comparing the results day by day, a good or excellent outcome was obtained during the first month in 80% irrespective of timing. Curiously the outcome was poor on day 2. The operative mortality was also the same whether operated on in the first week or delayed (Fig. 22.1).

Slightly better operative results were obtained in the younger patients below 50 (Table 22.6). The number of patients with multiple bleed (41%) was high in the early surgery group forming one of the indications for early attack. Twenty-nine percent had poor outcome as compared to 12% of patients with single bleed. Communicating hydrocephalus, requiring shunt treatment, was seen as frequently in the early as in the late surgery group. Surprisingly the frequency of intraoperative rupture of the aneurysm was not higher than in later surgery. Outcome in inadvertent intraoperative aneurysm ruptures was poor in 29% (without rupture 17%).

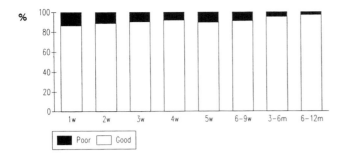

Figure 22.1. Outcome of surgery at different time intervals after SAH in 1018 good Grade (1, 2) patients with small or large vertebrobasilar artery aneurysms. *Poor* poor or dead, *Good* excellent or good, *w* week, *m* month

Re-operation and repositioning of the clip was carried out in four patients. Proximal vessel occlusion was performed in 18 patients (in 4 patients with tourniquet) where it proved to be impossible to directly clip the neck of the aneurysm.

Thirteen percent developed a delayed ischemic neurologic deficit as a consequence of reactive arterial narrowing or vasospasm. The onset of these ischemic symptoms ranged between 3 and 14 days following the last SAH.

Final Comments on Timing of Surgery

We have compared the results of early operation in patients with aneurysms arising from the anterior circulation and those with aneurysms arising from the posterior circulation. The results are equally good in those patients graded Botterell 1 or 2 at the time of surgery and equally poor in those graded 3 or 4. Thus, in our hands, the condition of the patient going into the operating room would appear to be the most powerful determinant of outcome (cf. Chapter 25, Fig. 25.1).

If the sac is of large or giant size, the technical complexity is markedly increased. Neck clipping may be difficult if not impossible and certainly hazardous for the patient. Proximal or Hunterian ligation in these circumstances is an effective and usually safe alternate method of treatment in those patients coming *electively* to surgery. But proximal vessel ligation attempted in 18 patients in the *acute* stage resulted in 5 deaths. These disappointing results in a few patients with complex lesions have made us cautious about attempting proximal vessel ligation in the immediate week following acute SAH.

In our hands, early surgery for a VBAA yields results similar to early surgery for aneurysms of the anterior circulation and not dissimilar to the results achieved in delayed operation of the VBAA in our unit. It is clear that early surgery, with the aneurysm appropriately clipped, will virtually eliminate the risk of rebleeding. It is our impression that vasospasm is not more common, less amenable to therapy or more severe in those patients who have been operated on early as in the patients *waiting for* delayed surgery. Volume expansion and elevation of blood pressure is more safely administered with the aneurysm surgically obliterated. Although early surgery more frequently presents a brain that is more swollen and tight with a confining exposure, the use of lumbar spinal fluid drainage, controlled ventilation and osmotic diuretics has made good exposure usual. Dissection of the aneurysm itself with removal of surrounding fresh clot, identification of the neck and separation of perforators, although somewhat more tedious in the acute case, is neither significantly more difficult nor more hazardous. Intraoperative aneurysm rupture was again not more frequent or apparently different in those cases operated on early or late.

We recommend early operation in those patients who are good grade (Botterell Grade 1-2, Hunt-Hess I-III), whose aneurysm does not present a particular technical difficulty because of size, configuration or location, and occasionally in those patients whose lives appear to be in jeopardy because of recurrent hemorrhage. However, review of this series makes us hesitant to recommend early surgery for aneurysms arising from the basilar trunk.

The most important factor in timing in surgery of good grade patients is the availability of an experienced, alert, surgical team. It is well shown by this series that results improve with experience. Patients with basilar bifurcation aneurysms, once held to be the most difficult aneurysms, had results comparable to patients with aneurysms at other locations whether in the anterior or posterior circulation. Centralizing the care of these challenging lesions in a few experienced hands with adequate surgical experience remains a factor for improved patient outcome.

In spite of improvements in surgical techniques, we are far away from ideal results. As there are now means to detect aneurysms before they rupture, there is progress toward the best timing of aneurysm surgery: operation before rupture. This will improve the management results more than any new technical innovation. The question also remains whether urgent early endovascular wire coiling of the dome of the ruptured sac can be used to tide the patient over the stormy time of vasospasm so that a definitive operation can be carried out later under a healed brain. If however intraoperative fibrinolysis proves effective for preventing vasospasm, endovascular treatment will seldom be possible.

Table 22.1. Patients with VBAAs operated upon (1767)

Operated upon 1959–1969	64
Operated upon 1970–1992	1703
Unruptured or remote (> 1 year) rupture	457
Early surgery (0–7 days)	206
Late surgery (8–365 days)	1040

Table 22.2. Baseline characteristics and timing of surgery in 1246 patients with VBAAs

Variable	Timing of surgery (0 = day of SAH)	
	Early surgery (0–7 days)	Late surgery (8–365 days)
No. of patients	206	1040
Mean preoperative grade	1.76	1.46
Females (%)	143 (69)	664 (64)
Age range (mean) years	8–80 (48)	4–77 (47)
Multiple bleeds (%)	40.8	24.5
Multiple aneurysms (%)	27.7	24.0
Redo aneurysm (%)	3.4	7.5
AVM (%)	1.5	3.0
Large and giant aneurysms (%)	41.8	38.5
Aneurysm location %		
Basilar bifurcation	54.9	53.4
Basilar SCA	14.1	14.9
Basilar trunk	4.4	7.0
Vertebrobasilar junction	6.8	6.2
Vertebral artery	15.1	13.6
Posterior cerebral artery	4.9	4.6

Table 22.3. Operative and perioperative factors and timing of surgery in 1246 patients with VBAAs

Variable	Timing of surgery (0 = day of SAH)	
	Early surgery (0–7 days)	Late surgery (8–365 days)
No. of patients	206	1040
Temporary clipping (%)	40.8	19.4
Use of hypotension (below 70 mm Hg) (%)	32.5	60.9
Intraoperative aneurysm rupture (%)	13.6	13.2
Inadvertent major vessel occlusion (%)	1.5	4.3
Perforator injury (%)	5.4	9.8
Cranial nerve injury (%)	0.5	1.8
Reoperation for postoperative hematoma (%)	4.4	2.9
Reclipping (%)	1.9	4.4
Shunt operation (%)	8.7	10.8
Symptomatic spasm (%)	15.0	6.9
Spasm contributing to death (%)	3.4	1.1

Table 22.4. Outcome as related to preoperative Grade in 206 patients with early operation on VBAAs (%)

Grade	Excellent	Good	Poor	Dead (%)	Total
1	85	12	6	4 (4)	107
2	34	17	6	5 (8)	62
3	9	7	2	4 (18)	22
4	0	3	4	3 (30)	10
5	1	0	0	4 (80)	5
Total	129	39	18 (9)	20 (10)	206

Table 22.5. Outcome as related to aneurysm site in 206 patients with early operation on VBAAs (%)

Site	Excellent	Good	Poor	Dead	Total
Basilar bif.	76	17	11	9 (8)	113
SCA	17	6	3	3 (10)	29
Basilar trunk	3	2	0	4 (44)	9
VB junction	8	4	1	1 (7)	14
Vertebral	19	7	3	2 (7)	31
PCA	6	3	0	1 (10)	10
Total	129	39	18 (9)	20 (10)	206

Table 22.6. Outcome as related to aneurysm size in 206 patients with early operation on VBAAs (%)

Aneurysm size	Excellent	Good	Poor	Dead	Total
Small	79	21	12	8 (7)	120
Large	39	13	3	9 (14)	64
Giant	11	5	3	3 (13)	22
Total	129	39	18 (9)	20 (10)	206

Table 22.7. Outcome as related to age in 206 patients with early operation on VBAAs (%)

Age group (years)	Excellent	Good	Poor	Dead	Total
0–9	1				1
10–19	2				2
20–29	9	2		1 (8)	12
30–39	29	6	1	3 (8)	39
40–49	42	8	5	3 (5)	58
50–59	27	12	2	7 (15)	48
60–69	16	9	7	6 (16)	38
70 or more	3	2	3		8
Total	129	39	18 (9)	20 (10)	206

Table 22.8. Operative method and outcome in 206 patients with early operation on VBAAs (%)

Operative method	Excellent	Good	Poor	Dead	Total
Clip	116	33	17 (10)	11 (6)	177
Silk ligature	1			1	2
Hunterian ligation	8	6	1	4	19
Trapping	3			1	4
Endovascular	1			2	3
Hematoma removed only				1	1
Total	129	39	18 (9)	20 (10)	206

Table 22.9. Operative method and completeness of aneurysm treatment in 206 patients with early operation on VBAAs (%)

Operative method	Total obliteration	Residual neck	Residual fundus	No obliteration	Total
Clip	162 (92)	12	3		177
Silk ligature	1		1		2
Hunterian ligation	13		5	1	19
Trapping	4				4
Endovascular			3		3
Hematoma removed				1	1
Total	180 (87)	12 (6)	12	2	206

Table 22.10. Outcome as related to timing of operation in 206 patients with early operation on VBAAs (%)

Timing of surgery	Excellent	Good	Poor	Dead	Total
0–1 day	20	6	5	6 (16)	37
2–3 day	34	10	8	7 (12)	59
4–6 day	55	17	3	3 (4)	78
7 day	20	6	2	4 (13)	32
Total	129	39	18 (9)	20 (10)	206

Table 22.11. Operative method and outcome in 113 patients with early operation on basilar bifurcation aneurysms (%)

Operative method	Excellent	Good	Poor	Dead	Total
Clip	73	16	11	6	106
Hunterian ligation	2	1		1	4
Endovascular	1			1	2
Hematoma removed				1	1
Total	76	17	11 (10)	9 (8)	113

Chapter 23
The Anesthetic Management of Patients During Posterior Fossa Aneurysm Surgery

By **P. H. Manninen** and **A. W. Gelb**

The goals of the anesthetic management of patients with cerebral aneurysms are to facilitate the operation and patient recovery while minimizing the risk of intraoperative rupture and the occurrence of neurological deficits. During posterior fossa aneurysm surgery, there are other factors to consider in the management of the patient. These include the positioning of the patient which may be sitting, park bench or prone, and the complications related to these positions. Second, potential complications may occur as a result of the manipulation of vital centers in the brain stem. This chapter will discuss the anesthetic management, positioning, complications and the monitoring of brain stem function during posterior fossa aneurysm surgery. We describe the techniques that we have used and found to be successful. More general reviews are available elsewhere.

Preoperative Preparation

The general status of the patient, including the neurological system, should be carefully assessed. A lesion in the posterior fossa may result in increased intracranial pressure (ICP) due to the size of the lesion or by the production of hydrocephalus by obstruction of the flow of cerebral spinal fluid. Cranial nerve involvement may occur resulting in bulbar palsy which may impair swallowing or normal glottic protective reflexes. This may result in aspiration pneumonia preoperatively or lead to an increased risk of pulmonary aspiration postoperatively.

Electrocardiographic changes are common in patients with subarachnoid hemorrhage (SAH) from ruptured cerebral aneurysms occurring in 50–80% of patients. The incidence of these changes is similar for patients with posterior fossa aneurysms as compared to anterior circulation aneurysms.

Premedication

Patients with lesions in the posterior fossa are particularly sensitive to respiratory depression caused by sedatives or opioids. If the patient has raised ICP or brain stem pathology, we give no preoperative sedation. A reassuring preoperative visit by the anesthesiologist is usually sufficient to relieve anxiety. In an alert patient who is very anxious, a small dose of a short-acting benzodiazepine is used.

Anesthesia Management

The goals of the anesthetic management can be accomplished by the control of the aneurysm's transmural pressure, control of ICP and the maintenance of cerebral oxygen delivery. The pressure within an aneurysm is equal to the systemic blood pressure so that transmural pressure is the difference between the blood pressure and ICP. The relationship between the transmural pressure and the wall tension of the aneurysm is linear so that an increase in mean arterial pressure (light anesthesia) or a fall in ICP by ventricular drainage or hyperventilation will increase the transmural pressure, the wall stress and the risk of aneurysm rupture. An increase in transmural pressure should be avoided. Cerebral perfusion pressure equals the difference between the mean arterial pressure and ICP. If while attempting to maintain low transmural pressure the cerebral perfusion pressure falls below the lower limit of autoregulation, a reduction in cerebral blood flow will occur.

Monitoring

During induction of anesthesia, pulse, blood pressure, oxygen saturation and end-tidal carbon dioxide are monitored. Blood pressure is monitored by an automated, rapidly cycling non-invasive cuff and the arterial cannula for intra-arterial blood pressure monitoring is inserted after the patient is asleep. Other monitors required after the induction of anesthesia include core temperature, central venous pressure, and urinary drainage. A central venous catheter is useful for volume measurement and for the treatment of air embolism if the patient is placed in the sitting position. We routinely use the internal or external jugular vein and if the sitting position is used, an x-ray is taken to confirm the location of the catheter at the junction of the superior vena cava and right atrium. A pulmonary artery catheter is only used in patients who have severe ischemic heart disease or cardiac dysfunction. Monitoring of brain stem function can be performed with the observation of changes in cardiovascular parameters, the use of spontaneous ventilation, and evoked potentials (vide infra).

Induction

Induction is a critical time and should be smooth and faultless. After preoxygenation, the induction of anesthesia is usually performed with an opioid such as fentanyl 2–5 µg/kg or sufentanil 0.5–1.0 µg/kg followed by the administration of thiopental or more recently propofol with or without lidocaine 1.0–1.5 mg/kg. These drugs result in a rapid loss of consciousness, a reduction in cerebral blood flow, ICP, cerebral metabolic rate and a desirable drop in blood pressure. For intubation muscle paralysis is obtained by either succinylcholine or a non-depolarizing agent. Succinylcholine produces a rapid onset of relaxation and excellent intubating conditions. Though some studies have shown succinylcholine to raise ICP and serum potassium, this has not been our experience. Additional doses of thiopental, propofol or gentle hyperventilation with isoflurane are administered prior to intubation to ensure that the patient is deeply anesthetized to attenuate the sympathetic response.

Maintenance

An anesthetic agent ideal for aneurysm surgery should have the properties of being able to quickly and reversibly lower blood pressure, control ICP, provide protection against cerebral ischemia, minimize the formation of vasogenic cerebral edema and allow for rapid awakening. There is no one ideal agent. Drugs we have most frequently used include combinations of nitrous oxide/oxygen, fentanyl or sufentanil, and isoflurane. Times of painful stimulation, for example the insertion of head pins, may result in marked hypertension. This should be anticipated and the response prevented by the administration of thiopental, propofol, opioids, or isoflurane.

Hyperventilation to a $PaCO_2$ of 25–30 mmHg is indicated in the presence of intracranial hypertension, otherwise $PaCO_2$ should remain between 32–35 mmHg. If spontaneous ventilation is to be used to monitor brain stem function, then the $PaCO_2$ will have to be allowed to increase to the patient's preoperative level or higher.

Fluid Administration

Fluids administered should not contain glucose as cerebral ischemia may be worsened by an above normal blood glucose. We use Ringer's Lactate as our standard solution. Although a modest degree of intravascular dehydration is accepted during the surgery, we aim to have the central venous pressure in the normal range or, more recently, slightly above by the end of the procedure.

We use mannitol (1.0 gm/kg) to decrease brain bulk. This is infused over 20–30 minutes starting at approximately the same time as the burr hole. At the surgeon's request a second 1 gm/kg is infused before temporary vessel occlusion. This results in a transient rise in serum potassium.

Induced Hypotension, Temporary Arterial Occlusion, and Cerebral Protection

We have used deliberate induced hypotension to decrease the risk of rupture during clipping of an aneurysm although objective evidence of such a benefit is lacking. Sodium nitroprusside was used until the introduction of isoflurane a decade ago.

More recently, it has become common surgical practice to use temporary occlusion of a feeding artery to produce an acute reduction of local blood flow in contrast to systemically induced hypotension. Moderate induced hypotension may be used during the dissection but whenever temporary occlusion is used the blood pressure is returned to the patient's preoperative normal level. Monitoring of brain stem function during temporary occlusion is critical and may be performed by cardiovascular and/or respiratory parameters and by the use of evoked potentials.

It has not been our practice to use special brain protective therapies such as barbiturate coma because there has been an absence of convincing rigorously performed clinical outcome studies. However, occasionally at the surgeon's request, we have given additional barbiturate or mannitol according to the prevailing fashion. In view of the recent evidence that mild hypothermia may offer some cerebral protection, it is worth noting that despite our efforts to maintain normothermia, most of our patients had intraoperative esophageal temperatures of 34.5–36°C.

Emergence and Recovery

The primary goals at the end of surgery are to avoid coughing, straining, hypoxia, hypercarbia and hypertension. We have used hydralazine with or without beta blockers and more recently esmolol or labetalol to control hemodynamic responses during emergence. Patients should be arousable and responsive as soon as possible after the termination of the operation to allow for clinical evaluation and ensure a patent airway. If the patient has any preoperative neurological deficits, particularly bulbar palsy with difficulty in swallowing and protecting the airway, the presence of a gag reflex needs to be evaluated to ascertain whether the patient can be safely extubated. If the patient has a reduced gag or is still drowsy, it is safer to keep the patient intubated (with or without ventilation) until they have fully recovered from anesthesia. Some patients may require a tracheostomy to protect their airway but this decision is usually deferred until the patient has required intubation for a few postoperative days.

The patient should be transferred fully monitored from the operating room to a recovery area staffed by personnel familiar with and skilled in the management of neurosurgical patients. Continuous, careful monitoring and control of blood pressure is required postoperatively. The patient should be nursed in an upright (30°) position to ensure good ventilation and decrease venous drainage.

Positioning

The position of the patient for posterior fossa aneurysm surgery can be park bench (semi-prone), prone, or sitting. The surgeon's preference usually determines the position. Over the past decade our use of the sitting position has steadily decreased because of concerns about air embolism and cervical cord injury so that now the park bench position is used almost exclusively.

Careful positioning to ensure patient safety is required for all positions. In the prone or park bench position, free movement of the abdomen is essential for good ventilation and decrease in intrathoracic pressure. In the park bench position, with flexion of the neck one has to ensure that there is not excessive pressure between the patient's chin and chest or shoulder to prevent obstruction of venous drainage from the head and the development of skin necrosis due to pressure. Migration and possible obstruction of the endotracheal tube may occur with extreme positions. Thus monitoring of airway pressures and ventilation by auscultation and end-tidal CO_2 during positioning and throughout the procedures is critical.

The sitting position allows for good surgical exposure and venous and cerebral spinal fluid drainage but, possible complications that may occur include hypotension, venous air embolism, pneumocephalus and spinal cord compression. We minimize the development of hypotension by ensuring that the patient is adequately hydrated, wrapping the legs to prevent pooling of blood in the lower extremities and by the slow placement of the patient into the upright position. Occasionally vasopressors may be required. Venous air embolism is a common complication in patients undergoing neurosurgical procedures in the sitting position with an incident of about 40%. Early detection of a venous air embolism is essential to successful treatment. The monitors we use are the precordial Doppler, end-tidal CO_2, SaO_2, and the esophageal stethoscope. We use a right atrial catheter for the aspiration of embolized air should this occur. The use of nitrous oxide when the risk of air embolism is present is an issue of debate. Nitrous oxide may enlarge the intravascular air bubbles due to difference in blood gas solubility between nitrous oxide and nitrogen. Arguments for the use of nitrous oxide are based on the fact that entrained air will expand rapidly allowing for earlier detection and therefore earlier treatment. In our practice, the use of nitrous oxide varies among the neuroanesthesiologist. As soon as detection of the air embolism occurs, the surgeon is alerted to identify and occlude the sites of air entry. Nitrous oxide, if used, is discontinued and the patient ventilated with 100% oxygen. If continuous or a large venous air embolism occurs, the patient's head should be lowered and cardiovascular support may be required. It has not been our practice to use positive end-expiratory pressure prophylactically or therapeutically. Positive end-expiratory pressure may raise central venous pressure which is helpful to prevent air embolism but it may also facilitate the passage of air through a patent foramen ovale which is known to occur in 20-25% of individuals with no known heart disease.

Monitoring of Brain Stem Function

Ischemia to vital areas of the brain stem may occur during posterior fossa surgery from manipulations such as retraction or from the temporary or permanent occlusion of a major feeding artery. Changes in cardiovascular parameters such as hypertension and/or bradycardia are considered by many to be the most useful clinical intraoperative indicators of brain stem ischemia. However, respiratory sequelae have been reported to occur without significant cardiovascular changes and thus spontaneous ventilation has been advocated as an important monitor of brain stem function during posterior fossa surgery. The use of spontaneous ventilation is controversial as it may result in hypercapnia leading to swelling of the brain and impairment of surgical conditions. In our institution we have frequently used spontaneous ventilation. Spontaneous ventilation is usually started after the dura has been opened and the aneurysm exposed. This is accomplished by lightening the anesthetic, reversing any muscle paralysis and opioids if needed and allowing the $PaCO_2$ to increase. In a recent review of patients from our institution where spontaneous ventilation was used during manipulation of the brain stem and/or the temporary or permanent occlusion of the vertebral basilar circulation we found that cardiovascular changes did not occur as frequently or as early as respiratory changes.

We have used evoked potentials as an additional monitor of brain stem function. We found brain stem auditory evoked potentials to be useful during basilar vertebral aneurysm surgery especially for the assessment of the safety of permanent occlusion of the vertebral or basilar artery. The value of somatosensory evoked potentials during posterior fossa surgery has been questioned and found not always to be helpful. In a series of patients from our institution, we found that using both modalities was feasible but found no difference between the ability of brain stem auditory compared to median nerve somatosensory evoked potentials in detecting intraoperative cerebral ischemia and predicting neurological deficits postoperatively. Both techniques had false positive and false negative results but using both modalities to monitor the patient was helpful in decreasing the incidence of false negative results. One limitation of evoked potential monitoring is that patients who have brain stem deficits preoperatively may have abnormal evoked potential waveforms which makes intraoperative interpretation difficult if not impossible.

Complications

Respiratory failure can occur following posterior fossa surgery presenting either as an abnormal pattern of breathing or apnea. This may be due to changes in the brain stem including edema, hematoma or acute hydrocephalus. Cranial nerve dysfunction may occur postoperatively. If there is loss of the function of the ninth, tenth and/or twelfth cranial nerves this may result in impaired swallowing and the loss of protective laryngeal reflexes. These patients will be at risk for aspiration. Pneumocephalus is a complication that may occur, particularly in patients who are in the sitting position. This involves an intracranial collection of air which raises intracranial pressure. These patients may have a delayed recovery, with slow return of consciousness and deterioration of neurological state. The latter has not been common in our experience and the possibility has not deterred us from using nitrous oxide.

Conclusion

The anesthetic management of patients during posterior fossa aneurysm surgery presents a real challenge to the anesthesiologist. All the principles of safe, careful neurosurgical anesthesia for patients with vascular lesions need to be considered, and in addition to this, the possible complications of positioning of the patient, especially in the sitting position, will require further attention to the patient and the procedure. Monitoring of brain stem function to detect cerebral ischemia as early as possible and thus prevent postoperative neurological deficits requires constant vigilance by the anesthesiologist. Monitoring techniques include the observation of cardiovascular parameters, the use of both brain stem auditory and somatosensory evoked potentials, and in select patients, respiratory monitoring by the use of spontaneous ventilation.

Chapter 24
Endovascular Saccular Treatment of Posterior Circulation Aneurysms

By **S. P. Lownie**

The first surgical approach to the direct treatment of an intracranial aneurysm was undertaken by Dott in 1931 who reinforced the outer wall of a ruptured aneurysm by wrapping it with strips of muscle. Later McConnell used muscle to pack the interior of an aneurysm which had been opened at surgery. Then in 1937, Dandy used a hemostatic clip to close off the neck of an aneurysm and arrest the blood flow within the sac. Over the next 30 years, surgical neck clipping became the consummate approach for the majority of cerebral aneurysms.

With the advent of catheter access to the intracranial vasculature, the notion developed that a cerebral aneurysm might be treated by approaching it from within the blood vessel rather than from outside the aneurysm sac. This was an enticing concept because it implied a potentially lower risk to the patient by precluding general anesthesia, retraction on the brain and dissection around the aneurysm.

Detachable Balloons

In 1974 Serbinenko introduced the use of balloon-tipped catheters for temporary or permanent occlusion of intracranial arteries. In three patients, he used a detachable balloon to directly occlude an aneurysm. One of these patients had a large basilar bifurcation aneurysm; the balloon was used to occlude most of the aneurysm cavity but unfortunately the patient died. The other two had internal carotid artery aneurysms; the balloon was used to occlude the aneurysm neck and both patients survived. Subsequently, Romodanov and Shcheglov reported their attempts at balloon occlusion of saccular aneurysms in 119 patients. In 93 of these, the aneurysm sac was occluded with a balloon and the parent artery was preserved. Only one aneurysm was on the posterior circulation, a reflection of their approach by direct carotid artery puncture in the neck. Seven patients died and there were three poor outcomes. Contraindications which emerged to the use of detachable balloons were the presence of a small-sized aneurysm, or a small aneurysm with a wide neck. Complications included rupture of the aneurysm by the balloon (one case) and stroke due either to balloon rupture, premature balloon detachment, or thromboembolism (five cases). Aneurysm recurrence was seen in three cases.

Debrun and colleagues reported their experience with detachable balloons in the treatment of surgically unclippable aneurysms in 1981. Three of the nine cases were cavernous carotid aneurysms, the only ones treated by balloon occlusion of the aneurysm rather than the parent artery. Two of the three experienced transient cerebral ischemia. Two ultimately required permanent carotid artery occlusion, one because of aneurysm recurrence and one because of local abscess formation. It was felt that occlusion of the aneurysm sac rather than the parent artery carried a significant risk of both cerebral ischemia and incomplete occlusion.

In North America, Hieshima was the first to report the direct occlusion of a posterior circulation aneurysm using a detachable balloon in 1986. The patient had a large basilar bifurcation aneurysm which had bled. Surgical treatment was considered risky due to the location and size of the aneurysm, and the presence of vasospasm. The aneurysm was completely occluded with a balloon containing liquid acrylic polymer with a good clinical result. In 1989, Hieshima and colleagues reported on 26 posterior circulation aneurysms treated with detachable balloon techniques. In 14 patients, 15 aneurysms were occluded with preservation of the parent artery. Complete angiographic occlusion was achieved in nine of these, incomplete occlusion in six. Two patients died immediately from procedure-related aneurysm rupture. Three patients had strokes. Aneurysm rebleeding occurred in three

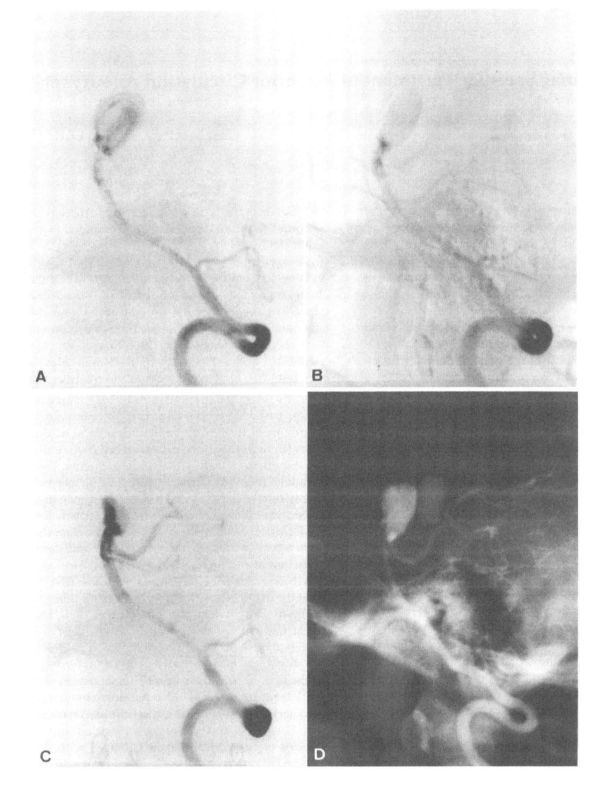

Figure 24.1. (Case 3) **A** Right vertebral angiogram, lateral projection. Large basilar bifurcation aneurysm which had ruptured. At surgery, the aneurysm proved to be larger than expected with mural thrombosis posteriorly. Attempts at clipping resulted in the clips slipping down onto the basilar bifurcation. **B** The aneurysm was embolized with a silastic detachable balloon filled with 0.85 cc of HEMA polymerizing mixture. **C** Early repeat angiography shows some contrast filling at the base of aneurysm anteriorly. **D** Follow-up angiogram 4 months later shows displacement of the balloon posteriorly into the mural thrombus and recanalization of the aneurysm. Two years later the patient was treated elsewhere with detachable platinum coils and did well

patients, two to four months after treatment, all of whom died. Death due to the procedure or to the failure of the procedure to protect against rebleeding thus occurred in 5 out of the 14 patients. One patient described as a "good" result later required surgery.

Other investigators have reported similar problems with saccular balloon occlusion including delayed aneurysm rupture or aneurysm recanalization and enlargement. The latter has been particularly noted following balloon occlusion of basilar aneurysms (Fig. 24.1). Few today consider detachable balloons a promising endovascular approach to saccular aneurysm occlusion.

Thrombosis with Coiled Wires

In the 1960s, the observation that aneurysms occasionally thrombose spontaneously, coupled with concerns about surgery in the setting of acute hemorrhage, led Mullan to attempt to occlude aneurysms by inducing thrombosis with electric current applied through a burr hole. However, the thrombosis proved to be only temporary on follow-up angiography. Stereotactically implanted metal needles were employed to act as a substrate for permanent thrombosis, but the results were not found to be superior to standard surgical methods. For giant aneurysms at high risk for surgical clipping, Mullan developed wires which could be inserted directly into the aneurysm sac at craniotomy. Beryllium copper wire was found to be a good packing material, which could be pre-shaped into the form of a coil thus preventing passage out of the aneurysm and into the parent artery.

Two of the 15 cases in Mullan's series involved the posterior circulation. The first was an intact giant basilar aneurysm, into which 32 feet of beryllium copper wire and 20 feet of copper wire were inserted. Follow-up angiography showed that the wire had become compressed into one corner of the aneurysm. Six weeks after treatment, the patient bled and died. The second case also involved the basilar artery. Despite a good angiographic result initially, the aneurysm recanalized and expanded and the patient succumbed to a combination of infarction and mass effect.

The development of the microcatheter in the mid 1980s led to the ability to catheterize aneurysms percutaneously. Platinum wire coils became used as embolic devices for the direct treatment of intracranial aneurysms.

Casasco et al. reported a series of 71 patients treated with platinum microcoils in 1993. The coils were coated with thrombogenic synthetic fibers. Forty-two aneurysms were located on the posterior circulation. Complete angiographic occlusion was accomplished in 85% of the 71 cases. Clinical outcome was good in 85%, moderate disability was seen in 4%, and 8 patients (11%) died. Two of the eight deaths occurred in good grade patients. Perforation of the aneurysm with the catheter guidewire or coil occurred in two patients resulting in nonfatal subarachnoid hemorrhage. Six treatment related strokes occurred, resulting in death in three and moderate disability in three. The strokes were due to inadvertent parent artery occlusion in four and embolism in two. Of the eight deaths in the series, five were either directly due to the procedure (stroke in three patients) or indirectly due to the failure of the treatment to protect against rebleeding (two cases). The other three deaths were due to vasospasm.

In the Casasco series, follow-up angiography showed that out of 54 aneurysms considered completely occluded, 3 showed aneurysm refilling at a mean of 13 months which required further treatment. Of 11 aneurysms incompletely occluded, 3 developed aneurysm enlargement. Two of these presented with rebleeding, in both cases fatal. The authors observed an apparently worse natural history for the aneurysm partially occluded with coils as compared to those partially clipped surgically.

A major development occurred with the development by Guglielmi and Viñuela of electrolytically detachable platinum coils. This innovation allowed the operator to retrieve the coil if its position was unsatisfactory, particularly if the coil extruded into the parent artery. It also allowed a more complete occlusion of the aneurysm at the level of the aneurysm neck. These improvements led to considerably more successful results: in a series of 42 posterior circulation aneurysm of all sizes treated in patients of all grades, less than 5% mortality occurred. The Guglielmi detachable coil is presently the superior device for the endovascular treatment of aneurysms.

In analyzing the completeness of aneurysm occlusion with detachable coils, it has been found that the degree of aneurysm occlusion is related to the width of the aneurysm neck. Defining a small aneurysm neck as 4 mm or less, and a large neck as greater than 4 mm, Zubillaga et al. noted a distinct difference in angiographic results. In their series of 74 aneurysms, complete occlusion was achieved in 85% of the small necked aneurysms, but only 15% of the wide necked aneurysms. Their findings emphasize the need for careful long term follow-up in patients with the potential for aneurysm recanalization or regrowth.

Experience at the University of Western Ontario, 1971 to 1994

Our experience over 23 years in the treatment of posterior circulation aneurysms using either coiled wire thrombosis, detachable balloons or glue has been comparatively small at 17 cases. This reflects the fact that the majority of aneurysms have been amenable to surgical neck clipping with acceptably low morbidity and mortality. Although Hunterian ligation of parent arteries using detachable balloons has frequently been employed in treating posterior circulation aneurysms, these cases are not included in this discussion which is restricted to those in which occlusion of the sac rather than the parent artery was the goal.

A variety of approaches have been taken depending largely upon the methods that were available at the time a patient was treated. Prior to 1971, two patients were treated using Gallagher's piloinjection technique. These have previously been reported. Neither aneurysm was completely thrombosed with the horsehair. One patient rebled from the inferior aspect of the aneurysm below the thrombosed portion and died at 3 1/2 months. The other patient did well with occlusion of the posterior loculus of a bilobed sac. The first patient treated with coils in 1971 underwent insertion of copper-beryllium and copper wire coils directly at craniotomy (one of two basilar aneurysms reported by Mullan and illustrated in Chapter 6, Fig. 6.3). The remaining 16 patients have been treated using endovascular techniques available since 1988. Eleven of these had saccular aneurysms, four aneurysms were fusiform, and one had a dissecting aneurysm. Each of the 16 patients underwent occlusion or attempted occlusion of the sac by coiled wire thrombosis (14 cases), detachable balloon (1 case, Fig. 24.1) or IBCA glue (1 case, Fig. 24.2). In the four with fusiform aneurysms, parent artery and aneurysm occlusion was the goal, in one instance to allow safe surgical evacuation of the mass.

The clinical indications for endovascular treatment included failed surgery, poor clinical grade, high risk medical condition, and anticipated surgical difficulty. Failed surgery was the reason in eight cases: either the aneurysm was unclippable due to neck width and/or thickness (three cases), perforating arteries were adherent to the aneurysm (two cases), scarring and adhesions from a previous surgery made adequate exposure impossible (two cases), or the sheer size of the aneurysm made access to the region difficult (1 case). Poor clinical grade was the primary reason in three patients. Two other patients had had recent myocardial infarctions. In two cases, it was the surgeon's opinion that clipping would be difficult and risky (Fig. 24.3).

Conventional non-detachable platinum coils were employed solely in six aneurysms, Guglielmi detachable coils in six, and a combination in two. For most patients, this was the extent of treatment. In 3 of the 10 saccular aneurysms treated with coils, angiographically complete occlusion of the aneurysm was accomplished at the initial treatment (Fig. 24.4). One of these was trapped (Fig. 24.5). Three out of 10 were left with a small aneurysm neck remnant, and 4 had a significant portion of the aneurysm (greater than 10%) still filling. Of the latter, dramatic splaying of the coils to the periphery of the aneurysm sac occurred in two patients, both having been treated with conventional coils. One underwent application of a Drake tourniquet to the basilar artery which was occluded uneventfully (illustrated in Chapter 6, Fig. 6.4). This was done in the hope that removal of the pounding axial stream directly into the aneurysm would prevent further radial dispersion and impaction of the wire. The second patient with incomplete occlusion had further endovascular treatment with detachable coils which led to a complete occlusion (Fig. 24.6). In the third patient, a second surgery was performed and the aneurysm was clipped. The fourth patient is being monitored, and follow-up angiography has shown some compaction of the Guglielmi coils (Fig. 24.3). Of the three with small neck remnants, one died related to the grade of the hemorrhage, one is angiographically unchanged at one year follow-up, and one has enlarged slightly at one year (Fig. 24.7).

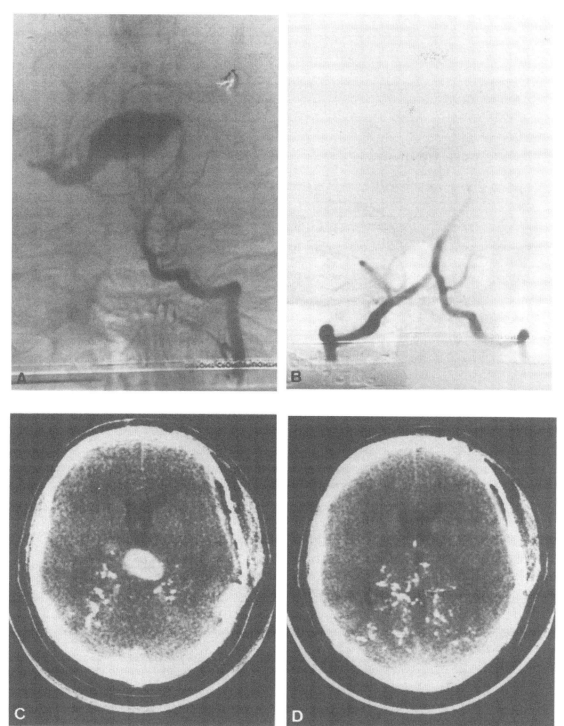

Figure 24.2. (Case 2) **A** Left vertebral angiogram, Towne projection. Giant fusiform aneurysm of the P1 segment of the right posterior cerebral artery. 38 year old man presenting with mass effect. Explored surgically from left to attempt clipping of P1 origin; not possible as it appeared to be included in the sac. An attempt at balloon occlusion failed. Cyanoacrylate injection through a calibrated leak balloon was done. **B** Post injection of isobutylcyanoacrylate. The glue blocked the aneurysm but diffused back into the basilar bifurcation occluding it as well. The patient became deeply comatose and subsequently brain dead. **C, D** CT scan post embolization. Diffuse embolization of glue throughout the upper basilar territory

290 Endovascular Saccular Treatment of Posterior Circulation Aneurysms

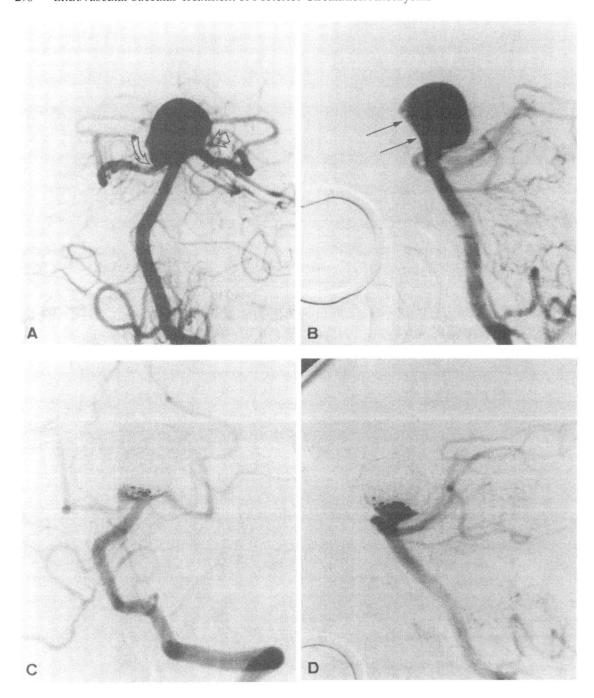

Figure 24.3 A–D

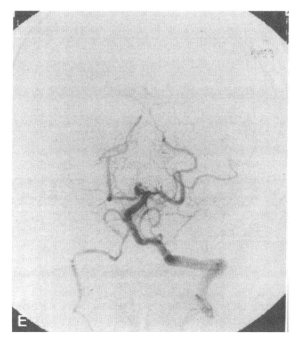
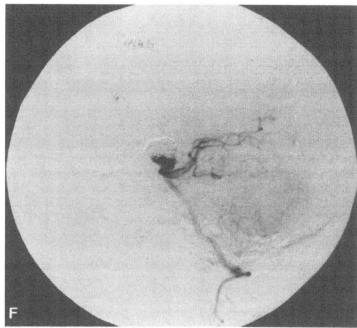

Figure 24.3 E, F

Figure 24.3. (Case 12) **A** Left vertebral angiogram, anteroposterior projection. Giant basilar bifurcation aneurysm which had caused a Grade 3 subarachnoid hemorrhage in a 70 year old woman. The aneurysm neck is wide, and the left posterior cerebral artery origin has been incorporated into the aneurysm wall (straight arrow). The right posterior cerebral artery origin is not distinctly separate from the aneurysm and may also be originating from it (curved arrow). **B** Same injection, lateral projection. There is mural thrombus anteriorly (arrows). **C** Left vertebral angiogram, Towne projection, following treatment with Guglielmi detachable coils. **D** Same injection, lateral projection. There is some filling of the aneurysm base. **E** Follow-up left vertebral angiogram at 7 months, Towne projection. Satisfactory appearance. **F** Same injection, lateral view. There has been some coil compaction within the aneurysm, but the majority remains occluded

Immediate complications occurred in 4 of the 16 patients. One patient had a stroke during catheter positioning prior to treatment. The microcatheter entered a long circumferential perforating artery resulting in thalamic infarction and a poor outcome. In the case treated with IBCA glue, the giant fusiform posterior cerebral aneurysm was successfully occluded, but the glue diffused back into the basilar bifurcation, occluding it and resulting in fatal brain stem infarction (Fig. 24.2). Among those treated with coils, catheter perforation of the aneurysm sac with contrast extravasation occurred in one (Fig. 24.8). This may have contributed to the death of the patient, who was already in Grade 4 condition. In another patient, the coil pusher penetrated the aneurysm wall causing a small subarachnoid hemorrhage, the patient sustaining a hemianopsia.

Technical complications without symptoms occurred in two patients. Small areas of infarction in the cerebellum and occipital lobes were seen on MR scan in one patient. Another had thrombus hanging off the coils at the origin of the posterior cerebral artery which resolved without incident (Fig. 24.9).

Clinical outcome was excellent or good in 12 of the 17 patients (71%), with 1 poor result and 4 deaths (24%).

292 Endovascular Saccular Treatment of Posterior Circulation Aneurysms

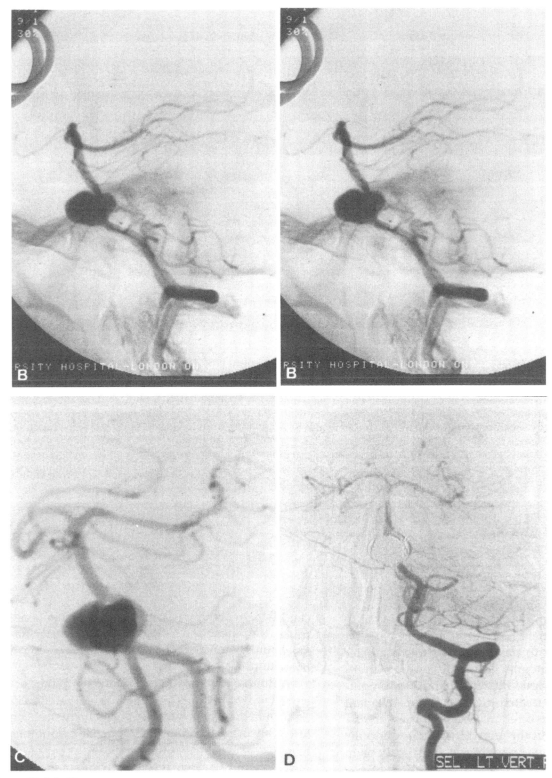

Figure 24.4 A–D

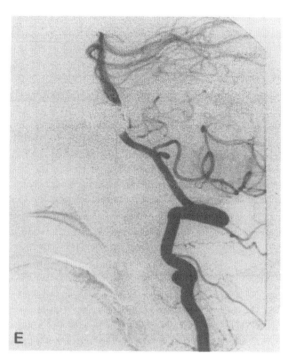 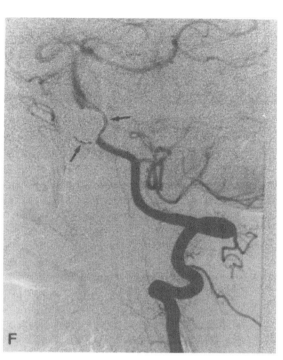

Figure 24.4 E, F

Figure 24.4. (Case 13) **A** Right vertebral angiogram, Towne projection. Large intact basilar aneurysm in a 53 year old woman. **B** Lateral projection. The aneurysm is lobulated, with a large lobule pointing anteriorly, and a smaller component pointing posteriorly. **C** Oblique projection confirms that the aneurysm arises in a fenestration of the basilar artery. The aneurysm was explored but could not be clipped. **D** Left vertebral angiogram, anteroposterior projection, 6 months after treatment with detachable coils. The aneurysm is completely occluded. **E** Same injection, lateral view. **F** Same injection, oblique view. Both limbs of the fenestration appear patent (arrows)

Endovascular Saccular Treatment of Posterior Circulation Aneurysms

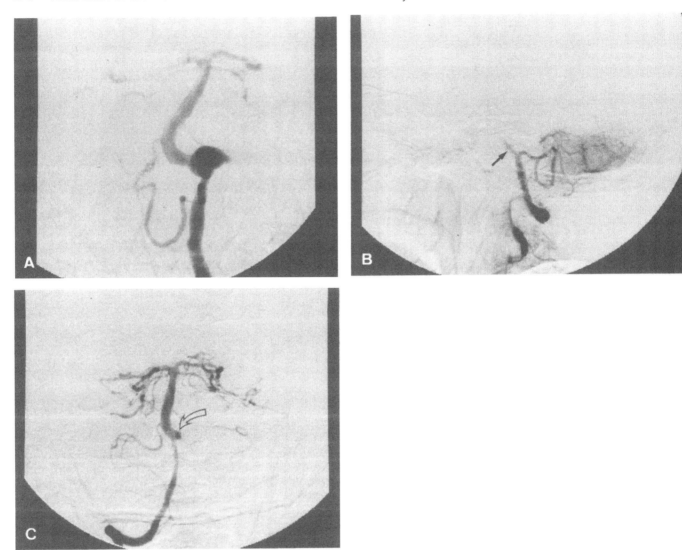

Figure 24.5. (Case 16) **A** Left vertebral angiogram, oblique projection. 72 year old man with Grade 3 subarachnoid hemorrhage and myocardial infarction with congestive failure. Hemorrhage due to a vertebral aneurysm without a well defined neck. **B** Left vertebral angiogram, lateral view, after trapping the aneurysm and adjacent artery with Guglielmi detachable coils. A short segment of artery fills distal to the posterior inferior cerebellar artery (arrow). **C** Right vertebral injection, anteroposterior projection. Reflux down the left vertebral artery to the level of the coils (arrow)

Endovascular Saccular Treatment of Posterior Circulation Aneurysms 295

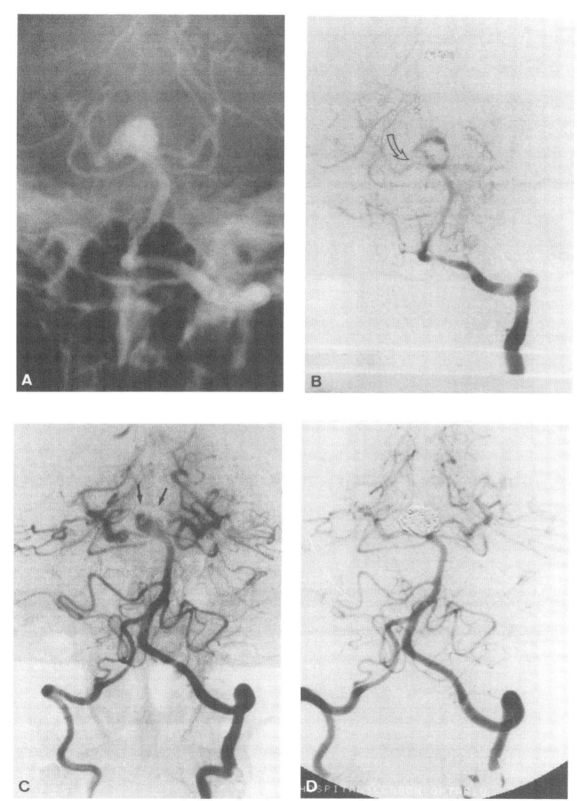

Figure 24.6. (Case 9) **A** Left vertebral angiogram, steep Towne projection. 42 year old woman with a large lobulated basilar bifurcation aneurysm. She rebled at the time of anesthetic induction. **B** Eleven conventional platinum coils have been used to partially occlude the aneurysm, particularly the lobule at the probable bleeding site (arrow). **C** Follow-up angiography at one year. Dramatic splaying of the coils to the periphery of the aneurysm (arrows). Further treatment undertaken with Guglielmi detachable coils. **D** Follow-up angiography 15 months later showing complete occlusion

296   Endovascular Saccular Treatment of Posterior Circulation Aneurysms

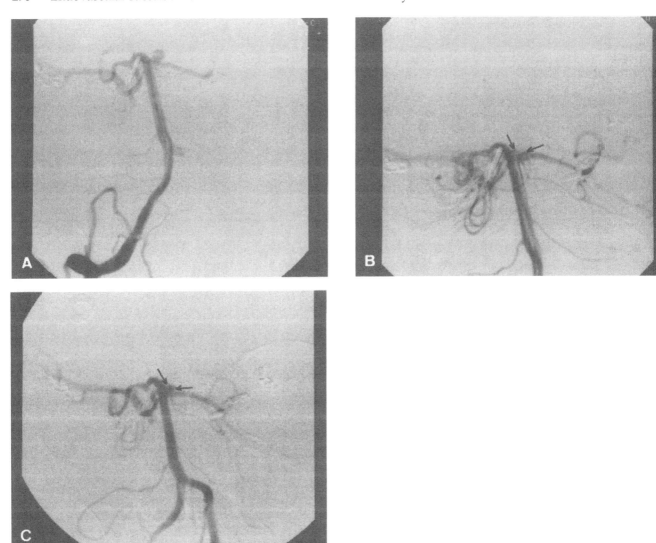

Figure 24.7. (Case 11) **A** Right vertebral angiogram, anteroposterior view. 46 year old woman with multiple aneurysms clipped previously. The small intact basilar bifurcation aneurysm could not be clipped due to adhesions from prior surgery. **B** After treatment with detachable coils, the aneurysm is almost completely occluded apart from a tiny neck remnant (arrows). **C** Follow-up angiography at one year shows coil compaction and a larger neck remnant (arrows)

Endovascular Saccular Treatment of Posterior Circulation Aneurysms

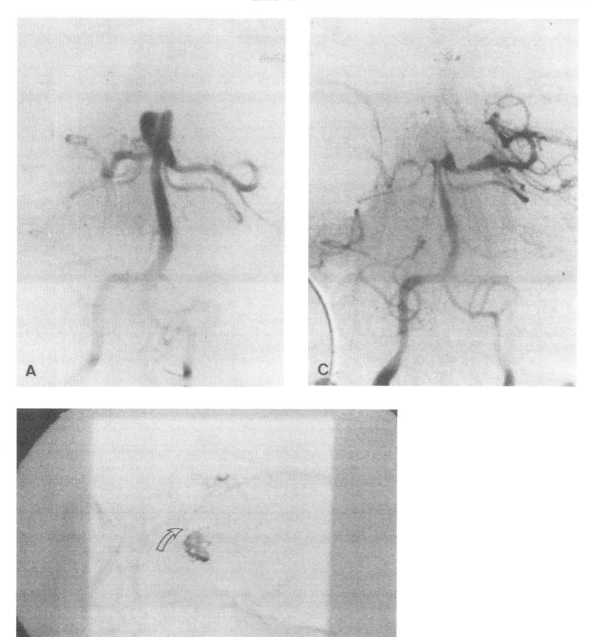

Figure 24.8. (Case 6) **A** Right vertebral angiogram, anteroposterior projection. Large basilar bifurcation in 52 year old man which had bled causing Grade 4 state. **B** Two treatment sessions using conventional platinum coils. During the second treatment after 10 coils had been deposited, the tip of the microcatheter was seen outside the coil mass (arrow). Contrast injection showed extravasation. A final coil was inserted as the catheter was being withdrawn. **C** Final angiogram. The patient suddenly deteriorated 2 days later and died. CT scan and postmortem examination did not indicate rebleeding. Death presumed due to raised intracranial pressure secondary to the severity of the initial bleed

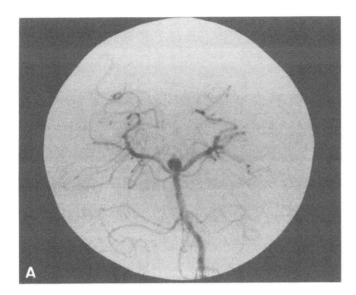 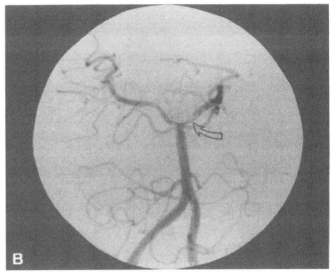

Figure 24.9. (Case 17) **A** Left vertebral angiogram, anteroposterior view. 42 year old man with remote subarachnoid hemorrhage. Failed surgery due to adherent perforators between the aneurysm neck and proximal P1 posterior cerebral artery segments. **B** Following treatment with Guglielmi coils. A tail of thrombus hangs into the proximal P1 segment on the left (arrow). No emboli occurred clinically. The thrombus partially resolved on follow-up angiography

Conclusions

Unlike surgery in which occlusion of the aneurysm neck is accomplished, endovascular treatment with coils or balloons generally results in packing of the aneurysm sac. In our experience and that of others, incomplete packing of an aneurysm carries a clear risk of aneurysm recanalization, regrowth and new or recurrent bleeding. Treatment with detachable balloons and conventional platinum coils has led to incomplete aneurysm occlusion in many patients. The Guglielmi detachable coils represent a significant advance due to the improved ability to pack the aneurysm sac down to the level of the neck. Recent studies indicate a high rate of complete occlusion in small necked aneurysms, but a reduced rate in aneurysms with necks greater than 4 mm in diameter. Follow-up studies will be necessary to determine whether the long term results of detachable coils are comparable to surgical neck clipping. Until then, endovascular treatment will continue to be reserved for patients in special circumstances.

Table 24.1. Saccular occlusion of posterior circulation aneurysms with coils, balloons or glue. Experience at the University of Western Ontario, 1971 to 1994 (continued on p. 299)

No.	Age	Sex	SAH grade	Type	Location	Size
1	53	F	2	saccular	basilar bif	giant
2	38	M	0	fusiform	post cerebral	giant
3	42	M	1	saccular	basilar bif	giant
4	56	F	2	saccular	basilar bif	large
5	50	M	0	fusiform	post cerebral	giant
6	52	M	4	saccular	basilar bif	large
7	47	F	4	dissect.	basilar trunk	large
8	41	F	1	saccular	sup cerebellar	small
9	42	F	3	saccular	basilar bif	large
10	49	M	1	saccular	basilar bif	small
11	46	F	0	saccular	basilar bif	small
12	70	F	3	saccular	basilar bif	giant
13	53	F	0	saccular	basilar fenest	large
14	62	F	1	fusiform	post cerebral	large
15	61	M	0	fusiform	post cerebral	giant
16	72	M	3	saccular	vertebral	small
17	42	M	1	saccular	basilar bif	small

Table 24.1. Continued from p. 298: Saccular occlusion of posterior circulation aneurysms with coils, balloons or glue. Experience at the University of Western Ontario, 1971 to 1994

No.	Indication	Treatment	Occlusion	Result	Outcome
1	failed surgery: beer belly aneurysm sac	beryllium copper coils (16.5') + copper coils (2')	incomplete	initially well; 9 months later coma; ?infarct/mass	dead
2	failed surgery: P1 origin could not be seen	isobutylcyanoaccrylate injection into aneurysm	complete	glue refluxed into basilar bifurcation	dead
3	failed surgery: clips slipped down on basilar	detachable HEMA filled balloon	incomplete	4 mos: balloon migration; GD coils used elsewhere	excellent
4	myocardial infarction	(1) platinum coils (2) Drake tourniquet	incomplete	8 mos: coils splayed out in aneurysm; tourniquet used	excellent
5	proximal control of PCA preoperatively	(1) platinum coils (2) surgical evacuation	complete	proximal occlusion permitted safe evacuation	good
6	grade	platinum coils	neck remnant	catheter perforation of sac during procedure	dead
7	grade and location	platinum coils	neck remnant	no postmortem obtained; death likely due to grade	dead
8	failed surgery: scarring from prior surgery	platinum coils	neck remnant	no change in minimal neck at 1 year	excellent
9	grade (bled on induction)	(1) platinum coils (2) GD coils	complete	6 mos: coils splayed out; GD coils used	excellent
10	failed surgery: adherent perforators on left side	(1) GD coils (2) repeat surgery	incomplete	GD coils allowed safe delayed surgery from left	good
11	failed surgery: scarring from prior surgery	GD coils	neck remnant	followup angios show enlarging neck remnant	excellent
12	surgical judgement: wide neck incorporating PCAs	GD coils	incomplete	some coil compaction on follow-up angio	excellent
13	failed surgery: confined exposure	GD coils	complete	remains complete on follow-up	excellent
14	surgical judgement: calcified mass under tent	GD and platinum coils	complete	coil pusher perforated aneurysm; small SAH	good
15	surgical judgement: test occlusion first	platinum coils	none	catheter got into PCA perforator; stroke resulted	poor
16	myocardial infarction	GD coils: trapping	complete	no problems	good
17	failed surgery: adherent perforators	GD coils	complete	asymptomatic thrombus in left P1 at neck	excellent

Chapter 25

Complications of Surgery for Vertebrobasilar Artery Aneurysms and Final Comments

With a Contribution of **M. Niskanen**

Specific and unique complications of vertebrobasilar aneurysm surgery were recognized by the senior author in the early 1960's: of the first 12 patients, only 5 had satisfactory results while 2 were poor and 5 died. In vertebrobasilar aneurysms, the difficulties with exposure and clip application may lead to the calamity of inadvertent major vessel occlusion, midbrain and/or thalamic infarction from perforator injury, problems in dealing with inadvertent intraoperative rupture, imperfect clipping with early rerupture, and frequent cranial nerve injuries.

In the following analysis, any, even short and transient, deterioration of cerebral function (consciousness, limb movement, speech) was counted as one complication and any new cranial nerve deficit(s) as one complication. In this very strict analysis, more than half (54.7%) of patients had no recorded complications or only minor or transient neurological deficits, but the rest were worse postoperatively (Table 25.6).

The aneurysms were grouped for this analysis as follows:

- basilar bifurcation (BB, 895 patients = 50.7%),
- superior cerebellar artery (SCA, 266 patients = 15.1%),
- basilar trunk (BT, 144 patients = 8.1%),
- vertebrobasilar junction (VBJ, 116 patients = 6.6%),
- vertebral artery (VA, 221 patients = 12.5%), and
- posterior cerebral artery (PCA, 125 patients = 7.1%).

Factors Increasing Complication Rates

The influence of pre-existing conditions on outcome, as preoperative Grade (Table 25.1), aneurysm site and size, patient's age and other diseases (especially those of cardiopulmonary system) are well known, and have been discussed in previous chapters. The influence on outcome of aneurysm configuration and the relationship of the sac to the skull base in non-giant basilar bifurcation aneurysms can be seen in Table 5.8. Aneurysms at the basilar bifurcation projecting forward and with a neck below the posterior clinoid process had the highest morbidity due to frequent intraoperative ruptures and inadvertent occlusions of major branch arteries.

Influence of Surgical Timing

Only 17% of patients with ruptured aneurysms were operated upon within seven days of subarachnoid hemorrhage (SAH), most in recent years (for rebleeding before operation and other details see Chapter 22). Fourteen out of 18 patients in Grades 4 and 5, all except 2 with recurrent hemorrhages, had a poor result when operated on urgently in the first week. Of 13 patients with basilar trunk aneurysms, 6 died and 1 remained poor when operated on in the same interval; 3 of the poor results occurred in 7 good risk patients.

Complications During Anesthesia

Problems with anesthesia accounted for six deaths and one poor result.

In total, eight patients had a rebleeding *during induction of anesthesia*, one without surgery died. Two operated upon remained poor and died later and two made excellent recoveries. Three others had good outcome after surgery was postponed.

Two patients had a rebleeding noted *during craniotomy*, both died.

One patient died with irreversible ventricular fibrillation when moderate hypothermia was allowed to drift below 25°C. Another remained in a vegetative state after induced hypotension fell below 20 torr MAP for more than 30 minutes.

Problems in Exposure

In 1353 patients (77%), the exposure was uncomplicated. A very tight brain was exposed in 23 patients, 18 of them had aneurysms at the basilar tip and 9 were operated on during the first week. The temporal lobe was injured in two patients but in most cases, the brain could be made slack and the operation could be continued. However, of the 23 patients, 5 died and 2 remained poor.

In 350 patients (20%), the surgeon noted and documented the dissection to be more difficult than usual. Technical difficulties were equally distributed between the specific aneurysm sites, sizes, and surgeons.

Serious retractor injury of the temporal lobe or laceration of temporal veins occurred in nine patients. Temporal lobe resection had to be used only three times, in two of them urgently when rerupture occurred during closure. In one patient with a very low neck of a basilar bifurcation aneurysm, a part of the posterior temporal lobe was excised, as the sac had ruptured during clipping. In this patient, a tic craniectomy was widened to a posterior temporal flap. Two further serious brain injuries were tragic: once a hemiplegia from a plunging burr during the craniotomy and in one case a middle cerebral artery branch adherent to the dura was avulsed when the bone flap was elevated with a fatal outcome. In 28 patients, the trochlear nerve at the tentorial edge was torn inadvertently in larger aneurysms of the basilar bifurcation, basilar-SCA or basilar trunk, often after the tentorium was divided to improve exposure. Trochlear paresis with diplopia on downward gaze (e.g. descending stairs) proved not to be a serious disability in daily life.

Intraoperative Aneurysm Rupture

Intraoperative aneurysm rupture always caused great stress for the surgical team and doubled the patients' morbidity and mortality. Inadvertent rupture of the sac, including minor bleedings, occurred in 181 patients (10%) during exposure, dissection or clip placement. Ten patients noted above rebled during the induction of anesthesia or craniotomy. Intraoperative rupture was *least* frequent in vertebral artery aneurysms (7%) and PCA aneurysms (8%), followed by VBJ aneurysms (10%) and the large group of basilar bifurcation aneurysms (10%). More frequently rupture occurred in aneurysms located on basilar trunk (13%) or basilar-SCA (14%). The highest morbidity of all sites was seen in intraoperative ruptures of VBJ aneurysms: 6 out of 12 patients had a poor result (3 poor outcomes and 3 deaths). The lowest morbidity of all sites was seen in intraoperative ruptures of basilar bifurcation aneurysms (18% poor outcomes and 10% deaths). Intraoperative rupture was rare (5.2%) in unruptured aneurysms, but ultimately most dangerous, maybe since so unexpected, equalling the results in poor grade patients: 6 poor results and 8 deaths in 25 patients. Half of the patients with giant aneurysms and inadvertent rupture had a poor result (8 poor results and 9 deaths in 33 patients). Intraoperative rupture doubled the morbidity and mortality in all sizes of aneurysms. Only half of the patients with inadvertent rupture had excellent outcome and 32% were poor (Table 25.2). With the routine use of temporary clipping, the incidence of this misadventure has decreased slightly in recent years.

Perforator Injury

Perforator injuries were identified if (1) perforator(s) were noted to be damaged or occluded by operative manipulation or by the clip irrespective of outcome, as well as (2) in patients developing postoperatively a thalamic, midbrain or pontine syndrome or a contralateral third nerve paresis. More recently, CT and MR scanning have defined the site and size of the midbrain and thalamic perforator infarctions.

Due to multiple perforators close to the basilar bifurcation, patients with aneurysms in this region were especially prone to this complication (14%). No perforator injuries occurred in the patients with forward projecting small basilar bifurcation aneurysms (61 patients), but did happen in 4 of 21 patients with large aneurysms. Perforators were injured in 20% of backward projecting sacs and only slightly less frequently in those sacs projecting upward (16%). Perforator injuries were seldom seen at other aneurysm sites: basilar-SCA 4%, PCA and basilar trunk 2%, and vertebral artery 1%. The frequency of perforator injuries doubled in large aneurysms (small 7%, large 14%). Assessment of perforator injuries in giant aneurysms is difficult due to the complexity of the lesions, and are not included in Table 25.3, but is certainly not less frequent than seen in smaller aneurysms. Perforator injuries were twice as common with intraoperative aneurysm rupture than without, and three times more common when a major branch artery was inadvertently occluded. Perforator injuries contributed to poor results by increasing the number of disabled patients but not the number of deaths (Table 25.3, cf. Table 5.3). Even so, it is remarkable how many patients with smaller midbrain or thalamic infarctions recovered to good outcomes.

Inadvertent Major Vessel Occlusion

Inadvertent arterial occlusion (83 patients = 4.8%) caused great misery as more than half of the patients had a poor outcome (Tables 25.4 to 25.11). A few were caused by spontaneous thrombosis of an adjacent artery near to an accurate aneurysm neck clipping, but most often the artery was inadvertently occluded by the clip, and occasionally avulsed or torn and then clipped. Inadvertent arterial occlusions were equally frequent at the various aneurysm sites except for the PCA aneurysms where the frequency was almost double. It was rare in small aneurysms (2.1%), and nearly equally frequent in large (7.0%) and giant (8.3%) aneurysms.

In basilar bifurcation aneurysms, the basilar bifurcation was inadvertently occluded with P1 or SCA uni- or bilaterally in 10 patients, P1 alone in 19 patients, P1 associated with SCA in 3 patients, P1 associated with SCA and basilar trunk in 1 patient and both P1s in 1 patient, SCA alone in 2 patients, PComA in 1 patient and two were thromboembolic in distal middle cerebral artery (MCA) and distal PCA (Table 25.6).

In superior cerebellar artery aneurysms, inadvertent vessel occlusion was always unilateral: P1 in five patients, SCA in two patients, P1 and SCA in three patients, and more distal thrombosis in PCA in one patient. One patient had occlusion of the distal anterior cerebral artery when an associated AComA aneurysm was operated on (Table 25.7).

In basilar trunk aneurysms, BT alone was inadvertently occluded in three patients and with SCA in one patient, and anterior-inferior cerebellar artery (AICA) alone in one patient (Table 25.8).

In vertebrobasilar junction aneurysms, VBJ with BT or VA was occluded three times, P1 in one patient with a ruptured associated basilar bifurcation aneurysm and MCA branches torn in one patient when opening the skull. The basilar artery was occluded by a clip in one patient (Table 25.9).

In vertebral artery aneurysms, the artery inadvertently occluded was proximal VA in one patient, VA at the level of PICA in four patients, VA with PICA in one patient, distal VA in two patients, and PICA in two patients (Table 25.10).

In posterior cerebral artery aneurysms, inadvertent occlusion of P1 with basilar bifurcation was seen in two patients, P1 with PComA or P1-P2 in two patients, P1 alone in one patient and distal PCA in four patients. In one patient proximal MCA was occluded, probably embolic from the heart (Table 25.11).

One-third of these arterial occlusions was associated with intraoperative ruptures and as well, was closely related to aneurysm size. They occurred in 20 patients with small aneurysms (2%), in 30 patients with large aneurysms (7%) and 33 patients with giant aneurysms (24% when those patients with deliberate arterial occlusion are excluded). Inadvertent arterial occlusions were best tolerated in VA aneurysms with only 1 death of 10 (Tables 25.5 and 25.10).

In one patient, inadvertent tear and thrombotic occlusion of the vein of Labbé was followed by fatal temporal lobe hemorrhagic infarction.

Postoperative Deterioration of Neurological State

Deterioration of consciousness, limb paresis or speech (usually dysarthria, infrequently dysphasia) from any cause noted during the first postoperative day had a very gloomy prognosis (Table 25.12). Postoperative deterioration of consciousness or limb movement was most common in BT aneurysms (one-third), followed by BB aneurysms (one-fourth), and least common in VA aneurysms (7%). Deterioration of consciousness or limb movement was most common in giant aneurysms (one-third), large (one-fourth), and only 15% in small aneurysms. Deterioration of speech was most common in patients with PCA aneurysms (19%) and least common in vertebral aneurysms (5%), and noted in 8% of small aneurysms, in 14% of large and in 22% of giant sacs.

New cranial nerve deficits were usually transient and most of them recovered, especially unilateral postoperative third nerve palsy which almost always recovered in 12 weeks, and only in a few patients had minor influence on their ultimate function (Table 25.13). Preoperative oculomotor palsies caused more often by hemorrhage into the nerve or stretch over a giant sac recovered in only half of the cases. Only half of the lower cranial nerve paresis recovered completely. Third nerve paresis caused by surgery was most common in BB aneurysms (70%), followed by SCA (51%), and PCA 27%; it was seldom in operations for BT aneurysms (19%). Lower cranial nerve deficits caused by surgery were understandably common in VBJ, BT and VA aneurysms (51%, 41% and 25%). As an example, all cranial nerve deficits at different time intervals in BT aneurysms are seen in Table 25.14. Preoperative oculomotor or lower cranial deficits were more common in large and giant aneurysms. Surprisingly, aneurysm size had little influence on new postoperative oculomotor or lower cranial deficits.

Memory Deficits

One-fourth of the patients were confused or drowsy preoperatively and one-third after operation. Most improved but tragically 9% were confused or had severe memory deficits at follow-up (more frequent in patients with basilar tip aneurysms), and was the major factor in the patient being listed as a poor result.

Postoperative Hematoma

Fifty-three (2.8%) postoperative, extracerebral clots occurred in the total series of more than 1900 approaches for aneurysms on the vertebrobasilar tree; 23 were extradural and 30 were subdural (Tables 25.15 and 25.16). Recovery was complete after removal of 15 extradural clots, but 5 died and 3 remained poor. Acute subdural hematoma carried a worse prognosis; only 12 patients had good outcomes, 10 were poor and 8 died. Patients with postoperative intracerebral clots fared still worse: of 24, 8 died and 8 remained poor. Three of these intracerebral clots occurred in 10 patients with basilar artery aneurysms, (including giant aneurysms) done under heparinization for deep hypothermia with cardiopulmonary bypass, resulting in 2 deaths. The other patient survived with only a mild hemiparesis even though the dominant temporal lobe was involved. Two of three patients with intraventricular clots had poor outcome. There was no difference in outcomes between supra- and infratentorial postoperative clots.

Before the CT era, six of seven acute subdural hematomas had a poor result (three died), after 1977 half of the patients were saved for independent life. In the same way, 5 of 9 extradural hematomas had a poor result (3 died) before CT era, after 1977 only 3 (2 died) of 14 were poor results. Outcome in intracerebral hematomas was not changed by the availability of CT.

Incomplete Occlusion and Re-operation (Failed Aneurysm Surgery)

In the total series of 1767 patients, 82.5% of the aneurysms were totally occluded and 6.5% had a small remnant of neck. Most common total occlusion was in PCA aneurysms (96%), and least frequent in VBJ aneurysms (72%). Three-fourths of the 1767 aneurysms (1340 patients) could be treated with neck clipping and 90% of these patients had their aneurysms totally occluded, 7% had a small residual neck and in the remainder, the aneurysm more or less filled.

One hundred and ninety-three (193) patients had a re-operation on their aneurysm (failed aneurysm surgery), 73 from referring institutions and 120 from our unit (16 patients with 3 operations and 4 patients with 4 operations). The outcome of these 193 patients is seen in Table 25.11. The most frequent aneurysm site to be re-operated was VBJ (21%), followed by BT (19%) and PCA (13%), the figure for BB aneurysms was 9.5%. Half (93) of repeat operations were done in giant aneurysms. In a few cases, the wrong (asymptomatic) aneurysm was operated on first necessitating a second exposure under the same anesthesia or delayed. The result of failed aneurysm surgery can be seen in Table 25.17.

Vasospasm

More than half (51%) of the 1305 patients with ruptured aneurysms were operated upon 11–30 days after SAH and 20% after one month. Severe symptoms of brain stem or cerebral ischemia thought to be caused by vasospasm were recorded in 109 patients (6%), and vasospasm alone was the main cause in 23 poor outcomes and 17 deaths (Table 25.18). Considering only the 1305 ruptured aneurysms, the incidence of recorded severe vasospasm was 8%. In early surgery (done during the first week of rupture), its recorded incidence was 15%, in late surgery 6% and in unruptured aneurysms 1%. Recently, maintaining higher levels of blood pressure (systolic 150–240) after volume expansion and occasionally angioplasty or intra-arterial papaverine infusion have undoubtedly saved several patients from this fate.

Rebleeding

Seventy-three patients (4%) had postoperative bleeding from their aneurysms. Thirty-seven of them had rebled and died and nine had rebled and were poor at three months follow-up. Two further patients died later in the first postoperative year, and 15 patients several years, up to 8 years, after surgery. In total, 54 patients died from rebleeding.

Incomplete clipping was the most frequent cause but only 2.5% of all aneurysms treated by direct clip ligation rebled, the frequency in proximal vessel occlusion was 7%. Surprisingly, only 2 (5%) of the 37 wrapped aneurysms rebled. In 10 patients, a clip slipped and was known to be the cause of hemorrhage. Twenty patients survived postoperative recurrences, and were re-operated: 12 made good recoveries, 7 died and 1 remained poor. Rebleedings were equally divided between different aneurysm sites. Twenty-three of the aneurysms with rebleeds were small, 19 large and 31 giant. Twenty-five of the 73 aneurysms with recurrent postoperative hemorrhage were angiographically judged postoperatively to be totally occluded. Yet there must have been some residual neck which enlarged to form a new aneurysm. In addition, 9 were known to have a residual neck, and 39 had some or complete filling of fundus.

Postoperative Infection
(Tables 25.19 to 25.22)

Prophylactic antibiotics were not used: the clean wound infection rate remained low (0.4%). Meningitis (including aseptic meningitis) was seen in 1.8% and accounted for five deaths and one poor result. Unfortunately, the organisms causing meningitis were not included in the database analysis. Three patients survived without deficit after removal of a temporal lobe abscess in two and a subdural empyema in the third. Fifteen of 50 patients with severe pulmonary infection or septicemia had a poor result, 5 of them died (1 with bleeding from a DIC syndrome). Postoperative infection (meningitis and septicemia) was most common in vertebral aneurysms (5%).

Medical Complications

Severe medical complications were infrequent but usually serious as nearly half of them contributed to or caused poor results (Table 25.20).

Hydrocephalus

The incidence of communicating hydrocephalus requiring shunting was 9%. It was used only in a small percentage of patients before discharge, since hydrocephalus often resolves without a shunting procedure. A number of patients returned to their referring surgeons for consideration of shunting, but their follow-up may be incomplete. Even so, this problem is probably no different than that occurring after SAH from anterior circulation aneurysms.

Of the 163 patients requiring shunting, 46% made excellent and 27% good recovery, 22% remained poor and 5% died. Shunting was more frequently needed in VBJ (14%) and BT aneurysms (16%), and very seldom in PCA aneurysms (4%). Only 12% of giant aneurysms were shunted. One-third of patients in Grades 3–4 needed a shunt. Early surgery did not influence the number of shunts.

Statistical Analysis for Predictors of Poor Outcome

To study the independent contribution of factors explaining outcome, multivariate statistical analy-

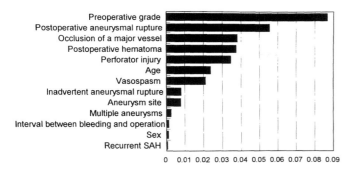

Figure 25.1. Independent contribution of the variable (R-square). Predictive value of different variables describing the pre-, peri- and postoperative course of 1340 patients with ruptured vertebrobasilar artery aneurysms

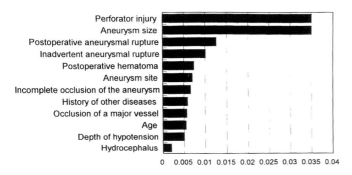

Figure 25.2. Independent contribution of the variable (R-square). Predictive value of different variables describing the pre-, peri- and postoperative course of 427 patients with unruptured vertebrobasilar artery aneurysms

sis (backward stepwise logistic regression model) was performed. A total of 24 predictor variables describing the pre-, peri- and postoperative course of the patient were included in the analysis, and after stepwise selection, 18 variables with the strongest contribution remained in the model (cf. Tables 25.21 and 25.22). The outcome was defined as good (excellent or good) or poor (poor or dead). The predictive value of these variables are presented in Figs. 25.1 and 25.2. "R" is the partial correlation coefficient in the logistic regression model, and "R^2" expresses the independent contribution of each predictor to the outcome. Among the patients with ruptured aneurysm, preoperative grade, postoperative aneurysmal rupture, occlusion of a major vessel, postoperative hematoma and perforator injury were the major determinants of outcome (Fig. 25.1). In patients with unruptured aneurysms, perforator injury and aneurysm size were the most powerful prognostic factors (Fig. 25.2).

Discussion

The most alarming intraoperative complication is aneurysm rupture. The fears and troubles associated with burst aneurysms are well described in numerous earlier reports on complications of aneurysm surgery. Experience, microsurgical techniques, hypotension and temporary clipping have partially reduced these anxieties. Even so, intraoperative rupture still occurs and results in a much more serious outcome in aneurysms of the posterior circulation than in aneurysms of the anterior circulation. A slight trend to fewer intraoperative ruptures was noted in the last decade coincidentally, we believe, with more routine use of temporary clipping. However, temporary clipping is technically not always possible or may come too late after rupture. There is still no sure way to prevent early rebleedings during induction of anesthesia, or exposure. Although infrequent, these early repeat hemorrhages before the aneurysm is exposed are known to be devasting, and often untreatable. Further development of temporary intravascular balloon occlusion may make temporary clipping seldom necessary. The fears of increasing the number of intraoperative ruptures by early surgery have been unfounded.

Earlier in the series, retractor injury of the temporal lobe and its veins was occasionally seen when the base of the temporal lobe was elevated from the middle fossa, even when a bone flap was used. The subtemporal "tic" craniectomy is much smaller and a hidden temporal vein can be partially torn at its insertion. Although a nuisance, it is controlled easily with hemostatic packing and has not been known to cause a major venous infarction or neurological deficit. We always endeavored to protect the veins, especially the vein of Labbé, which insertion is usually well posterior. Modern neuroanesthesia including mannitol and spinal drainage has produced slack brains routinely, and made retraction injury of the undersurface of the temporal lobe rare. Retractor pressures have been measured on many occasions and seldom exceed 10 torr with the final exposure.

Inadvertent major vessel occlusion is the most serious intraoperative complication. Its frequency before 1981 was 6.5% and after 3.5%. This improvement cannot be explained simply by the use of temporary clipping, but more likely due to increased experience. In giant aneurysms, deliberate proximal occlusion was frequently used (in two-thirds) and the specific complications of this treatment have been recently reported. Great care was taken always to preserve the integrity of the normal venous drainage in the exposure which we believe minimized the incidence of postoperative swelling and venous infarction.

In spite of our acute awareness of their importance and surgical anatomy, perforator injuries remain the most important cause for morbidity in basilar bifurcation aneurysms. A significant decline in major perforator infarction during the last five years of this experience was observed for reasons that are not clear.

Failed aneurysm surgery has been dealt earlier in the authors' experience: 193 patients had reoperations in this series. Postoperative rebleeding (4%) was clearly more common than in anterior circulation aneurysms. This reflects the very complex nature of these lesions treated with an exceptional number of large and giant aneurysms. It is also influenced by our early and at times ineffective methods of treatment – and the long follow-up. The frequency of early postoperative rebleedings, although low, has remained about the same in the recent years in spite of increasing experience and sophisticated methods: temporary clipping, careful inspection for the perfect position of the clip and proving complete obliteration by needling the sac. As well, nearly all patients had postoperative angiograms with a high frequency of obliteration in the total series; those with neck clipping had a 97% occlusion rate (includes 7% with only small remnants of neck). Sadly, one-third of those aneurysms known to rebleed were thought at the time of the postoperative angiograms to be completely obliterated, but some tag of neck must have remained open.

It is especially tragic to recall those patients injured by postoperative hematomas after otherwise successfully performed complex procedures. Most other postoperative complications common to all craniotomies, especially infections and swelling, were very infrequent even though prophylactic antibiotics or corticosteroids were not used.

The incidence of vasospasm was low. We do not think this is due to lower frequency than in anterior circulation but due to incomplete recording of often transient symptoms, a preponderance of late surgery and a relatively high number of unruptured aneurysms. The routine and early use of hypertension and volume expansion may also have resulted in fewer patients deteriorating from delayed ischemic deficits. A trivial number of these patients received calcium channel blocking agents.

Shunting was used only in a small percentage of patients before discharge, since hydrocephalus often resolves without a shunting procedure, without any treatment, or with recurrent lumbar punctures or spinal drainage. We do not think this problem is different from that occurring after SAH from anterior aneurysms. The number of patients with giant aneurysms needing a shunt was remarkably low.

Final Comments

There are many possible pitfalls in recording, saving and analyzing the data in a retrospective series over several decades: transient complications, e.g., transient ischemic deficits and minor medical complications are not necessarily always reported or recorded. However, we believe the complicated nature of vertebrobasilar aneurysm surgery is well demonstrated in this scrutiny: generally, a complicated course of recovery was more common than not. The main areas to improve results have been listed numerous times:

1. Technical: Minimizing the number of inadvertent major vessel occlusions, perforator injuries and intraoperative ruptures, and further by reducing the number of craniotomy related complications, especially postoperative hematomas.
2. Medical: Prevention, identification, and treatment of vasospasm and medical complications.
3. Prevention of SAH: Identification of aneurysms before rupture.

Surgery of vertebrobasilar aneurysms remains one of the most difficult tasks in neurosurgery. These rare patients should be referred to a few centers specialized in the treatment of complex cerebrovascular lesions to minimize technical and medical complications. Transfer of SAH patients by aircraft is safe. The importance of identifying patients with unruptured aneurysms was expressed 20 years ago and are now being slowly fulfilled. In our hands, incidental vertebral-basilar artery aneurysm could be treated with a high relative safety. Experience gathered with MRA in the last years gives some hope for meaningful screening to reduce the high management mortality, if the risk factors other than familial could be identified. Identification and treatment of aneurysms before rupture will likely improve management results more than any technical or medical advance.

Table 25.1. Influence of preoperative Grade on outcome in 1767 patients with VBAAs, all sites and sizes

Grade	No. of patients	Excellent %	Good %	Poor %	Dead %
0[a]	462	65.8	13.2	13.2	7.8
1	841	81.2	10.5	4.5	3.8
2	289	62.3	21.5	9.3	6.9
3	139	30.2	38.1	22.3	9.4
4	30	6.7	20.0	40.0	33.3
5	6	16.7			83.3
Total	1767	1212	270	169	116
	100.0	68.6	15.3	9.6	6.6

[a] 0 Unruptured aneurysm or remote hemorrhage (> 1 year).

Table 25.2. Influence of intraoperative aneurysm rupture on outcome in 1767 patients with VBAAs

Intraoperative aneurysm rupture	Excellent	Good	Poor	Dead
No rupture 1586 pts = 89.8%	71%	15%	9%	6%
Rupture 181 pts = 10.2%	50%	18%	16%	16%
Total 1767 pts	68.6%	15.3%	9.6%	6.6%

Table 25.3. Influence of perforator injury on outcome in 1370 small and large VBAAs (cf. with Table 5.3)

Perforator injury	Excellent	Good	Poor	Dead
No perforator injury 1241 pts (90.6%)	78%	12%	5.5%	4.5%
Perforator injury 129 pts (9.4%)	41%	28%	25%	6%
Total 1370 pts	74.7	13.4	7.3	4.7

Table 25.4. Influence of inadvertent arterial occlusion on outcome in 1767 VBAAs

Arterial occlusion	Excellent	Good	Poor	Dead
No arterial occlusion 1349 pts = 76.3%	74%	14%	7%	5%
Planned arterial occlusion 335 pts = 19.0%	58%	19%	13%	11%
Inadvertent arterial occlusion 83 pts = 4.7%	30%	16%	32%	22%
Total 1767 pts	68.6%	15.3%	9.6%	6.6%

Table 25.5. Aneurysm site and outcome in 83 patients with inadvertent arterial occlusion. For artery occluded, see text and Tables 25.6 to 25.11

Location	Total	E	G	P	D
Basilar bifurcation (BB)	39	11	7	16	5
Basilar SCA	13	1	3	5	4
Basilar trunk (BT)	5	2		1	2
Vertebrobasilar junction (VBJ)	6	2		1	3
Vertebral artery (VA)	10	6	1	2	1
Posterior cerebral artery (PCA)	10	3	2	2	3
Total	83	25	13	27	18

E Excellent, G good, P poor, D dead.

Table 25.6. Outcome in 39 patients with basilar bifurcation aneurysms and inadvertent arterial occlusion

Vessel(s) occluded	Total	E	G	P	D
BB with P1 or SCA uni- or bilaterally	10	1	1	7	1
P1 alone	19	8	4	5	2
P1 with SCA	3			3	
P1 with SCA and BT	1				1
Both P1s	1				1
SCA	2	1	1		
PCom	1	1			
Distal MCA (thromboembolic)	1		1		
Distal PCA (thromboembolic)	1			1	
Total	39	11	7	16	5

Table 25.7. Outcome in 13 patients with basilar SCA aneurysms and inadvertent arterial occlusion

Vessel(s) occluded	Total	E	G	P	D
P1 alone	5		1	3	1
P1 with SCA	4			1	3
SCA	2		1	1	
PCom					
Distal ACA	1	1			
Distal PCA (thrombosis)	1		1		
Total	13	1	3	5	4

Table 25.8. Outcome in 5 patients with basilar trunk aneurysms and inadvertent arterial occlusion

Vessel(s) occluded	Total	E	G	P	D
BT alone	3	2		1	
BT with SCA	1				1
AICA	1				1
Total	5	2		1	2

Table 25.9. Outcome in 6 patients with vertebrobasilar junction aneurysms and inadvertent arterial occlusion

Vessel(s) occluded	Total	E	G	P	D
VBJ with BT or VA	3	1		1	1
P1	1				1
BT with VA	1	1			
MCA	1				1
Total	6	2		1	3

Table 25.10. Outcome in 10 patients with vertebral artery aneurysms and inadvertent arterial occlusion

Vessel(s) occluded	Total	E	G	P	D
Proximal VA	1		2		
VA at the level of PICA	4	4			
VA with PICA	1				1
PICA	2			2	
Distal VA	2	2			
Total	10	6	2	2	1

Table 25.11. Outcome in 10 patients with PCA aneurysms and inadvertent arterial occlusion

Vessel(s) occluded	Total	E	G	P	D
P1 with BB	2			1	1
P1 with PCom or P1–P2	2	1	1		
P1 alone	1			1	
Distal PCA	4	1	1		2
MCA (thromboembolic)	1	1			
Total	10	3	2	2	3

Table 25.12. Outcome in 1744 patients with VBAAs with or without postoperative deterioration of neurological state

Immediate post-operative state	No.	%	E	G	P	Dead
Same as before	407	23.3%	89%	8%	2%	1%
Minor or transient neurological deficit	547	31.4%	86%	11%	3%	0%
Worse	790	45.3%	46%	22%	18%	14%
Total	1744	100.0%				

Table 25.13. Cranial nerve deficits (%) in 1767 patients with VBAAs

Cranial nerves paralyzed	Pre-operatively	Post-operatively	Follow-up
CNIII unilateral	11%	52%	8%
CNIII bilateral	0.6%	5%	2%
One other cranial nerve, uni- or bilateral	8%	13%	4%
Several other cranial nerves, uni- or bilateral	3%	9%	4%

Table 25.14. Cranial nerve paresis preoperatively, postoperatively and at follow-up in 144 patients with basilar trunk aneurysms

Cranial nerve paresis	Preoperative Unilat-Bilat	Postoperative Unilat-Bilat	Follow-up Unilat-Bilat
CNIII	9–1	34–3	8–1
CNIV	1–1	18–1	12–1
CNV	5–0	11–0	4–0
CNVI	17–7	43–13	13–2
CNVII	10–0	23–0	9–0
CNVIII	8–0	16–1	16–1
CNIX–X	4–2	10–4	3–1
CNXI	0–0	0–0	0–0
CNXII	0–0	1–2	1–0
Number of patients with cranial nerve deficit (%)	40 (28%)	99 (69%)	39 (31%)

Unilat Unilateral cranial nerve paresis, *Bilat* bilateral cranial nerve paresis.

Table 25.15. Postoperative hematoma in 1767 patients with VBAAs

Type of hematoma	No.	Percent
Intracerebral	21	1.2
Intraventricular	3	0.2
Subdural[a]	33	1.9
Extradural	23	1.3
Total	80	4.4
Removed	51	

[a] Includes significant hygromas.

Table 25.16. Influence of postoperative hematoma on outcome in 1767 VBAAs

Hematoma	Excellent	Good	Poor	Dead
No hematoma 1687 pts = 95.5%	70%	15%	9%	6%
Hematoma 80 pts = 4.5%	33%	13%	28%	28%
Total 1767 pts	68.6%	15.3%	9.6%	6.6%

Table 25.17. Outcome in 193 patients with incomplete occlusion and reoperation for VBAAs (failed aneurysm surgery)

Outcome	No.	Percent
Excellent	115	59.6
Good	36	18.7
Poor	24	12.4
Dead	18	9.3
Total	193	100.0

Table 25.18. Influence of postoperative vasospasm on outcome in 1767 VBAAs

Vasospasm	Excellent	Good	Poor	Dead
No vasospasm 1658 pts = 93.8%	71%	15%	9%	6%
Vasospasm 109 pts = 6.2%	38%	26%	21%	16%
Total 1767 pts	68.6%	15.3%	9.6%	6.6%

Table 25.19. Postoperative infection in 1767 patients with VBAAs

Type of infection	No.	Percent
Wound infection	7	0.4
Subdural empyema	1	0.1
Brain abscess	2	0.1
Meningitis	31	1.8
Severe pulmonary infection or septicaemia	54	3.0

Table 25.20. Medical complications in 1767 patients with VBAAs

Nature	No.	Percent (of 1767)	Poor	Dead
Severe electrolyte disturbances	14	0.7	2	0
Cardiac	10	0.6	2	3
Respiratory	33	1.9	5	4
Gastrointestinal	11	0.6	0	3
Genitourinary	6	0.3	1	0
Bleeding diathesis	4	0.2	0	3
Pulmonary embolus/DVT	17	1.0	5	1
Combined medical	60	3.4	24	17
Total	155	8.8	39	31

Table 25.21. Mean age and frequency of variables among patients with good (n = 1482) and poor (n = 285) outcome in 1767 patients with VBAAs

Variable	Good outcome 1482 pts	Poor outcome 285 pts
Age (years) (mean±SD)	45.7 ± 12.9	50.9 ± 11.8
Grade (0–5) (mean±SD)	1.41 ± 0.68	2.18 ± 1.14
Hypertension	269 (18.2%)	71 (24.9%)
Multiple bleedings	334 (22.5%)	82 (28.8%)
Coma by SAH	458 (30.9%)	110 (38.6%)
Preoperative cranial nerve symptoms	222 (15.0%)	84 (29.5%)
Mass effect	196 (13.2%)	93 (32.6%)
AVM	53 (3.6%)	6 (2.1%)
Multiple aneurysms	378 (25.5%)	84 (29.5%)
2 or more operations	107 (7.2%)	37 (13.0%)
Intraoperative aneurysm rupture	139 (9.4%)	58 (20.4%)
Perforator injury	93 (6.3%)	49 (17.2%)
Inadvertent arterial occlusion	39 (2.6%)	45 (15.8%)
Postoperative recurrent bleeding	27 (1.8%)	46 (16.3%)
Nonsaccular aneurysm	143 (9.6%)	44 (15.4%)
Giant aneurysm	276 (18.6%)	121 (42.5%)
Postop. hematoma	36 (2.4%)	44 (15.4%)
Postop. infection	68 (4.6%)	27 (9.5%)
Shunt dependent hydrocephalus	119 (8.1%)	44 (15.4%)

Table 25.22. Main cause of poor result in 285 patients with VBAAs

Variable	Poor 169 patients	Dead 116 patients
Poor preoperative Grade (4 or 5)	12	15
Recurrent postop. bleed	6	40
Vasospasm	20	13
Intraoperative aneurysm rupture	22	16
Inadvertent major vessel occlusion	16	6
Perforator injury	22	3
Postoperative hematoma	9	5
Postop. infection	4	5
Medical complications	21	13
Varia	37	0

References

References for Chapter 1

1. Bassett RC: Intracranial aneurysms. Some clinical observations concerning their development. J Neurosurg 6: 216–221, 1949
2. Dandy WE: Intracranial arterial aneurysms. Ithaca, New York: Comstock, 1944, 147 pp
3. DeSaussure RL, Hunter SE, Robertson JT: Saccular aneurysms of the posterior fossa. J Neurosurg 15: 385–391, 1958
4. Drake CG: Bleeding aneurysms of the basilar artery. Direct surgical management in four cases. J Neurosurg 23: 230–238, 1961
5. Drake CG: Surgical treatment of ruptured aneurysms of the basilar artery. Experience with 14 cases. J Neurosurg 23: 457–473, 1965
6. Drake CG: Further experience with surgical treatment of aneurysms of the basilar artery. J Neurosurg 29: 372–392, 1968
7. Drake CG: The surgical treatment of aneurysms of the basilar artery. J Neurosurg 29: 436–446, 1968
8. Drake CG: The surgical treatment of the vertebral-basilar aneurysms. Clin Neurosurg 16: 114–169, 1969
9. Drake CG: Ligation of the vertebral (unilateral or bilateral) or basilar artery in the treatment of large intracranial aneurysms. J Neurosurg 43: 255–74, 1975
10. Drake CG: Giant intracranial aneurysms: Experience with surgical treatment in 174 patients. Clin Neurosurg 26: 12–95, 1979
11. Drake CG: The treatment of aneurysms of the posterior circulation. Clin Neurosurg 26: 96–144, 1979
12. Drake CG, Peerless SJ, Ferguson GG: Hunterian proximal arterial occlusion for giant aneurysms on the carotid circulation. J Neurosurg 81: 656–665, 1994
13. Falconer MA: Surgical treatment of spontaneous intracranial hemorrhage. BMJ 1: 790–792, 1958
14. Fox JL: Intracranial aneurysms, vol I–III. New York, Berlin, Heidelberg, Tokyo: Springer, 1983, 1463 pp
15. Friedman AH, Drake CG. Subarachnoid hemorrhage from intracranial dissecting aneurysms. J Neurosurg 60: 325–334, 1984
16. Gillingham FJ: The management of ruptured intracranial aneurysms. Ann R Coll Surg Engl 23: 89–117, 1958
17. Guthkelch AN: Large saccular aneurysm of the intracranial part of the vertebral artery. Br J Surg 37: 107–108, 1949
18. Hamby WB: Intracranial aneurysms. Springfield, Illinois: Thomas, 1952, 564 pp
19. Höök O, Norlen G, Guzman J: Saccular aneurysms of the vertebrobasilar system. Acta Neurol Scand 39: 271–304, 1963
20. Jamieson KG: Aneurysms of the vertebrobasilar system. Surgical intervention in 19 cases. J Neurosurg 21: 781–797, 1964
21. Jamieson KG: Aneurysms of the vertebrobasilar system: Further experience with 9 cases. J Neurosurg 28: 544–555, 1967
22. Krayenbühl H: Das Hirnaneurysma. Schweiz Arch Neurol Psychiat 47: 155–236, 1941
23. Logue V: The surgical treatment of aneurysms of the posterior fossa. J Neurol Neurosurg Psychiatry 21: 66–77, 1958
24. Logue V: Posterior fossa aneurysms. Clin Neurosurg 11: 183–207, 1964
25. Moniz E: Die Cerebrale Arteriographie und Phlebographie. Berlin: Springer, 1940
26. Mount LA, Taveras JM: Ligation of basilar artery in treatment of an aneurysm at the basilar artery bifurcation. J Neurosurg 19: 167–170, 1962
27. Paulson G, Nashold BS Jr, Margolis G: Aneurysms of the vertebral artery; report of 5 cases. Neurology (Minneap) 9: 590–598, 1959
28. Peerless SJ, Drake CG: Management of aneurysms of posterior circulation. In: Youmans JR (ed) Neurological surgery, vol 3, 2nd ed. Philadelphia: Sounders, 1982, pp 1715–1763
29. Poppen JL: Vascular surgery of the posterior fossa. Proc Congr Neurol Surg 6: 198–209, 1969
30. Radner S: Intracranial angiography via the vertebral artery: preliminary report of a new technique. Acta Radiol 28: 838–842, 1947
31. Sahs AL, Perret GE, Locksley HB, Nishioka H: Intracranial aneurysms and subarachnoid hemorrhage: A cooperative study. Philadelphia, Toronto: Lippincott, 1969
32. Schwartz HG: Arterial aneurysms of the posterior fossa. J Neurosurg 5: 312–316, 1948
33. Steelman HF, Hayes GJ, Rizzoli HV: Surgical treatment of saccular intracranial aneurysms. J Neurosurg 10: 564–576, 1953
34. Steinberg GK, Drake CG, Peerless SJ: Deliberate basilar or vertebral artery occlusion in the treatment of intracranial aneurysms. J Neurosurg 79: 161–173, 1993
35. Tönnis W: Zur Behandlung intrakranieller Aneurysmen. Arch Klin Chir 189: 474–476, 1937
36. Walsh FB, Hoyt WF: Clinical neuro-opthalmology, vol 2. Baltimore: Williams and Wilkins, 1969, pp 1110, 1737–1774

37. Yaşargil MG: Vertebrobasilar aneurysms. In: Microneurosurgery in 4 volumes, vol II. Stuttgart, New York: Thieme, 1986, pp 232–295

References for Chapter 2

1. Botterell EH, Lougheed WM, Scott JW, Vandewater SL: Hypothermia, and interruption of carotid, or carotid and vertebral circulation, in the surgical management of intracranial aneurysms. J Neurosurg 13: 1–42, 1956
2. Drake CG: Report of World Federation of Neurological Surgeons Committee on a universal subarachnoid haemorrhage grading scale. J Neurosurg 68: 985–986, 1988
3. Drake CG: On the surgical treatment of ruptured intracranial aneurysms. Clin Neurosurg 13: 122–155, 1966
4. Gallagher JP: Pilojection for intracranial aneurysms. Report of progress. J Neurosurg 21: 129–134, 1964
5. Kassell NF, Torner JC, Jane JA, Haley EC Jr, Adams HP: The International Cooperative Study on the Timing of Aneurysm Surgery. Part II: surgical results. J Neurosurg 73: 37–47, 1990
6. Minielli R, Yuzbe A, Drake CG: Subarachnoid hemorrhage secondary to ruptured cerebral aneurysm in pregnancy. Obst Gyn 53: 64–70, 1979
7. Peerless SJ: Pre- and postoperative management of cerebral aneurysms. Clin Neurosurg 26: 209–231, 1979
8. Peerless SJ, Wallace MC, Drake CG: Giant intracranial aneurysms. In: Youmans JR (ed) Neurological surgery, vol 3, 3rd ed. Philadelphia: Saunders, 1990, pp 1742–1763
9. Peerless SJ, Hernesniemi JA, Gutman FB, Drake CG: Early surgery for ruptured posterior circulation aneurysms. J Neurosurg 80: 643–649, 1994

References for Chapters 3–5

1. Abe T, Sugishita M, Yatsuzuka S, Tashibu K, Onoue H, Suzuki T, Nakamura N: Transcallosal interforniceal approach for a posteriorly projecting high basilar bifurcation aneurysm. J Neurosurg 78: 970–973, 1993
2. Al-Mefty O, Anand VK: Zygomatic approach to skull base lesions. J Neurosurg 73: 668–673, 1990
3. Batjer HH, Samson DS: Causes of morbidity and mortality from surgery of aneurysms of the distal basilar artery. Neurosurgery 25: 904–916, 1989
4. Clark K: Complications of aneurysm surgery. Clin Neurosurg 23: 342–356, 1976
5. de los Reyes RA, Kantrowitz AB, Boehm FH, Spatola MA: Transcallosal, transventricular approach to a basilar apex aneurysm. Neurosurgery 31: 597–602, 1992
6. Dolenc VV, Skrap M, Sustersic J, Skrbec M, Morina A: A transcavernous-transsellar approach to the basilar tip aneurysms. Br J Neurosurg 1: 251–259, 1987
7. Drake CG, Friedman AH, Peerless SJ: Failed aneurysm surgery. Reoperation in 115 cases. J Neurosurg 61: 848–856, 1984
8. Drake CG: Bleeding aneurysms of the basilar artery. Direct surgical management in four cases. J Neurosurg 23: 230–238, 1961
9. Drake CG: Further experience with surgical treatment of aneurysms of the basilar artery. J Neurosurg 29: 372–392, 1968
10. Drake CG: Surgical treatment of ruptured aneurysms of the basilar artery. Experience with 14 cases. J Neurosurg 23: 457–473, 1965
11. Drake CG: The surgical treatment of aneurysms of the basilar artery. J Neurosurg 29: 436–446, 1968
12. Drake CG: The surgical treatment of the vertebralbasilar aneurysms. Clin Neurosurg 16: 114–169, 1969
13. Drake CG: The treatment of aneurysms of the posterior circulation. Clin Neurosurg 26: 96–144, 1979
14. Ferguson GG: Physical factors in the initiation, growth and rupture of human intracranial saccular aneurysms. J Neurosurg 37: 666–677, 1972
15. Fox JL: Intracranial aneurysms, vol I–III. New York, Berlin, Heidelberg, Tokyo: Springer, 1983, 1463 pp
16. Hakuba A, Liu S, Nishimura S: The orbitozygomatic infratemporal approach: A new surgical technique. Surg Neurol 26: 271–276, 1986
17. Harsh GR 4th, Sekhar LN: The subtemporal, transcavernous, anterior transpetrosal approach to the upper brain stem and clivus. J Neurosurg 77: 709–717, 1992
18. Hernesniemi J, Vapalahti M, Niskanen M, Tapaninaho A, Kari A, Luukkonen M, Puranen M, Saari T, Rajpar M: One-year outcome in early aneurysm surgery: a 14 years experience. Acta Neurochir (Wien) 122: 1–10, 1993
19. Hernesniemi JA, Vapalahti MP, Niskanen M, Kari A: Management outcome in vertebrobasilar artery aneurysms by early surgery. Neurosurgery 31: 857–862, 1992
20. Heros RC, Lee SH: The combined pterional/anterior temporal approach for aneurysms of the upper basilar complex. Technical article. Neurosurgery 33: 244–251, 1993
21. Ikeda K, Yamashita J, Hashimoto M, Futami K: Orbitozygomatic temporopolar approach for a high basilar tip aneurysm associated with a short intracranial internal carotid artery: a new surgical approach. Neurosurgery 28: 105–110, 1991
22. Kassel NF, Torner JC, Haley EC Jr, Jane JA, Adams HP, Kongable GL: The International Cooperative Study on the Timing of Aneurysm Surgery. Part I: Overall management results. J Neurosurg 73: 18–36, 1990
23. Kassell NF, Torner JC, Jane JA, Haley EC Jr, Adams HP: The International Cooperative Study on the Timing of Aneurysm Surgery. Part II: Surgical results. J Neurosurg 73: 37–47, 1990
24. Kodama N, Sasaki T, Yamanobe K, Kikuchi Y, Kurashima Y: High position basilar top aneurysm treated via third ventricle. Neurol Surg(Tokyo) 14: 1277–1281, 1986

25. Lam AM, Gelb AW: Cardiovascular effects of isoflurane-induced hypotension for cerebral aneurysm surgery. Anesth Analg 64: 742–748, 1983
26. Marinkovic SV, Gibo H: The surgical anatomy of the perforating branches of the basilar artery. Neurosurgery 33: 80–87, 1993
27. Matsuno H, Rhoton AL Jr, Peace D: Microsurgical anatomy of the posterior fossa cisterns. Neurosurgery 23: 58–80, 1988
28. Mizoi K, Takahashi A, Yoshimoto T, Fujiwara S, Koshu K: Combined endovascular and neurosurgical approach for paraclinoid internal carotid artery aneurysms. Neurosurgery 33: 986–992, 1993
29. Mizoi K, Yoshimoto T, Takahashi A, Ogawa A: Direct clipping of basilar trunk aneurysms usink temporary balloon occlusion. J Neurosurg 80: 230–236, 1994
30. Neil-Dwyer G, Sharr M, Haskell R, Currie D, Hosseini M: Zygomaticotemporal approach to the basis cranii and basilar artery. Neurosurgery 23: 20–22, 1988
31. Norrgård O, Ängqvist KA, Fodstad H, Forssell A, Lindberg M: Coexistence of abdominal aortic aneurysms and intracranial aneurysms. Acta Neurochir (Wien) 87: 34–39, 1987
32. Pedrozo A, Dujovny M, Ausman JI, Diaz FG, Artero JC, Berman SK, Mirchandani HG, Umansky F: Microvascular anatomy of the posterior fossa. J Neurosurg 64: 484–493, 1986
33. Peerless SJ, Drake CG: Management of aneurysms of posterior circulation. In: Youmans JR (ed) Neurological surgery, vol 3, 3rd ed. Philadelphia: Saunders, 1990, pp 1764–1806
34. Peerless SJ, Hernesniemi JA, Gutman FB, Drake CG: Early surgery for ruptured posterior circulation aneurysms. J Neurosurg 80: 643–649, 1994
35. Peerless SJ: Pre- and postoperative management of cerebral aneurysms. Clin Neurosurg 26: 209–231, 1979
36. Pool JL, Potts DG: Aneurysms and arteriovenous anomalies of the brain. Diagnosis and treatment. New York: Harper and Row, 1965
37. Rice BJ, Peerless SJ, Drake CG: Surgical treatment of unruptured aneurysms of the posterior circulation. J Neurosurg 73: 165–173, 1990
38. Saeki N, Rhoton AL Jr: Microsurgical anatomy of the upper basilar artery and the posterior circle of Willis. J Neurosurg 46: 563–578, 1977
39. Samson DS, Hodosh RM, Clark WK: Microsurgical evaluation of the pterional approach to aneurysms of the distal basilar circulation. Neurosurgery 3: 135–141, 1978
40. Sano K: Temporopolar approach to aneurysms of the basilar artery at and around the distal bifurcation: Technical note. Neurol Res 2: 361–367, 1980
41. Shiokawa Y, Saito I, Aoki N, Mizutani H: Zygomatic temporopolar approach for basilar artery aneurysms. Neurosurgery 24: 385–391, 1989
42. Solomon RA, Stein BM: Surgical approaches to aneurysms of the vertebral and basilar arteries. Neurosurgery 23: 203–208, 1988
43. Sugita K, Kobayashi S, Shintani A, Mutsuga N: Microneurosurgery for aneurysms of the basilar artery. J Neurosurg 51: 615–620, 1979
44. Suzuki J, Kwak R, Okudaira Y: The safe time limit of temporary clamping of cerebral arteries in the direct surgical treatment of intracranial aneurysm under moderate hypothermia. In: Suzuki J (ed) Cerebral aneurysms: experiences with 1000 directly operated cases. Tokyo: Tokyo Press, 1979, pp 325–329
45. Toyota BD, Ferguson GG: Basilar artery dissection: An early postoperative complication of aneurysm clipping. J Neurosurg 81: 139–142, 1994
46. Yaşargil MG, Antic J, Lagica R, Jain KK, Hodosh RM, Smith RD: Microneurosurgical pterional approach to aneurysms of the basilar bifurcation. Surg Neurol 6: 83–91, 1976
47. Yaşargil MG: Vertebrobasilar aneurysms. In: Microneurosurgery in 4 volumes, vol II. Stuttgart, New York: Thieme, 1986, pp 232–295
48. Yoshimoto T, Uchida K, Kaneko U, Kayama T, Suzuki J: An analysis and follow-up results of 1000 intracranial saccular aneurysms with definitive surgical treatment. J Neurosurg 50: 152–157, 1979

References for Chapter 6

1. Alksne JF, Smith RW: Stereotactic occlusion of 22 consecutive anterior communicating artery aneurysms. J Neurosurg 52: 790–793, 1980
2. Drake CG, Barr HWK, Coles JC, Gergely NF: The use of extracorporeal circulation and profound hypothermia in the treatment of ruptured intracranial aneurysm. J Neurosurg 21: 575–581, 1964
3. Drake CG: On the surgical treatment of ruptured intracranial aneurysms. Clin Neurosurg 13: 122–155, 1966
4. Drake CG: Ligation of the vertebral (unilateral or bilateral) or the basilar artery in the treatment of large intracranial aneurysms. J Neurosurg 43: 255–274, 1975
5. Drake CG: Giant intracranial aneurysms: Experience with surgical treatment in 174 patients. Clin Neurosurg 26: 12–95, 1979
6. Drake CG, Peerless SJ, Ferguson GG: Hunterian proximal arterial occlusion for giant aneurysms on the carotid circulation. J Neurosurg 81: 656–665, 1994
7. Gallagher JP: Pilojection for intracranial aneurysms. Report of progress. J Neurosurg 21: 129–134, 1964
8. Mullan S, Reyes C, Dawlwy J, Dobben G: Stereotactic copper electric thrombosis of intracranial aneurysms. In: Krayenbühl H, Maspes P, Sweet W (eds) Progress in neurological surgery, vol 3. Basel: Karger, 1969, pp 212–229
9. Peerless SJ, Wallace MC, Drake CG: Giant intracranial aneurysms. In: Youmans JR (ed) Neurological surgery, vol 3, 3rd ed. Philadelphia: Saunders, 1990, pp 1742–1763
10. Pelz DM, Vinuela F, Fox AJ, Drake CG: Vertebrobasilar occlusion therapy of giant aneurysms. Significance of angiographic morphology of the posterior communicating arteries. J Neurosurg 60: 560–5, 1984

11. Roach MR: A model study of why some intracranial aneurysms thrombose but others rupture. Stroke 9: 583–587, 1978
12. Rush JA, Balis GA, Drake CG: Bitemporal hemianopsia in basilar artery aneurysm. J Clin Neuroophthalmol 1: 129–33, 1981
13. Spetzler RF, Hadley MN, Rigamonti D, Carter LP, Raudzens PA, Shedd SA, Wikinson E: Aneurysms of the basilar artery treated with circulatory arrest, hypothermia, and barbiturate cerebral protection. J Neurosurg 68: 868–879, 1988
14. Steinberg GK, Drake CG, Peerless SJ: Deliberate basilar or vertebral artery occlusion in the treatment of intracranial aneurysms. J Neurosurg 79: 161–173, 1993

References for Chapters 7–8

1. Batjer HH, Samson DS: Causes of morbidity and mortality from surgery of aneurysms of the distal basilar artery. J Neurosurg 25: 904–915, 1989
2. Drake CG: Bleeding aneurysms of the basilar artery. Direct surgical management in four cases. J Neurosurg 23: 230–238, 1961
3. Drake CG: Further experience with surgical treatment of aneurysms of the basilar artery. J Neurosurg 29: 372–392, 1968
4. Drake CG: Surgical treatment of ruptured aneurysms of the basilar artery. Experience with 14 cases. J Neurosurg 23: 457–473, 1965
5. Drake CG: The surgical treatment of aneurysms of the basilar artery. J Neurosurg 29: 436–446, 1968
6. Drake CG: The surgical treatment of the vertebral-basilar aneurysms. Clin Neurosurg 16: 114–169, 1969
7. Drake CG: Ligation of the vertebral (unilateral or bilateral) or basilar artery in the treatment of large intracranial aneurysms. J Neurosurg 43: 255–74, 1975
8. Drake CG: Giant intracranial aneurysms: Experience with surgical treatment in 174 patients. Clin Neurosurg 26: 12–95, 1979
9. Drake CG: The treatment of aneurysms of the posterior circulation. Clin Neurosurg 26: 96–144, 1979
10. Drake CG, Friedman AH, Peerless SJ: Failed aneurysm surgery. Reoperation in 115 cases. J Neurosurg 61: 848–856, 1984
11. Ferguson GG: Physical factors in the initiation, growth and rupture of human intracranial saccular aneurysms. J Neurosurg 37: 666–677, 1972
12. Fox JL: Intracranial aneurysms, vol I–III. New York, Berlin, Heidelberg, Tokyo: Springer, 1983, 1463 pp
13. Gacs G, Vinuela F, Fox AJ, Drake CG: Peripheral aneurysms of the cerebellar arteries. Review of 16 cases. J Neurosurg 58: 63–68, 1983
14. Marinkovic SV, Gibo H: The surgical anatomy of the perforating branches of the basilar artery. Neurosurgery 33: 80–87, 1993
15. Matsuno H, Rhoton AL Jr, Peace D: Microsurgical anatomy of the posterior fossa cisterns. Neurosurgery 23: 58–80, 1988
16. Peerless SJ, Drake CG: Management of aneurysms of posterior circulation. In: Youmans JR (ed) Neurological surgery, vol 3, 3rd ed. Philadelphia: Saunders, 1990, pp 1764–1806
17. Peerless SJ, Hernesniemi JA, Drake CG: Surgical techniques of terminal basilar and posterior cerebral artery Aneurysms. In: Schmidek H, Sweet H (eds) Operative neurosurgical techniques, 3rd ed. Philadelphia: Saunders, 1995, pp 1071–1086
18. Peerless SJ, Hernesniemi JA, Gutman FB, Drake CG: Early surgery for ruptured posterior circulation aneurysms. J Neurosurg 80: 643–649, 1994
19. Pool JL, Potts DG: Aneurysms and arteriovenous anomalies of the brain. Diagnosis and treatment. New York: Harper and Row, 1965
20. Saeki N, Rhoton AL Jr: Microsurgical anatomy of the upper basilar artery and the Posterior circle of Willis. J Neurosurg 46: 563–578, 1977
21. Samson DS, Hodosh RM, Clark WK: Microsurgical evaluation of the pterional approach to aneurysms of the distal basilar circulation. Neurosurgery 3: 135–141, 1978
22. Solomon RA, Stein BM: Surgical approaches to aneurysms of the vertebral and basilar arteries. Neurosurgery 23: 203–208, 1988
23. Steinberg GK, Drake CG, Peerless SJ: Deliberate basilar or vertebral artery occlusion in the treatment of intracranial aneurysms. J Neurosurg 79: 161–173, 1993
24. Sugita K, Kobayashi S, Shintani A, Mutsuga N: Microneurosurgery for aneurysms of the basilar artery. J Neurosurg 51: 615–620, 1979
25. Yaşargil MG: Vertebrobasilar aneurysms. In: Microneurosurgery in 4 volumes, vol II. Stuttgart, New York: Thieme, 1986, pp 232–295

References for Chapters 9–11

1. Abe M, Uetsuki T: Clinico-pathological study of diseases of the central nervous system. VII. Autopsied case of a large aneurysm in the left anterior inferior cerebellar artery. No To Shinkei 20: 933–939, 1968
2. Crockard HA, Koksel T, Watkin N: Transoral transclival clipping of anterior inferior cerebellar artery aneurysm using new rotating applier. Technical note. J Neurosurg 75: 483–485, 1991
3. Drake CG: Surgical treatment of ruptured aneurysms of the basilar artery. Experience with 14 cases. J Neurosurg 23: 457–473, 1965
4. Drake CG: The surgical treatment of vertebral-basilar aneurysms. Clin Neurosurg 16: 114–69, 1969
5. Drake CG: Management of aneurysms of the posterior circulation. In: Youmans JR (ed) Neurological surgery, 1st ed, vol 2. Philadelphia: Saunders, 1973, pp 787–806
6. Drake CG: Ligation of the vertebral (unilateral or bilateral) or the basilar artery in the treatment of large intracranial aneurysms. J Neurosurg 43: 255–274, 1975
7. Drake CG: Giant intracranial aneurysms: Experience with surgical treatment in 174 patients. Clin Neurosurg 26: 12–95, 1979

8. Drake CG: The treatment of aneurysms of the posterior circulation. Clin Neurosurg 26: 96–144, 1979
9. Drake CG, Friedman AH, Peerless SJ: Failed aneurysm surgery. Reoperation in 115 cases. J Neurosurg 61: 848–856, 1984
10. Eguchi T, Fuchinoue T, Yahagi Y: Posterior subtemporal transtentorial approach for a lower basilar trunk aneurysm. No Shinkei Geka 7: 513–517, 1979
11. Fox JL: Intracranial aneurysms, vol I–III. New York, Berlin, Heidelberg, Tokyo: Springer, 1983, pp 63–117
12. Gacs G, Vinuela F, Fox AJ, Drake CG: Peripheral aneurysms of the cerebellar arteries. Review of 16 cases. J Neurosurg 58: 63–68, 1983
13. Hori T, Watanabe T, Numata H, Ishii T, Teraoka A: Basilar trunk aneurysms – operative and clinical experiences of 9 cases. In: Sugita K, Shibuya M (eds) Intracranial aneurysms and arteriovenous malformations – state of art. Proceeding of the 2nd International Workshop on Intracranial Aneurysms (IWIA) IV/1989 Toba. Nagoya: Nagoya University Coop Press, 1990, pp 243–250
14. Johnson JH Jr, Kline DG: Anterior inferior cerebellar artery aneurysms. Case report. J Neurosurg 48: 455–460, 1978
15. Kaech D, de Tribolet N, Lasjaunias P: Anterior inferior cerebellar artery aneurysm, carotid bifurcation aneurysm, and dural arteriovenous malformation of the tentorium in the same patient. Neurosurgery 21: 575–582, 1987
16. Kamii H, Ogawa A, Sakurai Y, Kayama T: Anterior inferior cerebellar artery aneurysm with a sudden onset of caudal cranial nerve symptoms. No Shinkei Geka 17: 387–91, 1989
17. Kawase T, Toya S, Shiobara R, Mine T: Transpetrosal approach for aneurysms of the lower basilar artery. J Neurosurg 63: 857–61, 1985
18. Krayenbühl HA, Yaşargil MG: The cerebral arteries. In: Cerebral angiography. London: Butterworths, 1968, pp 20–84
19. Marinkovic SV, Gibo H: The surgical anatomy of the perforating branches of the basilar artery. Neurosurgery 33: 80–87, 1993
20. Peerless SJ, Drake CG: Posterior circulation aneurysms. In: Wilkins RH, Rengachary SS (eds) Neurosurgery. New York: McGraw-Hill, 1985, pp 1422–1437
21. Pia HW: Classification of vertebro-basilar aneurysms. Acta Neurochir (Wien) 47: 3–30, 1979
22. Russegger L, Furtschegger A: Aneurysms of the anterior inferior cerebellar artery. A case report and review of the literature. Nervenarzt 61: 499–503, 1990
23. Santucci N, Gazzeri G, Magliocco C: Aneurysm of the anterior inferior cerebellar artery (AICA). 18th case in the literature. Riv Neurol 55: 30–37, 1985
24. Sugita K, Kobayashi S: Basilar trunk aneurysms. In: Kikuchi H, Fukushima T, Watanabe K (eds) Intracranial aneurysms. Surgical timing and techniques. Proceeding of the First International Workshop on Intracranial Aneurysms (IWIA) IV/1986 Tokyo. Tokyo: Nishimura, 1986, pp 350–352
25. Uede T, Matsumura S, Ohtaki M, Kurokawa Y, Tanabe S, Hashi K: Aneurysm of the anterior inferior cerebellar artery at the internal auditory meatus: report of two cases. No Shinkei Geka 14: 1263–1268, 1986
26. Yaşargil MG: Vertebrobasilar aneurysms. In: Microneurosurgery in 4 volumes, vol II. Stuttgart, New York: Thieme, 1986, pp 232–295

References for Chapters 12–13

1. Andrews BT, Brant-Zawadzki M, Wilson CB: Variant aneurysms of the fenestrated basilar artery. Neurosurgery 18: 204–207, 1986
2. Beck DW, Boarini DJ, Kassell NF: Surgical treatment of giant aneurysm of vertebral-basilar junction. Surg Neurol 12: 283–285, 1979
3. Bohmfalk GL, Story JL: Aneurysms of the persistent hypoglossal artery. Neurosurgery 1: 291–296, 1977
4. Botterell EH, Lougheed WM, Scott JW, Vandewater SL: Hypothermia, and interruption of carotid, or carotid and vertebral circulation, in the surgical management of intracranial aneurysms. J Neurosurg 13: 1–42, 1956
5. Campos J, Fox AJ, Vinuela F, Lylyk P, Ferguson GG, Drake CG, Peerless SJ: Saccular aneurysms in basilar artery fenestration. AJNR 8: 233–236, 1987
6. Drake CG: Ligation of the vertebral (unilateral or bilateral) or basilar artery in the treatment of large intracranial aneurysms. J Neurosurg 43: 255–274, 1975
7. Drake CG: The treatment of aneurysms of the posterior circulation. Clin Neurosurg 26: 96–144, 1979
8. Drake CG: Giant intracranial aneurysms: Experience with surgical treatment in 174 patients. Clin Neurosurg 26: 12–95, 1979
9. Drake CG, Friedman AH, Peerless SJ: Failed aneurysm surgery. Reoperation in 115 cases. J Neurosurg 61: 848–856, 1984
10. Ferguson GG, Drake CG, Peerless SJ: Basilar fenestration aneurysms. In: Sugita K, Shibuya M (eds) Intracranial aneurysms and arteriovenous malformations – state of art. Proceeding of the 2nd International Workshop on Intracranial Aneurysms (IWIA) IV/1989 Toba. Nagoya: Nagoya University COOP Press, 1990, pp 251–254
11. Fox JL: Intracranial aneurysms, vol I. New York, Berlin, Heidelberg, Tokyo: Springer, 1983, pp 63–117
12. Giannotta SL, Maceri DR: Retrolabyrinthine transsigmoid approach to basilar trunk and vertebrobasilar artery junction aneurysms. J Neurosurg 69: 461–466, 1988
13. Guha A, Montanera W, Hoffman HJ: Congenital aneurysmal dilatation of the petrous-cavernous carotid artery and vertebral basilar junction in a child. Neurosurgery 26: 322–327, 1990
14. Hoffman WF, Wilson CB: Fenestrated basilar artery with an associated saccular aneurysm. Case report. J Neurosurg 50: 262–264, 1979

15. Hudgins RJ, Day AL, Quisling RG, Rhoton AL Jr, Sypert GW, Garcia-Bengochea F: Aneurysms of the posterior inferior cerebellar artery. A clinical and anatomical analysis. J Neurosurg 58: 381–387, 1983
16. Kalia KK, Pollack IF, Yonas H: A partially thrombosed, fenestrated basilar artery mimicking an aneurysm of the vertebrobasilar junction: case report. Neurosurgery 30: 276–278, 1992
17. Kawase T, Toya S, Shiobara R, Mine T: Transpetrosal approach for aneurysms of the lower basilar artery. J Neurosurg 63: 857–861, 1985
18. Kempe LG: Aneurysms of the vertebral artery. In: Pia HW, Langmaid C, Zierski J (eds) Cerebral aneurysms. Advances in diagnosis and therapy. Berlin, Heidelberg, New York: Springer, 1979, pp 199–120
19. Nagao S, Kinugasa K, Bukeo T, Nishimoto A, Harada Y: Giant, fusiform and dissecting aneurysms at the vertebro-basilar junction-report of five cases and their clinical pathophysiological aspects. No Shinkei Geka 15: 1093–1100, 1987
20. Peerless SJ, Drake CG: Posterior circulation aneurysms. In: Wilkins RH, Rengachary SS (eds) Neurosurgery. New York: McGraw-Hill, 1985, pp 1422–1437
21. Pelz DM, Vinuela F, Fox AJ, Drake CG: Vertebrobasilar occlusion therapy of giant aneurysms. Significance of angiographic morphology of the posterior communicating arteries. J Neurosurg 60: 560–565, 1984
22. Pia HW: Classification of vertebro-basilar aneurysms. Acta Neurochir(Wien) 47: 3–30, 1979
23. Salcman M, Rigamonti D, Numaguchi Y, Sadato N: Aneurysms of the posterior inferior cerebellar artery-VA complex: variations on a theme. Neurosurgery 27: 12–21, 1990
24. Sekhar LN, Estonillo R: Transtemporal approach to the skull base: an anatomical study. Neurosurgery 19: 799–808, 1986
25. Steinberg GK, Drake CG, Peerless SJ: Deliberate basilar or vertebral artery occlusion in the treatment of intra-cranial aneurysms. Immediate results and long-term outcome in 201 patients. J Neurosurg 79: 161–173, 1993
26. Yamada K, Hayakawa T, Ushio Y, Iwata Y, Koshino K, Bitoh S, Takimoto N: Therapeutic occlusion of the VA for unclippable vertebral aneurysm: relationship between site of occlusion and clinical outcome. Neurosurgery 15: 834–838, 1984
27. Yamaura A: Diagnosis and treatment of vertebral aneurysms. J Neurosurg 69: 345–349, 1988
28. Yaşargil MG: Vertebrobasilar aneurysms. In: Microneurosurgery in 4 volumes, vol II. Stuttgart, New York: Thieme, 1986, pp 232–295

References for Chapters 14–15

1. Andoh T, Itoh T, Yoshimura S, Shirakami S, Nakashima T, Nishimura Y, Sakai N, Yamada H, Ohkuma A, Tanabe Y: Peripheral aneurysms of the posterior inferior cerebellar artery; analysis of 15 cases. No Shinkei Geka 20: 683–90, 1992
2. Azzam CJ: Growth of multiple peripheral high flow aneurysms of the posterior inferior cerebellar artery associated with a cerebellar arteriovenous malformation. Neurosurgery 21: 934–939, 1987
3. Beyerl BD, Heros RC: Multiple peripheral aneurysms of the posterior inferior cerebellar artery. Neurosurgery 19: 285–289, 1986
4. Crockard HA, Koksel T, Watkin N: Transoral transclival clipping of anterior inferior cerebellar artery aneurysm using new rotating applier. Technical note. J Neurosurg 75: 483–485, 1991
5. Dernbach PD, Sila CA, Little JR: Giant and multiple aneurysms of the distal posterior inferior cerebellar artery. Neurosurgery 22: 309–312, 1988
6. Drake CG: The surgical treatment of vertebral-basilar aneurysms. Clin Neurosurg 16: 114–169, 1969
7. Drake CG: Management of aneurysms of the posterior circulation. In: Youmans JR (ed) Neurological surgery, 1st ed, vol 2. Philadelphia: Saunders, 1973, pp 787–806
8. Drake CG: Ligation of the vertebral (unilateral or bilateral) or basilar artery in the treatment of large intracranial aneurysms. J Neurosurg 43: 255–274, 1975
9. Drake CG: Giant intracranial aneurysms: Experience with surgical treatment in 174 patients. Clin Neurosurg 26: 12–95, 1979
10. Drake CG: The treatment of aneurysms of the posterior circulation. Clin Neurosurg 26: 96–144, 1979
11. Fox JL: Intracranial aneurysms, vol I–III. New York, Berlin, Heidelberg, Tokyo: Springer, 1983, pp 63–117
12. Friedman AH, Drake CG: Subarachnoid hemorrhage from intracranial dissecting aneurysms. J Neurosurg 60: 325–334, 1984
13. Gacs G, Vinuela F, Fox AJ, Drake CG: Peripheral aneurysms of the cerebellar arteries. Review of 16 cases. J Neurosurg 58: 63–68, 1983
14. Hammon WM, Kempe LG: The posterior fossa approach to aneurysms of the vertebral and basilar arteries. J Neurosurg 37: 339–347, 1972
15. Hernesniemi JA, Vapalahti MP, Niskanen M, Kari A: Management outcome in vertebrobasilar artery aneurysms by early surgery. Neurosurgery 31: 857–862, 1992
16. Hiscott P, Crockard A: Multiple aneurysms of the distal posterior inferior cerebellar artery. Neurosurgery 10: 101–102, 1982
17. Hudgins RJ, Day AL, Quisling RG, Rhoton AL Jr, Sypert GW, Garcia-Bengochea F: Aneurysms of the posterior inferior cerebellar artery. A clinical and anatomical analysis. J Neurosurg 58: 381–387, 1983
18. Karasawa J, Kikuchi H, Furuse S, Sakaki T, Yoshida Y: Surgery of vertebral aneurysms at the origin of PICA. No Shinkei Geka 4: 1157–1163, 1976
19. Kempe LG: Aneurysms of the vertebral artery. In: Pia HW, Langmaid C, Zierski J (eds) Cerebral aneurysms. Advances in diagnosis and therapy. Berlin, Heidelberg, New York: Springer, 1979, pp 199–120
20. Krayenbühl HA, Yaşargil MG: The cerebral arteries. In: Cerebral angiography. London: Butterworths, 1968, pp 20–84

21. Meguro K, Rowed DW: Traumatic aneurysm of the posterior inferior cerebellar artery caused by fracture of the clivus. Neurosurgery 16: 666–668, 1985
22. Morard M, de Tribolet N: Traumatic aneurysm of the posterior inferior cerebellar artery: case report. Neurosurgery 29: 438–441, 1991
23. Nishino A, Sakurai Y, Satoh H, Niizuma H, Kayama T, Ogawa A, Ohtoh T: Aneurysms of the distal posterior inferior cerebellar artery; the report of 10 cases. No Shinkei Geka 19: 925–932, 1991
24. Nishizaki T, Tamaki N, Nishida Y, Fujita K, Matsumoto S: Aneurysms of the distal posterior inferior cerebellar artery: experience with three cases and review of the literature. Neurosurgery 16: 829–832, 1985
25. Ogura K, Hara M, Kageyama N: Distal aneurysm of the posterior inferior cerebellar artery – report of 3 cases. No Shinkei Geka 13: 211–215, 1985
26. Peerless SJ, Drake CG: Posterior circulation aneurysms. In: Wilkins RH, Rengachary SS (eds) Neurosurgery. New York: McGraw-Hill, 1985, pp 1422–1437
27. Pelz DM, Vinuela F, Fox AJ, Drake CG: Vertebrobasilar occlusion therapy of giant aneurysms. Significance of angiographic morphology of the posterior communicating arteries. J Neurosurg 60: 560–565, 1984
28. Pia HW: Classification of vertebro-basilar aneurysms. Acta Neurochir (Wien) 47: 3–30, 1979
29. Quattrocchi KB, Nielsen SL, Poirier V, Wagner FC Jr: Traumatic aneurysm of the superior cerebellar artery: case report and review of the literature. Neurosurgery 27: 476–479, 1990
30. Rhoton AL Jr, Saeki N, Perlmutter D, Zeal A: Microsurgical anatomy of common aneurysm sites. Clin Neurosurg 26: 248–306, 1979
31. Salcman M, Rigamonti D, Numaguchi Y, Sadato N: Aneurysms of the posterior inferior cerebellar artery-vertebral artery complex: variations on a theme. Neurosurgery 27: 12–21, 1990
32. Sasaki O, Ogawa H, Koike T, Koizumi T, Tanaka R: A clinicopathological study of dissecting aneurysms of the intracranial vertebral artery. J Neurosurg 75: 874–882, 1991
33. Shintani A, Zervas NT: Consequence of ligation of the vertebral artery. J Neurosurg 36: 447–450, 1972
34. Yamada K, Hayakawa T, Ushio Y, Iwata Y, Koshino K, Bitoh S, Takimoto N: Therapeutic occlusion of the vertebral artery for unclippable vertebral aneurysm: relationship between site of occlusion and clinical outcome. Neurosurgery 15: 834–838, 1984
35. Yamamoto I, Tsugane R, Ohya M, Sato O, Ogura K, Hara M: Peripheral aneurysms of the posterior inferior cerebellar artery. Neurosurgery 15: 839–845, 1984
36. Yamaura A: Diagnosis and treatment of vertebral aneurysms. J Neurosurg 69: 345–349, 1988
37. Yaşargil MG: Vertebrobasilar aneurysms. In: Microneurosurgery in 4 volumes, vol II. Stuttgart, New York: Thieme, 1986, pp 232–295
38. Yasui T, Yagura H, Komiyama M, Fu Y, Nagata Y, Tamura K, Kim A: Therapeutic occlusion of unilateral vertebral artery for unclippable aneurysms; special reference to postoperative brainstem ischemia. No Shinkei Geka 20: 325–32, 1992
39. Yeh HS, Tomsick TA, Tew JM Jr: Intraventricular hemorrhage due to aneurysms of the distal posterior inferior cerebellar artery. Report of three cases. J Neurosurg 62: 772–775, 1985

References for Chapters 16–17

1. Amacher AL, Drake CG, Ferguson GG: Posterior circulation aneurysms in young people. Neurosurgery 8: 315–320, 1981
2. Chang HS, Fukushima T, Takakura K: Aneurysms of the posterior cerebral artery: Report of ten cases. Neurosurgery 19: 1006–1011, 1986
3. Drake CG, Amacher AL: Aneurysms of the posterior cerebral artery. J Neurosurg 30: 468–474, 1969
4. Drake CG: Giant intracranial aneurysms: Experience with surgical treatment in 174 patients. Clin Neurosurg 26: 12–95, 1979
5. Drake CG: The treatment of aneurysms of the posterior circulation. Clin Neurosurg 26: 96–144, 1979
6. Krayenbühl HA, Yaşargil MG: The cerebral arteries. In: Cerebral angiography. London: Butterworths, 1968, pp 20–84
7. Pia HW, Fontana H: Aneurysms of the posterior cerebral artery. Acta Neurochir (Wien) 38: 13–35, 1977
8. Sakata S, Fujii K, Matsushima T, Fujiwara S, Fukui M, Matsubara T, Nagatomi H, Kuromatsu C, Kamikaseda K: Aneurysms of the posterior cerebral artery: report of eleven cases – surgical approaches and procedures. Neurosurgery 32: 163–168, 1993

References for Chapters 18

1. af Björkesten G, Halonen V: Incidence of intracranial vascular lesions in patients with subarachnoid hemorrhage investigated by four-vessel angiography. J Neurosurg 23: 29–32, 1965
2. af Björkesten G, Troupp H: Multiple intracranial aneurysms. Acta Chir Scand 118: 387–391, 1960
3. Andrews RJ, Spiegel PK: Intracranial aneurysms. Age, sex, blood pressure and multiplicity in an unselected series of patients. J Neurosurg 51: 27–32, 1979
4. Cervoni L, Delfini R, Santoro A, Cantore G: Multiple intracranial aneurysms: Surgical treatment and outcome. Acta Neurochir (Wien) 124: 66–70, 1993
5. Fox JL: Multiple intracranial aneurysms occurring in adults. In: Intracranial aneurysms, vol I. New York, Berlin, Heidelberg, Tokyo: Springer, 1983, pp 36–43
6. Hamby WB: Multiple intracranial aneurysms. J Neurosurg 16: 558–563, 1959
7. Heiskanen O: Risk of bleeding from unruptured aneurysms in cases with multiple intracranial aneurysms. J Neurosurg 55: 524–526, 1981
8. Heiskanen O: Risks of surgery for unruptured intracranial aneurysms. J Neurosurg 65: 451–453, 1986

9. Hernesniemi J, Tapaninaho A, Vapalahti M, Niskanen M, Kari A, Luukkonen M: Saccular aneurysms of the distal anterior cerebral artery and its branches. Neurosurgery 31: 994–999, 1992
10. Hernesniemi J, Vapalahti M, Niskanen M, Tapaninaho A, Kari A, Luukkonen M, Puranen M, Saari T, Rajpar M: One-year outcome in early aneurysm surgery: A 14 years experience. Acta Neurochir (Wien) 122: 1–10, 1993
11. Inagawa T: Multiple intracranial aneurysms in elderly patients. Acta Neurochir(Wien) 106: 119–126, 1990
12. Inagawa T: Surgical treatment of multiple intracranial aneurysms. Acta Neurochir(Wien) 108: 22–29, 1991
13. Juvela S, Porras M, Heiskanen O: Natural history of unruptured intracranial aneurysms: A long-term follow-up study. J Neurosurg 79: 174–182, 1993
14. Kassel NF, Torner JC, Haley EC Jr, Jane JA, Adams HP, Kongable GL: The International Cooperative Study on the Timing of Aneurysm Surgery. Part I: Overall management results. J Neurosurg 73: 18–36, 1990
15. King JT Jr, Berlin JA, Flamm ES: Morbidity and mortality from elective surgery for asymptomatic, unruptured, intracranial aneurysms: a meta-analysis. J Neurosurg 81: 837–842, 1994
16. Koos WT, Perneczky A: Timing of surgery for ruptured aneurysms – experience from 800 consecutive cases. Acta Neurochir (Wien) 63: 125–133, 1982
17. Locksley HB: Natural history of subarachnoid hemorrhage, intracranial aneurysms and arteriovenous malformations. Based on 6368 cases on cooperative study. In: Sahs AL, Perret GE, Locksley HB, Nishioka H (eds) Intracranial aneurysms and subarachoid hemorrhage. A cooperative study. Philadelphia, Toronto: Lippincott, 1969, pp 37–109
18. McKissock W, Richardson A, Walsh L, Owen E: Multiple intracranial aneurysms. Lancet 1: 623–626, 1964
19. Mizoi K, Suzuki J, Yoshimoto T: Surgical treatment of multiple aneurysms. Acta Neurochir(Wien) 96: 8–14, 1989
20. Nakstad P, Nornes H, Hauge HN, Kjartansson O: Cerebral panangiography in spontaneous subarachnoid hemorrhage from intracranial aneurysms. Acta Radiol 29: 633–636, 1988
21. Nehls DG, Flom RA, Carter PL, Spetzler RF: Multiple intracranial aneurysms: Determining the site of rupture. J Neurosurg 63: 342–348, 1985
22. Nishimoto A, Ueta K, Onbe H, Kitamura K, Omae T, Goto F, Ohneda G, Chigasaki H, Tsuru M, Suzuki J, Wada T, Sano K, Mannen T, Yoshioka M, Nakai O, Kageyama N, Nomura T, Handa H, Tanaka K: Nationwide co-operative study of intracranial aneurysm surgery in Japan. Stroke 16: 48–52, 1985
23. Nyström SHM: Psychodynamics in subarachnoid hemorrhage. A study based on 1183 patients. Helsinki: Sahalan kirjapaino, 1973, pp 1–114
24. Østergaard JR, Hog E: Incidence of multiple intracranial aneurysms. J Neurosurg 63: 49–55, 1985
25. Pasqualin A, Bazzan A, Cavazzani P, Scienza R, Licata C, Da Pian R: Intracranial hematomas following aneurysmal rupture: Experience with 309 cases. Surg Neurol 25: 6–17, 1986
26. Poppen JL, Fager CA: Multiple intracranial aneurysms. J Neurosurg 16: 581–589, 1959
27. Reynolds AF, Shaw C-M: Bleeding patterns from ruptured intracranial aneurysms: An autopsy study series of 205 patients. Surg Neurol 15: 232–235, 1981
28. Rice BJ, Peerless SJ, Drake CG: Surgical treatment of unruptured aneurysms of the posterior circulation. J Neurosurg 73: 165–173, 1990
29. Rinne JK, Hernesniemi JA: Formation of de novo aneurysms: Special multiple intracranial aneurysms. Neurosurgery 33: 981–985, 1993
30. Rinne J, Hernesniemi J, Puranen M, Saari T: Multiple intracranial aneurysms in a defined population: prospective angiographic and clinical study. Neurosurgery 35: 803–808, 1994
31. Rinne J, Hernesniemi J, Niskanen M, Vapalahti M: Management outcome for multiple intracranial aneurysms. Neurosurgery, 36: 31–38, 1995
32. Rosenørn J, Eskesen V, Schmidt K, Espersen JO, Haase J, Harmsen A, Hein O, Knudsen V, Midholm S, Marcussen E, Rasmussen P, Rønde F, Voldby B, Hansen L: Clinical features and outcome in 1076 patients with ruptured intracranial saccular aneurysms: A prospective consecutive study. Br J Neurosurg 1: 33–46, 1987
33. Shephard RH: Ruptured cerebral aneurysms: Early and late prognosis with surgical treatment. A personal series, 1958–1980. J Neurosurg 59: 6–15, 1983
34. Vajda J, Juhasz J, Orosz E, Pasztor E, Toth S, Horvath M: Surgical treatment of multiple intracranial aneurysms. Acta Neurochir (Wien) 82: 14–23, 1986
35. Vajda J: Multiple intracranial aneurysms: A high risk condition. Acta Neurochir(Wien) 118: 59–75, 1992
36. Wiebers DO, Whisnant JP, O'Fallon WM: The natural history of unruptured intracranial aneurysms. N Engl J Med 304: 696–698, 1981
37. Wilson FMA, Jaspan T, Holland IM: Multiple cerebral aneurysms – a reappraisal. Neuroradiology 31: 232–236, 1989
38. Wirth F: Surgical treatment of incidental intracranial aneurysms. Clin Neurosurg 33: 125–135, 1986
39. Yamaki T, Takeda M, Takayama H, Nakagaki Y: Treatment of multiple intracranial aneurysms in the anterior circulation. Neurol Med Chir (Tokyo) 30: 47–50, 1990
40. Yaşargil MG: Multiple aneurysms. In: Microneurosurgery in 4 volumes, vol I. Stuttgart, New York: Thieme, 1986, pp 305–328

References for Chapter 19

1. Batjer H, Suss RA, Samson D: Intracranial arteriovenous malformations associated with aneurysms. Neurosurgery 18: 29–35, 1986
2. Brown RD Jr, Wiebers DO, Forbes GS: Unruptured intracranial aneurysms and arteriovenous malformations: frequency of intracranial hemorrhage and relationship of lesions. J Neurosurg 73: 859–863, 1990

3. Cronqvist S, Troupp H: Intracranial arteriovenous malformation and arterial aneurysm in the same patient. Acta Neurol Scand 42: 307–316, 1966
4. Cunha e Sa MJ, Stein BM, Solomon RA, McCormick PC: The treatment of associated intracranial aneurysms and arteriovenous malformations. J Neurosurg 77: 853–859, 1992
5. Deruty R, Mottolese C, Soustiel JF, Pelissou-Guyotat I: Association of cerebral arteriovenous malformation and cerebral aneurysm. Diagnosis and management. Acta Neurochir (Wien) 107: 133–139, 1990
6. Drake CG: Surgical removal of A.V. malformations of the "brain stem": a report of 3 cases. In: Handa H (ed) Microneurosurgery. Tokyo: Igaku Shoin, 1975, pp 21–25
7. Drake CG, Friedman AH, Peerless SJ: Posterior fossa arteriovenous malformations. J Neurosurg 64: 1–10, 1986
8. Fox JL: Intracranial arteriovenous malformations and aneurysms (Appendix 3). In: Fox JL (ed) Intracranial aneurysms. New York: Springer, 1983, pp 1389–1400
9. Gacs G, Vinuela F, Fox AJ, Drake CG: Peripheral aneurysms of the cerebellar arteries: review of 16 cases. J Neurosurg 58: 63–68, 1983
10. Hernesniemi J, Keränen T: Microsurgical treatment of arteriovenous malformations of the brain in a defined population. Surg Neurol 33: 384–390, 1990
11. Kikuchi K, Kowada M, Yonea M: Association of arteriovenous malformation and intracranial aneurysm in the posterior fossa. Surg Neurol 22: 499–502, 1984
12. Lasjaunias P, Piske R, Terbrugge K, Willinsky R: Cerebral arteriovenous malformations (CAVM) and associated arterial aneurysms (AA). Acta Neurochir (Wien) 91: 29–36, 1988
13. Miysaka K, Wolpert SM, Prager RJ: The association of cerebral aneurysms, infundibula, and intracranial arteriovenous malformations. Stroke 13: 196–203, 1982
14. Noterman J, Georges P, Brotchi J: Arteriovenous malformation associated with multiple aneurysms in the posterior fossa: A case report with a review of the literature. Neurosurgery 21: 387–391, 1987
15. Okamoto S, Handa H, Hashimoto N: Location of intracranial aneurysms associated with cerebral arteriovenous malformation: statistical analysis. Surg Neurol 22: 335–340, 1984
16. Ondra SL, Troupp H, George ED, Schwab K: The natural history of symptomatic arteriovenous malformations of the brain: a 24-year follow-up assessment. J Neurosurg 73: 387–391, 1990
17. Peerless SJ, Hernesniemi JA, Drake CG: Arteriovenous malformations of the posterior fossa. In: Wilkins RH, Rengachary SS (eds) Neurosurgery, 2nd ed. New York: McGraw-Hill, 1995, in press
18. Suzuki J, Onuma T: Intracranial aneurysms associated with AV malformations. J Neurosurg 50: 742–746, 1979
19. Wilkins RH: Multiple aneurysms and associated arteriovenous malformations. Operative considerations. In: Hopkins LN, Long DM (eds) Clinical management of intracranial aneurysms. New York: Raven, 1982, pp 193–200

References for Chapter 20

1. Heiskanen O: Risks of surgery for unruptured intracranial aneurysms. J Neurosurg 65: 451–453, 1986
2. Juvela S, Porras M, Heiskanen O: Natural history of unruptured intracranial aneurysms: a long-term follow-up study. J Neurosurg 79: 174–182, 1993
3. King JT Jr, Berlin JA, Flamm ES: Morbidity and mortality from elective surgery for asymptomatic, unruptured, intracranial aneurysms: a meta-analysis. J Neurosurg 81: 837–842, 1994
4. Rice BJ, Peerless SJ, Drake CG: Surgical treatment of unruptured aneurysms of the posterior circulation. J Neurosurg 73: 165–173, 1990
5. Wiebers DO, Whisnant JP, O'Fallon WM: The natural history of unruptured intracranial aneurysms. N Engl J Med 304: 696–698, 1981
6. Wirth F: Surgical treatment of incidental intracranial aneurysms. Clin Neurosurg 33: 125–135, 1986

References for Chapter 21

1. Amacher AL, Drake CG, Ferguson GG: Posterior circulation aneurysms in young people. Neurosurgery 8: 315–320, 1981
2. Drake CG, Amacher AL: Aneurysms of the posterior cerebral artery. J Neurosurg 30: 468–474, 1969
3. Drake CG: Giant intracranial aneurysms: Experience with surgical treatment in 174 patients. Clin Neurosurg 26: 12–95, 1979
4. Drake CG: The treatment of aneurysms of the posterior circulation. Clin Neurosurg 26: 96–144, 1979
5. Fox JL: Intracranial aneurysms, vol I–III. New York, Berlin, Heidelberg, Tokyo: Springer 1983, 1463 pp

References for Chapter 22

1. Batjer HH, Samson DS: Causes of morbidity and mortality from surgery of aneurysms of the distal basilar artery. Neurosurgery 25: 904–916, 1989
2. Botterell EH, Lougheed WM, Scott JW, Vandewater SL: Hypothermia, and interruption of carotid, or carotid and vertebral circulation, in the surgical management of intracranial aneurysms. J Neurosurg 13: 1–42, 1956
3. Dandy WE: Intracranial arterial aneurysms. Ithaca, New York: Comstock, 1944, 147 pp
4. Drake CG: Bleeding aneurysms of the basilar artery. Direct surgical management in four cases. J Neurosurg 23: 230–238, 1961
5. Drake CG: Surgical treatment of ruptured aneurysms of the basilar artery. Experience with 14 cases. J Neurosurg 23: 457–473, 1965
6. Drake CG: Further experience with surgical treatment of aneurysms of the basilar artery. J Neurosurg 29: 372–392, 1968
7. Drake CG: The treatment of aneurysms of the posterior circulation. Clin Neurosurg 26: 96–144, 1979

8. Falconer MA: Surgical treatment of spontaneous intracranial hemorrhage. BMJ 1: 790–792, 1958
9. Fisher CM, Kistler JP, Davis JM: Relation of cerebral vasospasm to subarachnoid hemorrhage visualized by computer tomography scanning. Neurosurgery 1: 245–248, 1977
10. Hernesniemi JA, Vapalahti MP, Niskanen M, Kari A: Management outcome in vertebrobasilar artery aneurysms by early surgery. Neurosurgery 31: 857–862, 1992
11. Hunt WE, Hess RM : Surgical risks as related to time of intervention in repair of intracranial aneurysms. J Neurosurg 28: 14–20, 1968
12. Jamieson KG: Aneurysms of the vertebrobasilar system. Surgical intervention in 19 cases. J Neurosurg 21: 781–797, 1964
13. Kassel NF, Torner JC, Haley EC Jr, Jane JA, Adams HP, Kongable GL: The International Cooperative Study on the Timing of Aneurysm Surgery. Part I: Overall management results. J Neurosurg 73: 18–36, 1990
14. Kassell NF, Torner JC, Jane JA, Haley EC Jr, Adams HP: The International Cooperative Study on the Timing of Aneurysm Surgery. Part II: Surgical results. J Neurosurg 73: 37–47, 1990
15. Logue V: Posterior fossa aneurysms. Clin Neurosurg 11: 183–207, 1964,
16. MacFarlane MR, McAllister VL, Whitby DJ, Sengupta RR: Posterior circulation aneurysms. Results of direct operations. Surg Neurol 20: 399–413, 1983
17. Öhman J, Heiskanen O: Timing of operation for ruptured supratentorial aneurysms: A prospective randomized study. J Neurosurg 70: 55–60, 1989
18. Peerless SJ, Drake CG: Posterior circulation aneurysms. In: Wilkins RH, Rengachary SS (eds) Neurosurgery. New York: McGraw-Hill, 1985, pp 1422–1437
19. Peerless SJ, Nemoto S, Drake CG: Acute surgery for ruptured posterior circulation aneurysms. In: Symon L et al (eds) Advances and technical standards in neurosurgery, vol 15. Wien, New York: Springer, 1987, pp 115–129
20. Peerless SJ: Pre- and post-operative management of intracranial aneurysms. Clin Neurosurg 26: 209–231, 1979
21. Poppen JL: Vascular surgery of the posterior fossa. Proc Congr Neurol Surg 6: 198, 1969
22. Schwartz HG: Arterial aneurysms of the posterior fossa. J Neurosurg 5: 312–316, 1948
23. Sugita K, Kobayashi S, Shintani A, Mutsuga N: Microneurosurgery for aneurysms of the basilar artery. J Neurosurg 51: 615–620, 1979
24. Steinberg GK, Drake CG, Peerless SJ: Deliberate basilar or vertebral artery occlusion in the treatment of intracranial aneurysms. Immediate results and long-term outcome in 201 patients. J Neurosurg 79: 161–173, 1993
25. Tönnis W: Zur Behandlung intrakranieller Aneurysmen. Arch Klin Chir 189: 474–476, 1937
26. Troupp H: The natural history of aneurysms of the basilar bifurcation. Acta Neurol Scand 47: 350–356, 1971
27. Vapalahti M, Ljunggren B, Säveland H, Hernesniemi J, Brandt L, Tapaninaho A: Early aneurysm operation and outcome in two remote Scandinavian populations. J Neurosurg 60: 1160–1162, 1984
28. Yaşargil MG, Antic J, Lagica R, Jain KK, Hodosh RM, Smith RD: Microneurosurgical pterional approach to aneurysms of the basilar bifurcation. Surg Neurol 6: 83–91, 1976
29. Yaşargil MG: Vertebrobasilar aneurysms. In: Microneurosurgery in 4 volumes, vol II. Stuttgart, New York: Thieme, 1986, pp 232–295

References for Chapter 23

1. Black S, Cucchiara RF, Nishimura RA, Michenfelder JD: Parameters affecting occurrence of paradoxical air embolism. Anesthesiology 71: 235–241, 1989
2. Craen R, Gelb AW: Applications in neurosurgery. In: Ornstein E (ed) Problems in anesthesia: Deliberate hypotension in anesthesia and curgery. Philadelphia: Lippincott, 1993, pp 23–30
3. Domino KB, Hemstad JR, Lam AM, Laohaprasit V, Mayberg TA, Harrison SD, Grady MS, Winn HR: Effect of nitrous oxide on intracranial pressure after cranial– dural closure in patients undergoing craniotomy. Anesthesiology 77: 421–425, 1992
4. Ferguson GG: Direct measurement of mean and pulsatile blood pressure at operation in human intracranial saccular aneurysms. J Neurosurg 36: 560–563, 1972
5. Halldin M, Wahlin A: Effect of succinylcholine on intraspinal fluid pressure. Acta Anaesthesiol Scand 3: 155–161, 1959
6. Hamill JF, Bedford RF, Weaver DC, Colohan AR: Lidocaine before endotracheal intubation: intravenous or laryngotracheal? Anesthesiology 55: 578, 1981
7. Lam AM, Gelb AW: Cardiovascular effects of isoflurane induced hypotension for cerebral aneurysm surgery. Anesth Analg 62: 742-, 1983
8. Lam AM, Keane JF, Manninen PH: Monitoring of brainstem auditory evoked potentials during basilar artery occlusion in man. Br J Anaesth 57: 924–928, 1985
9. Lam AM, Manninen PH: Induced hypotension for cerebral aneurysm – isoflurane or sodium nitroprusside. Can J Anaesth 34: 121–122, 1987
10. Lanier WL, Milde JH, Michenfelder JD: Cerebral stimulation following succinylcholine in dogs. Anesthesiology 64: 551–559, 1986
11. Lanier WL, Stangland KJ, Scheithauer BW, Milde JH, Michenfelder JD: The effects of dextrose infusion and head position on neurological outcome after complete cerebral ischemia in primates: examination of a model. Anesthesiology 66: 39–48, 1987
12. Little JR, Lesser RP, Luders H: Electrophysiological monitoring during basilar aneurysm operation. Neurosurgery 20: 421–427, 1987
13. Losasso TJ, Muzzi DA, Dietz NM, Cucchiara RF: Fifty percent nitrous oxide does not increase the risk of

venous air embolism in neurosurgical patients operated upon in the sitting position. Anesthesiology 77: 21–30, 1992
14. Macnab MSP, Manninen PH, Lam AM, Gelb AW: The stress response to induced hypotension for cerebral aneurysm surgery: A comparison of two hypotensive techniques. Can J Anaesth 35: 111–115, 1988
15. Manninen PH, Cuillerier DJ, Nantau WE, Gelb AW: Monitoring of brainstem function during vertebral basilar aneurysm surgery. Anesthesiology 77: 681–685, 1992
16. Manninen PH, Gelb AW, Lam AM, Moote CA: Perioperative monitoring of the electrocardiogram during cerebral aneurysm surgery. J Neurosurg Anesthesiol 2: 16–22, 1990
17. Manninen PH, Gelb AW: Anesthesia for cerebral aneurysms and arteriovenous malformations. Problems in anesthesia. Neuroanesthesia 4: 81–93, 1990
18. Manninen PH, Lam AM, Gelb AW, Brown SC: The effect of high dose mannitol on serum and urine electrolytes and osmolality in neurosurgical patients. Can J Anaesth 34: 442–446, 1987
19. Manninen PH, Lam AM, Nantau WE: Monitoring of somatosensory evoked potentials during temporary arterial occlusion in cerebral aneurysm surgery. J Neurosurg Anesthesiol 2: 97–104, 1990
20. Manninen PH, Mahendran B, Gelb AW, Merchant RN: Succinylcholine does not increase serum potassium levels in patients with acutely ruptured cerebral aneurysms. Anesth Analg 70: 172–175, 1990
21. Manninen PH, Mahendran B, Merchant RN: Low dose sufentanil and isoflurane for cerebral aneurysm surgery. Anesthesiol Rev 19: 43–47, 1992
22. Manninen PH, Patterson S, Lam AM, Gelb AW, Nantau WE: Evoked potential monitoring during posterior fossa aneurysm surgery: a comparison of two modalities. Can J Anaesth 41: 92–7, 1994
23. Matjasko J, Petrozza P, Cohen M, Steinberg P: Anesthesia and surgery in the seated position: analysis of 554 cases. Neurosurgery 17: 695–702, 1985
24. Pearl RG, Larson CP Jr: Hemodynamic effects of positive end-expiratory pressure during continuous venous air embolism in the dog. Anesthesiology 64: 724–729, 1986
25. Pilato MA: New developments in the treatment of subarachnoid hemorrhage. In: Bissonnette B (ed) Anesthesiology clinics of North America. Philadelphia: Saunders, 1992, pp 521–536
26. Pulsinelli WA, Levy DE, Sigsbee B, Scherer P, Plum F: Increased damage after ischemic stroke in patients with hyperglycemia with or without established diabetes mellitus. Am J Med 74: 540, 1983
27. Rosomoff HL: Adjunct to neurosurgical anaesthesia. Br J Anaesth 37: 246–261, 1965
28. Schramm J, Koht A, Schmidt G, Pechstein V, Taniguchi M, Fahlbusch R: Surgical and electrophysiological observations during clipping of 134 aneurysms with evoked potential monitoring. Neurosurgery 26: 61–70, 1990
29. Sellery GR, Aitken RR, Drake CG: Anesthesia for intracranial aneurysms with hypotension and spontaneous respiration. Can Anaesth Soc J 20: 468–478, 1973
30. Warren JE, Tsuedak K, Young B: Respiratory pattern changes during repair of posterior fossa arteriovenous malformations. Anesthesiology 45: 690–693, 1976
31. Whitby JD: Electrocardiography during posterior fossa operations. Br J Anaesth 35: 624–630, 1963
32. Wilder BL: Hypothesis: The etiology of mid-cervical quadriplegia after operation with patients in the sitting position. Neurosurgery 11: 530–531, 1982
33. Young ML, Smith DS, Murtagh F, Vasquez A, Levitt J: Comparison of surgical and anesthetic complications in neurosurgical patients experiencing venous air embolism in the sitting position. Neurosurgery 18: 157–161, 1986

References for Chapter 24

1. Casasco AE, Aymard A, Gobin YP, Houdart E, Rogopoulos A, George B, Hodes JE, Cophignon J, Merland JJ: Selective endovascular treatment of 71 intracranial aneurysms with platinum coils. J Neurosurg 79: 3–10, 1993
2. Dandy WE: Intracranial aneurysm of the internal carotid artery: cured by operation. Ann Surg 107: 654–659, 1938
3. Debrun G, Fox A, Drake C, Peerless S, Girvin J, Ferguson G: Giant unclippable aneurysms: treatment with detachable balloons. AJNR 2: 167–173, 1981
4. Drake CG: On the surgical treatment of ruptured intracranial aneurysms. Clin Neurosurg 13: 122–155, 1965
5. Drake CG: Earlier times in aneurysm surgery. Clin Neurosurg 32: 41–50, 1985
6. Guglielmi G, Viñuela F, Sepetka I, Macellari V: Electrothrombosis of saccular aneurysms via endovascular approach. Part 1: Electrochemical basis, technique and experimental results. J Neurosurg 75: 1–7, 1991
7. Guglielmi G, Viñuela F, Duckwiler G, Dion J, Lylyk P, Berenstein A, Strother C, Graves V, Halbach V, Nichols D: Endovascular treatment of posterior circulation aneurysms by electrothrombosis using electrically detachable coils. J Neurosurg 77: 515–524, 1992
8. Hieshima GB, Higashida RT, Wapenski J, Halbach VV, Cahan L, Bentson JR: Balloon embolization of a large distal basilar artery aneurysm. Case report. J Neurosurg 65: 413–416, 1986
9. Higashida RT, Halbach VV, Cahan LD, Hieshima GB, Konishi Y: Detachable balloon embolization therapy of posterior circulation intracranial aneurysms. J Neurosurg 71: 512–519, 1989
10. Hilal SK, Khandji AG, Chi TL, Stein BM, Bello JA, Silver AJ: Synthetic fiber-coated platinum coils successfully used for the endovascular treatment of arteriovenous malformations, aneurysms and direct arteriovenous fistulas of the CNS (abstract). AJNR 9: 1030, 1988

11. Hodes JE, Fox AJ, Pelz DM, Peerless SJ: Rupture of aneurysms following balloon embolization. J Neurosurg 72: 567–571, 1990
12. Kwan ES, Heilman CB, Shucart WA, Klucznik RP: Enlargement of basilar artery aneurysms following balloon occlusion – "water-hammer effect." J Neurosurg 75: 963–968, 1991
13. Mullan S, Raimondi AJ, Dobben G, Vailati G, Hekmatpanah J: Electrically induced thrombosis in intracranial aneurysms. J Neurosurg 22: 539–547, 1965
14. Mullan S, Reyes C, Dawley J, Dobben G: Stereotactic copper electric thrombosis of intracranial aneurysms. Progr Neurol Surg 3: 193–211, 1969
15. Mullan S: Experiences with surgical thrombosis of intracranial berry aneurysms and carotid cavernous fistulas. J Neurosurg 41: 657–670, 1974
16. Romodanov AP, Shcheglov VI: Intravascular occlusion of saccular aneurysms of the cerebral arteries by means of a detachable balloon catheter. In: Krayenbühl H (ed) Advances and technical standards in neurosurgery, vol 9. Wien, New York: Springer, 1982, pp 25–49
17. Serbinenko FA: Balloon catheterization and occlusion of major cerebral vessels. J Neurosurg 41: 125–145, 1974
18. Strother CM, Lunde S, Graves V, Toutant S, Hieshima GB: Late paraophthalmic aneurysm rupture following endovascular treatment. Case report. J Neurosurg 71: 777–780, 1989
19. Taki W, Nishi S, Yamashita K, Sadatoh A, Nakahara I, Kikuchi H, Iwata H: Selection and combination of various endovascular techniques in the treatment of giant aneurysms. J Neurosurg 77: 37–42, 1992
20. Yang PJ, Halbach VV, Higashida RT, Hieshima GB: Platinum wire: a new transvascular embolic agent. AJNR 9: 547–550, 1988
21. Zubillaga AF, Guglielmi G, Viñuela F, Duckwiler GR: Endovascular occlusion of intracranial aneurysms with electrically detachable coils: correlation of aneurysm neck size and treatment results. AJNR 15: 815–820, 1994

References for Chapter 25

1. Batjer HH, Samson DS: Causes of morbidity and mortality from surgery of aneurysms of the distal basilar artery. J Neurosurg 25: 904–915, 1989
2. Botterell EH, Lougheed WM, Scott JW, Vandewater SL: Hypothermia, and interruption of carotid, or carotid and vertebral circulation, in the surgical management of intracranial aneurysms. J Neurosurg 13: 1–42, 1956
3. Clark K: Complications of aneurysm surgery. Clin Neurosurg 23: 342–356, 1976
4. Drake CG: Bleeding aneurysms of the basilar artery. Direct surgical management in four cases. J Neurosurg 23: 230–238, 1961
5. Drake CG: Surgical treatment of ruptured aneurysms of the basilar artery. Experience with 14 cases. J Neurosurg 23: 457–473, 1965
6. Drake CG: Further experience with surgical treatment of aneurysms of the basilar artery. J Neurosurg 29: 372–392, 1968
7. Drake CG: The surgical treatment of aneurysms of the basilar artery. J Neurosurg 29: 436–446, 1968
8. Drake CG: The surgical treatment of the vertebral-basilar aneurysms. Clin Neurosurg 16: 114–169, 1969
9. Drake CG: Ligation of the vertebral (unilateral or bilateral) or basilar artery in the treatment of large intracranial aneurysms. J Neurosurg 43: 255–74, 1975
10. Drake CG: Giant intracranial aneurysms: Experience with surgical treatment in 174 patients. Clin Neurosurg 26: 12–95, 1979
11. Drake CG: The treatment of aneurysms of the posterior circulation. Clin Neurosurg 26: 96–144, 1979
12. Drake CG, Friedman AH, Peerless SJ: Failed aneurysm surgery. Reoperation in 115 cases. J Neurosurg 61: 848–856, 1984
13. Drake CG, Peerless SJ, Ferguson GG: Hunterian proximal arterial occlusion for giant aneurysms on the carotid circulation. J Neurosurg 81: 656–665, 1994
14. Fox JL: Intracranial aneurysms, vol I–III. New York, Berlin, Heidelberg, Tokyo: Springer, 1983, 1463 pp
15. Hernesniemi J, Vapalahti M, Niskanen M, Tapaninaho A, Kari A, Luukkonen M, Puranen M, Saari T, Rajpar M: One-year outcome in early aneurysm surgery: A 14 years experience. Acta Neurochir (Wien) 122: 1–10, 1993
16. Hernesniemi JA, Vapalahti MP, Niskanen M, Kari A: Management outcome in vertebrobasilar artery aneurysms by early surgery. Neurosurgery 31: 857–862, 1992
17. Kassel NF, Torner JC, Haley EC Jr, Jane JA, Adams HP, Kongable GL: The International Cooperative Study on the Timing of Aneurysm Surgery. Part I: Overall management results. J Neurosurg 73: 18–36, 1990
18. Kassell NF, Torner JC, Jane JA, Haley EC Jr, Adams HP: The International Cooperative Study on the Timing of Aneurysm Surgery. Part II: Surgical results. J Neurosurg 73: 37–47, 1990
19. Muizelaar JP: The use of electroencephalography and brain protection during operation for basilar aneurysms. Neurosurgery 25: 899–903, 1989
20. Niskanen MM, Hernesniemi JA, Vapalahti MP, Kari A: One-year outcome in early aneurysm surgery: prediction of outcome. Acta Neurochir (Wien) 123: 25–32, 1993
21. Niskanen MM: Prediction of outcome from critical illness in specific diagnostic categories. Academic dissertation, University of Kuopio. Kuopio: Kuopio University Printing Office, 1994
22. Peerless SJ: The surgical approach to middle cerebral and posterior communicating aneurysms. Clin Neurosurg 21: 151–165, 1974
23. Peerless SJ, Drake CG: Management of aneurysms of posterior circulation. In: Youmans JR (ed) Neurological surgery, 3rd ed, vol 3. Philadelphia, Saunders, 1990, pp 1764–1806
24. Peerless SJ, Wallace MC, Drake CG: Giant intracranial aneurysms. In: Youmans JR (ed) Neurological surgery

vol 3, 3rd ed. Philadelphia: Saunders, 1990, pp 1742–1763
25. Peerless SJ, Hernesniemi JA, Drake CG: Surgical techniques of terminal basilar and posterior cerebral artery aneurysms. In: Schmidek H, Sweet H (eds) Operative neurosurgical techniques, 3rd ed. Philadelphia: Saunders, 1995, pp 1071–1086
26. Peerless SJ, Hernesniemi JA, Gutman FB, Drake CG: Early surgery for ruptured vertebrobasilar aneurysms. J Neurosurg 80: 643–649, 1994
27. Peerless SJ: Pre- and postoperative management of cerebral aneurysms. Clin Neurosurg 26: 209–231, 1979
28. Rice BJ, Peerless SJ, Drake CG: Surgical treatment of unruptured aneurysms of the posterior circulation. J Neurosurg 73: 165–173, 1990
29. Spetzler RF, Hadley MN, Rigamonti D, Carter LP, Raudzens PA, Shedd SA, Wilkinson E: Aneurysms of the basilar artery treated with circulatory arrest, hypothermia, and barbiturate cerebral protection. J Neurosurg 68: 868–879, 1988
30. Ronkainen A, Hernesniemi J, Ryynänen M, Puranen M, Kuivaniemi H: A ten percent prevalence of asymptomatic familial intracranial aneurysms: Preliminary report on 110 magnetig resonance angiography studies in members of 21 Finnish familial intracranial aneurysm families. Neurosurgery 35: 208–213, 1994
31. Ronkainen A, Hernesniemi J, Puranen M, Vanninen R, Vainio P, Ryynänen M: MR angiographic screening for incidental intracranial aneurysms: Experience with 400 asymptomatic individuals with increased familial risk. Radiology, 195: 25–40, 1995
32. Steinberg GK, Drake CG, Peerless SJ: Deliberate basilar or vertebral artery occlusion in the treatment of intracranial aneurysms. J Neurosurg 79: 161–173, 1993
33. Sugita K, Kobayashi S, Shintani A, Mutsuga N: Microneurosurgery for aneurysms of the basilar artery. J Neurosurg 51: 615–620, 1979
34. Troupp H: The natural history of aneurysms of the basilar bifurcation. Acta Neurol Scand 47: 350–356, 1971
35. Vajda J, Pasztor E, Orosz E, Nyary I, Juhasz J, Horvath M, Czirjak S, Futo J: Early surgery for ruptured cerebral aneurysm. Int Surg 75: 123–126, 1990
36. Yaşargil MG, Antic J, Lagica R, et al: Microneurosurgical pterional approach to aneurysms of the basilar bifurcation. Surg Neurol 6: 83–91, 1976
37. Yaşargil MG: Vertebrobasilar aneurysms. In: Microneurosurgery in 4 volumes, vol II. Stuttgart, New York: Thieme, 1986, pp 232–295
38. Yoshimoto T, Uchida K, Kaneko U, Kayama T, Suzuki J: An analysis and follow-up results of 1000 intracranial saccular aneurysms with definitive surgical treatment. J Neurosurg 50: 152–157, 1979

Subject Index[*]

A
Age 7, 14
- mean ages in patients with VBA aneurysms 7
- related to outcome 14; see for each specific aneurysm sites

AICA aneurysms 133
Allcock's test 42, 81
Anatomy, basilar bifurcation 17, 18, 21, 35, 42
Anatomy, see for each specific aneurysm sites
Anesthesia management 280
- circulatory arrest 75, 112
- complications 283
- conclusion 283
- emergence and recovery 282
- fluid administration 281
- hypothermia 75, 112
- induced hypotension, systemic 27, 44, 65, 262
- induction 281
- maintenance 27, 281
- monitoring 280
- monitoring of brainstem function 283
- positioning 282
- premedication 280
- preoperative preparation 280
- temporary arterial occlusion, and cerebral protection 27, 281

Aneurysm
- alternative treatments 8, 9, 51, 52
- anterior circulation 254
- asymptomatic 267
- atherosclerotic 1, 8, 11, 143, 207
- bilateral 137
- bilobular 18, 44, 48, 87
- butterfly 121, 137, 138, 167–169
- children 269
- dissecting 119, 128, 195, 197, 203
- distal 95, 117, 137, 140, 195
- enlargement 7, 69, 89, 200
- fusiform 8, 11, 68, 119, 140, 143, 177, 269
- giant 68, 110, 143, 167, 207, 230
- incidental 8, 17, 249, 267
- multiple 249
- mycotic 8, 11
- projection 18
- recurrence 7, 89
- ruptured 8, 17

---

[*] The chapters of the book are arranged according the various aneurysm origins from the vertebrobasilar tree. For additional information see for each specific chapter and its tables.

- saccular 8, 11, 17
- side 95
- sites 7, 11, 17
- sizes 4, 8, 11
- traumatic 8, 11, 121, 123
- type 8, 11, 131, 206, 273
- unoperated 69, 254, 255
- unruptured 8, 17, 249, 262, 267

Approach initial 4, 21
- contralateral 96, 97, 98, 146, 201, 250, 251
- half and half 29
- occipital 222
- pterional 28, 29, 36
- rare approaches 23, 29
- side 22, 96
- suboccipital lateral 135, 170-174, 177, 201, 202, 203
- subtemporal 21, 22, 26, 42, 96
- subtemporal transtentorial 134, 135, 167, 177
- temporopolar 30
- transclival 201
- transmastoid transpetrosal 37, 135, 172, 173, 177
- transsylvian pterional 28, 29, 36

Arteriovenous malformations (AVMs), associated 8, 95, 133, 141, 249, 256
- embolization intraoperative 259
- general principles of treatment 256
- natural history 259
- operative method 266
- patients 262
- poor results 263
- treatment 262

B
Balloon occlusion 209
Basilar anterior inferior cerebellar artery (AICA) aneurysms 133
- anatomical features 133
- approaches 135
- clinical features 133
- results 141

Basilar artery occlusion, deliberate 3, 5, 38, 51, 72, 89, 91, 92, 112, 143, 269
Basilar bifurcation anatomy 18, 21, 35, 42
Basilar bifurcation aneurysms
- giant 68
-- anatomical features 68
-- basilar artery occlusion 81, 84, 92, 93
-- clinical features 68
-- explorative treatment 69
-- intra-aneurysmal occlusion 69
-- morbidity 92

Basilar bifurcation aneurysms
- giant
-- mortality 92
-- neck clipping 75, 92
-- treatment 69, 94
-- vertebral artery occlusion 80
- large (or bulbous) 42
-- clinical features 42
-- final comments 65
-- operative morbidity 55
-- perforator injury or occlusion 51, 55, 58
-- results 51
- small 17
-- anatomical features 18
-- backward projecting aneurysms 18, 37, 58
-- clinical features 17
-- dolichocephalic 21, 30
-- early surgical experience 17
-- final comments 65
-- forward projecting aneurysms 18, 37, 58
-- high basilar bifurcation 21, 36
-- induced intraoperative hypotension 27
-- low basilar bifurcations 21, 36
-- operative morbidity 55
-- perforator injury or occlusion 17, 30, 55, 58–60, 301
-- rare surgical approaches 29
-- results 38, 39
-- subtemporal approach 21
-- transsylvian (pterional) approach 28
-- upward projecting basilar bifurcation aneurysms 18, 30, 58
Basilar superior cerebellar artery aneurysms
- giant 110
-- anatomical features 110
-- basilar artery occlusion 112
-- clinical features 110
-- explored only 110
-- inadvertent arterial occlusion 110
-- neck clipping 112
- non-giant 95
-- anatomical features 95
-- clinical features 95
-- projection 95
-- side 95
-- treatment 96
Basilar trunk aneurysms 119, 143
- giant 143
-- anatomical features 143
-- clinical features 143
-- neck clipping 145
-- parent artery occlusion 145
-- trapping 162
-- treatment 143
- non-giant 119
Beer belly 18, 42, 46
Botterell Grading 9, 12

C
Children with vertebrobasilar aneurysms 269
- clinical features 269
- treatment 269

Clinical material general 7–16, 277
Clip
- Drake-Kees 8
- Drake-Sugita 203
- encircling (Sundt clip graft) 27, 101, 22
- fenestrated 4, 8, 9, 31, 32, 44, 65, 99
- malpositioned 31, 47
- Olivecrona 2
- Scoville 5
- slipped 62, 303
- Sugita 9, 31
- temporary 27
- Weck 5
Clipping
- bilateral 34
- blind 100, 101
- contralateral 98, 139
- incomplete 7, 31, 32, 36, 303
- gathered 47
- piggy back 9
- tandem 9, 31, 32, 34, 36, 47, 49, 75, 79, 177, 222
- temporary 27
Coagulation of aneurysmal neck 9, 36, 101
Coating of aneurysm 9, 15
Complications, medical 62, 67, 304, 310
Complications of surgery 66, 206, 277, 300
- complications during anesthesia 39, 300
- factors increasing complication rates 300
- hydrocephalus 304
- inadvertent major vessel occlusion 44, 67, 75, 80, 127, 302
- incomplete occlusion and reoperation (failed aneurysm surgery) 55, 303
- influence of surgical timing 300
- intracranial hematoma 55, 310
- intraoperative aneurysm rupture 35, 55, 137, 301
- medical complications 304
- memory deficits 303
- perforator injury 31, 36, 55, 58, 66, 75, 127, 301
- postoperative deterioration of neurological state 302
- postoperative hematoma 55, 262, 303, 310
- postoperative infection 304, 310
- problems in exposure 301
- rebleeding 55, 56, 57, 66, 304
- statistical analysis for predictors of poor outcome 304, 311
- vasospasm 10, 55, 130, 228, 253, 277, 304, 310
Cranial nerve deficit
- as complications of surgery (permanent vs. transient) 138, 277, 309
- preoperative 17, 66, 91, 95, 96, 121, 124, 133, 143, 167, 177, 197, 207, 221, 230, 309
- trochlear nerve injury 26, 301
Craniotomy, see Approach
Cushing 1

D
Dandy 1
Database, description 10
Direction of aneurysm fundus 67
Dissecting aneurysms 119, 128, see basilar trunk, vertebral artery

Division of tentorium 26, 36, 121, 134, 135
Dog ears 29

E
Early surgery 275
Early surgical experience 17
Endovascular saccular treatment 9, 52, 73, 77, 285
- conclusions 298
- detachable balloons 285
- experience at the University of Western Ontario, 1971 to 1994 288
- thrombosis with coiled wires 287
Epidural hematoma 55, 126, 303
Experience, influence of surgical 6, 65
Explorative surgery 9, 15, 38, 52, 69, 110, 143, 177

F
Facial nerve preservation in tic approach 23
Fenestration 167, 177
Frequency of vertebrobasilar aneurysms 1
Final comments 5, 65, 276, 305, 306
Follow-up 11
Fox 1, 256

G
General condition related to timing of surgery 275
Giant aneurysms 68, 110, 143, 167, 207, 230
Grading clinical 9
- Botterell 9
- WFNS 9

H
Hamby 1
Hematoma 55, 303
- cisternal 17, 25
- epidural 55, 126, 303
- intracerebral 8, 55, 303
- intraventricular 17
- subdural 55, 303
Hemianopia 244, 248
Hemifacial spasm 188, 267
Historical notes 1, 17
Hunterian parent artery occlusion 4, 9, 80, 223
Hydrocephalus 304
Hypertension, arterial 8
Hypertension, induced 55
Hypoglossal artery 167, 170, 174
Hypotension, induced 27, 39

I
Incidence of VBA aneurysms 1, 13, 17
Incidental VBA aneurysms 267
Infection after aneurysm surgery 304, 310
Intra-aneurysmal occlusion 69
Intraoperative rupture 35, 301
Ischemia and infarction after aneurysmal surgery 301, 302, 304

J
Jamieson 3
Juvenile aneurysms 269

K
Krayenbühl 1
Kees 8
Kuopio 256

L
Laterality of aneurysms 95, 195
Ligation of aneurysms 8
Ligation of arteries, see for specific aneurysm sites
Liljequist's membrane 23
Local anesthesia 5
Logue 3
Lumbal drainage 23

M
Mannitol 23, 27
Mayfield 8
Meningitis 51, 201, 304, 310
Method of aneurysm treatment 8, 15
Miami 7
Mid basilar trunk aneurysms 119
- anatomical features 119
- approach 121
- clinical features 121
- results 128
Moniz 1
Morbidity 7, 12, 65, 300, 311, see for specific aneurysm sites
Mortality 7, 12, 65, 300, 311, see for specific aneurysm sites
Mullan 9
Multiplicity 8, 249
Multiple aneurysms 8, 64, 95, 249
- butterfly aneurysms 121, 137, 138, 167–169
- incidence 249
- multiplicity, see for specific aneurysm sites
- operative results 250
- treatment 23, 249

N
Norlèn 2

O
Oculomotor nerve 18, 96, see for specific aneurysm sites
- identification 22, 23
- outcome 24
- palsy 24, 91, 95
- surgical anatomy 26, 37
Olivecrona 1, 2
Outcome 7–16, see for specific aneurysm sites
- and age 14
- categorization of 10
- Grade 12
- location 11, 12, 13
- sex 14, 197
- size 12
- operative method 8, 9, 15, 16
- timing 16, 275
- type 11
Operative complications, see for complications of surgery 300

P

Perforators 17, 18, 30, 31, 36, 37, 55, 58, 143
PICA aneurysms 195
Pilo-injection of aneurysms 9, 69
Pool 27
Poppen 2, 3
Postoperative rebleeding 56, 57, 304
Pregnancy and SAH 8
Preoperative rebleeding 275
Posterior cerebral artery aneurysms 221, 230
– giant 230
– – anatomical features 230
– – – P1 aneurysms 230
– – – P1-P2 junction aneurysms 230
– – – P2 and P3-4 aneurysms 230
– – clinical features 230
– – – P1 and P1-P2 junction aneurysms 230
– – – P2-4 aneurysms 230
– – treatment 232
– – – treatment P1 aneurysms 232
– – – treatment P1/P2-posterior communicating aneurysms 239
– – – treatment P2-4 aneurysms 239
– non-giant 221
– – anatomical features 221
– – clinical features 221
– – results 228
– – subtemporal approach 221
Posterior cerebral artery occlusion 222, 232
Posterior clinoid process, relationship to aneurysm neck 18, 21, 37
Posterior communicating artery 81, 150, 231
– aneurysm of 239
– division of 25
– identification of 25
Proximal control, see for temporary clipping 27
Psycho-organic syndrome 303
Pterional approach 28
Pulmonary embolism 310
Puncture of aneurysm 31, 37, 44, 101

R

Radner 1
Rebleeding, postoperative 32, 56, 57, 304
Rebleeding, preoperative 275
Recurrent hemorrhage, preoperative (prevention of) 55, 275
Redo-operations 7, 8, 36, 303
References 312
Retractor pressure 23
Rhoton 18, 36
Risk of hemorrhage in unruptured aneurysms 39, 69, 254, 255
Rupture intraoperative 35, 55, 137, 301

S

Schwartz 2
Scoville 5, 8
Selverstone 185, 207
Sex 7, 14
Silk ligature 8, 15, 17, 118
Sites of aneurysmal formation 11–13
Size of aneurysms 4, 8, 11, see for specific aneurysm sites
Slipped clip 129, 175
Statistical analysis 304, 311
Steelman 2
Subarachnoid hemorrhage, number of 8
Sundt 27
Superior cerebellar artery aneurysms 95, 110

T

Temporary clipping 26, 27, 30, 44, 75, 137
Tentorium cerebellii 23, 26, 37
Thrombus evacuation 75, 98, 112, 192, 193, 211, 216, 232
Thrombus in aneurysm 51
Tic craniectomy 21–23
Timing of surgery 10, 16, 275, 300
– early versus late surgery 275
– final comments on timing of surgery 276
– rebleeding, transfer of patients 275
– vasospasm, relationship to 276, 277
Tourniquet 4, 5, 42, 81, 92, 93, 145, 191
Towne's projection 21
Track sheet 10
Trapping 9, 15, 162–165, 192, 193, 211, 216, 226, 232, 244
Trochlear nerve 37
Tönnis 2
Transfer of patients 275
Turnbull 17, 18

U

Unclipped aneurysms 8, 15
Unoperated aneurysm 15, 250, 254, 275

V

Vasospasm, postoperative 10, 55, 130, 228, 253, 277, 304, 310
Veins
– Labbé 23, 128, 135
– Sylvian 23, 29
– venous thrombosis 29
Vertebral aneurysms 195, 207
– giant 207
– – anatomical features 207
– – clinical features 207
– – treatment 207
– non-giant 195
– – anatomical features 195
– – approaches 201
– – classification 195
– – clinical features 197
– – results 203
Vertebral artery occlusion, deliberate 2, 80, 145, 152–161, 165, 166, 180, 203, 207, 271
Vertebral-basilar junction aneurysms 167
– giant 177
– – bilateral vertebral occlusion 180
– – trapping and evacuation 192
– – treatment 177
– – unilateral vertebral occlusion 180
– – vertebral artery occlusion 180

Vertebral-basilar junction aneurysms
- non-giant 167
-- anatomical features 167
-- approach 167
-- clinical features 167
-- results 174

W
Warning leak 8
Weber's syndrome 63, 106, 110, 113, 115, 116, 143, 230
WFNS 9
Wrapping 9, 15, 174

Springer Neurosurgery

Advances and Technical Standards in Neurosurgery

Volume 22

Edited by L. Symon (Editor-in-Chief), L. Calliauw, F. Cohadon, V. V. Dolenc,
J. Lobo Antunes, H. Nornes, J. D. Pickard, H.-J. Reulen, A. J. Strong, N. de Tribolet

1995. 149 partly coloured figures. XV, 381 pages.
Cloth DM 298,–, öS 2086,–, approx. US $ 198.00
ISBN 3-211-82634-3

This series, sponsored by the European Association of Neurosurgical Societies, has already become a classic. In general, one volume is published per year. The Advances section presents fields of neurosurgery and related areas in which important recent progress has been made. The Technical Standards section features detailed descript of standard procedures to assist young neurosurgeons in their post-graduate training. The contributions are written by experienced clinicians and are reviewed by all members of the Editorial Board.

Contents:
Advances: K. Thapar, K. Kovacs, E. R. Laws: The Classification and Molecular Biology of Pituitary Adenomas.
J. P. Chirossel, G. Vanneuville, J. G. Passagia, J. Chazal, Ch. Coillard, J. J. Favre, J. M. Garcier, J. Tonetti, M. Guillot: Biomechanics and Classification of Traumatic Lesions of the Spine.
U. Ebeling, H.-J. Reulen: Space-Occupying Lesions of the Sensori-Motor Region.
Technical Standards: J. P. Houtteville: The Surgery of Cavernomas Both Supra-Tentorial and Infra-Tentorial.
A. Bricolo, S. Turazzi: Surgery for Gliomas and Other Mass Lesions of the Brainstem.
M. Samii, C. Matthies: Hearing Preservation in Acoustic Tumour Surgery.

Springer Wien New York

P.O.Box 89, A-1201 Wien • New York, NY 10010, 175 Fifth Avenue
Heidelberger Platz 3, D-14197 Berlin • Tokyo 113, 3-13, Hongo 3-chome, Bunkyo-ku

SpringerNeurosurgery

Advances and Technical Standards in Neurosurgery

Volume 21

Edited by L. Symon (Editor-in-Chief), L. Calliauw, F. Cohadon, J. Lobo Antunes, F. Loew, H. Nornes, E. Pásztor, J. D. Pickard, A. J. Strong, M. G. Yasargil

1994. 69 partly coloured figures. XIII, 286 pages.
Cloth DM 228,–, öS 1596,–, approx. US $ 149.00
ISBN 3-211-82482-0

This series, sponsored by the European Association of Neurosurgical Societies, has already become a classic. In general, one volume is published per year. The Advances section presents fields of neurosurgery and related areas in which important recent progress has been made. The Technical Standards section features detailed descript of standard procedures to assist young neurosurgeons in their post-graduate training. The contributions are written by experienced clinicians and are reviewed by all members of the Editorial Board.

Contents:
Advances: G. J. Pilkington, P. L. Lantos: Biological Markers for Tumours of the Brain.
C. Daumas-Duport: Histoprognosis of Gliomas.
F. Cohadon: Brain Protection.
Technical Standards: S. F. Ciricillo, M. L. Rosenblum: AIDS and the Neurosurgeon – an Update.
M. Choux, G. Lena, L. Genitori, M. Foroutan: The Surgery of Occult Spinal Dysraphism.
P. Cosyns, J. Caemaert, W. Haaijman, C. van Veelen, J. Gybels, J. van Manen, J. Ceha: Functional Stereotactic Neurosurgery for Psychiatric Disorders: an Experience in Belgium and The Netherlands.

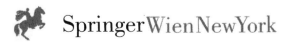

P.O.Box 89, A-1201 Wien • New York, NY 10010, 175 Fifth Avenue
Heidelberger Platz 3, D-14197 Berlin • Tokyo 113, 3-13, Hongo 3-chome, Bunkyo-ku